Assaults within
Psychiatric Facilities

Assaults within Psychiatric Facilities

Edited by

John R. Lion, M.D.
Professor of Psychiatry
Institute of Psychiatry and Human Behavior
University of Maryland School of Medicine
Baltimore, Maryland

William H. Reid, M.D., M.P.H.
Associate Professor of Psychiatry
Director of Education and Training
Nebraska Psychiatric Institute
University of Nebraska Medical Center
Omaha, Nebraska

Grune & Stratton
A Subsidiary of Harcourt Brace Jovanovich, Publishers
New York   London
Paris   San Diego   San Francisco   São Paulo
Sydney   Tokyo   Toronto

Library of Congress Cataloging in Publication Date
Main entry under title:

Assaults within psychiatric facilities.

    Includes bibliographies and index.
    1. Violence in psychiatric hospitals. 2. Psychiatric
hospital patients—Psychology. 3. Psychiatric
hospitals—Employees—Psychology. I. Lion, John R.
II. Reid, William H., 1945–
RC439.4.A77   1983   362.2′1   83-18362
ISBN 0-8089-1559-2

Grune & Stratton, Inc.
111 Fifth Avenue
New York, New York 10003

Distributed in the United Kingdom by
Grune & Stratton, Inc. (London) Ltd.
24/28 Oval Road, London NW 1

Library of Congress Catalog Number 83-18362
International Standard Book Number 0-8089-1559-2

Printed in the United States of America

Contents

PART I: PHENOMENOLOGY AND EPIDEMIOLOGY

Acknowledgments

The editors gratefully acknowledge time and facility support from the Nebraska Psychiatric Institute, Merrill T. Eaton, M.D., Professor and Director; and the University of Maryland School of Medicine, Russell R. Monroe, M.D., Chairman. Many thanks are due to Edna Brooks-Pittman and Beth Dawson for considerable administrative assistance and typing of the final manuscript.

Preface

Violence has always been a problem in mental hospitals, but the discipline of psychiatry has been curiously indifferent to it. Bengt Ekblom wrote a definitive monograph on the subject in 1970. His book, *Acts of Violence by Patients in Mental Hospitals* (Scandinavian University Books, Uppsala), describes a 10-year study of acts of violence within the Swedish hospital system. Among some 27,000 patients, Ekblom found 25 cases of assault, eight of which were fatal.

Ekblom's work seems paradoxical—so many patients, so few cases of assault, so serious the outcome in those few cases. In personal communication Ekblom indicates that assaults were probably underreported; this is consistent with expectations and data in this country. For instance, unpublished data from the VA hospital system indicate that over 12,000 assaults occurred in a five-year period. Published works cited within this volume show that assaults within a typical American hospital are found in the hundreds and thousands. Both patients and mental health staff are injured; indeed, the January 1982 issue of *Psychiatric News* from the American Psychiatric Association devoted the cover story to the finding that three psychiatrists had been victims of homicide. Two of these dramatic cases occurred in outpatient settings.

During the preparation of this work, we also became aware of assaults in other health care settings, such as emergency rooms and medical and surgical wards of general hospitals. While the bulk of writings herein cover mainly the latter, chapters on violence in nonpsychiatric settings are also included.

The number of psychiatrists and nurses or patients seriously harmed in the United States and the profiles of those injured—or those who assault—are largely unknown. We hope that the data and policy chapters in this book spur the systematic collection of information and help to make the mental health workplace a safer one.

John R. Lion, M.D.
William H. Reid, M.D., M.P.H.

Contributors

WOLFE N. ADLER, M.D.
Director, Division of Adult Inpatient Programs, Sheppard and Enoch Pratt Hospital, Baltimore, Maryland

PAUL S. APPELBAUM, M.D.
Assistant Professor of Psychiatry and Co-Director, Law and Psychiatry Program, Western Psychiatric Institute and Clinic, University of Pittsburgh School of Medicine; Adjunct Associate Professor of Law, University of Pittsburgh School of Law, Pittsburgh, Pennsylvania

STEPHEN ARMSTRONG, Ph.D.
Department of Psychiatry, Baystate Medical Center, Springfield, Massachusetts; Associate Clinical Professor, Tufts University School of Medicine; Adjunct Assistant Professor, School of Public Health, University of Massachusetts at Amherst, Amherst, Massachusetts

LOIS M. CONN, M.D.
Assistant Professor, Institute of Psychiatry and Human Behavior, University of Maryland School of Medicine, Baltimore, Maryland; Medical Director, Drug Detoxification Program, Maryland Correctional Institution for Women, Jessup, Maryland

FREDERICK C. DEPP, Ph.D.
Chief, The Clinical Studies and Support Section, The Dixon Implementation Office, Saint Elizabeths Hospital, Washington, D.C.

PARK ELLIOTT DIETZ, M.D., M.P.H.
Associate Professor of Law and of Behavioral Medicine and Psychiatry, University of Virginia Schools of Law and Medicine, Charlottesville, Virginia

J. GUY EDWARDS, M.B., B.Ch., F.R.C.Psych., D.P.M.
Consultant Psychiatrist, Royal South Hants Hospital; Clinical Teacher in Psychiatry, University of Southampton Medical School, Southampton, England

ERNEST A. HAFFKE, M.D.
Clinical Director, Preventive and Social Psychiatry, and Associate Professor of Psychiatry, Nebraska Psychiatric Institute, University of Nebraska College of Medicine, Omaha, Nebraska

JOSEPH A. IONNO, M.D.
Senior Staff Psychiatrist, The Institute of Living, Hartford, Connecticut

CHRISTOPHER KREEGER, M.A.
Quality Assurance Analyst, Sheppard and Enoch Pratt Hospital, Baltimore, Maryland

MARY ELLEN KRONBERG, M.S.N.
Assistant Professor, Creighton University School of Nursing, Omaha, Nebraska

JOHN R. LION, M.D.
Professor of Psychiatry, Institute of Psychiatry and Human Behavior, University of Maryland School of Medicine, Baltimore, Maryland

DENIS J. MADDEN, Ph.D.
Director, Clinical Research Program for Violent Behavior, and Clinical Associate Professor of Psychiatry, Institute of Psychiatry and Human Behavior, University of Maryland School of Medicine, Baltimore, Maryland

KAREN J. MERRIKIN
Research Assistant, Battelle Human Affairs Research Centers, Seattle, Washington

BARRY J. NIGROSH, Ph.D.
Assistant Professor of Psychiatry, Psychiatric Regional Resource Unit, University of Massachusetts Medical School, Northampton, Massachusetts

GARY W. NYMAN, M.D., M.B.A.
Clinical Associate Professor of Psychiatry, Institute of Psychiatry and Human Behavior, University of Maryland School of Medicine, and Chief, Department of Psychiatry, Loch Raven Veterans Administration Hospital, Baltimore, Maryland

HERBERT N. OCHITILL, M.D.

Director, Consultation Liason Service, Department of Psychiatry, San Francisco General Hospital; Assistant Professor of Psychiatry, University of California, San Francisco, California

THOMAS D. OVERCAST, J.D., Ph.D.

Research Scientist, Battelle Human Affairs Research Centers, Seattle, Washington

MANOEL W. PENNA, M.D.

Clinical Associate Professor of Psychiatry, Institute of Psychiatry and Human Behavior, University of Maryland School of Medicine, Baltimore, Maryland

RICHARD T. RADA, M.D.

Medical Director, College Hospital, Cerritos, California; Clinical Professor, Department of Psychiatry, University of New Mexico School of Medicine, Albuquerque, New Mexico

WILLIAM H. REID, M.D., M.P.H.

Associate Professor of Psychiatry, Director of Education and Training, and Clinical Research Coordinator, Nebraska Psychiatric Institute, University of Nebraska College of Medicine, Omaha, Nebraska

BRUCE DENNIS SALES, Ph.D., J.D.

Professor of Psychology and Director, Law-Psychology Program, Department of Psychology, University of Arizona, Tucson, Arizona

WILLIAM SNYDER, III, Ph.D.

Staff Psychologist, Springfield Hospital Center, Sykesville, Maryland

PAUL H. SOLOFF, M.D.

Associate Professor of Psychiatry, University of Pittsburgh School of Medicine, Pittsburgh, Pennsylvania

KENNETH TARDIFF, M.D., M.P.H.

Associate Dean for Student Affairs, Associate Professor of Psychiatry, and Assistant Professor of Public Health, Cornell University Medical College, New York, New York

PENELOPE ZIEGLER, M.D.

Assistant Clinical Professor, Department of Psychiatry, University of Maryland School of Medicine, Baltimore, Maryland

PART I

Phenomenology and Epidemiology

Kenneth Tardiff

A Survey of Assault by Chronic Patients in a State Hospital System

There is a growing concern that assaultive psychiatric patients pose a danger to professionals responsible for their care as well as to patients and other health care workers. There is evidence that this concern is justified and that being assaulted is an occupational hazard for personnel in psychiatric institutions. Two studies have found that approximately 40 percent of psychiatrists have been assaulted at least once in their careers,[21,30] and a third has shown that 48 percent of psychiatric residents in one program were assaulted at least once in the several years of their training.[24] Vulnerability is not restricted to psychiatrists. In another study 24 percent of mental health professionals in several disciplines (34 percent of whom were psychiatrists) reported being assaulted at least once in the past year.[40]

Psychopathology is likely to be most severe in inpatient settings. This author will review some attempts to study assaultive behavior among psychiatric inpatients and will present the results of his own large, systematic survey of assault in state hospitals.

REVIEW OF THE LITERATURE ON ASSAULTS BY
PSYCHIATRIC INPATIENTS

There have been four studies that examined small numbers of schizo-phrenic patients and reported conflicting findings in rates of assaultive behavior and in association of particular subtypes of schizophrenia with increased risk. Three studies found increased verbal or physical aggression in paranoid schizophrenics,[1,5,23] while the fourth found no statistically significant increase of physical aggression in such patients.[25] In a study by Bach-Y-Rita and Veno, 13 out of 62 habitually violent patients from a prison population merited a diagnosis of paranoid schizophrenia in spite of the fact that inmates perceived by the correctional authorities as psychotic were excluded from the unit studied.[3] Another subgroup of habitually violent patients had a high incidence of self-destructive behavior and self-mutilation.

Fareta focused on age in her study of aggressive behavior.[12] She assessed 438 patients in a state psychiatric hospital who were 5–15 years old. She found that 66 patients (15 percent), all at least 12 years old, had a history of serious violence directed toward themselves or others. Those patients with such a history were most likely to have been boys from minority groups, diagnosed as schizophrenic, with low intelligence. Follow-up of 18 subjects for 18 years suggested a high degree of continued antisocial and criminal behavior.

Some researchers have attempted to survey assaultive behavior in hos-pitals by using incident reports. Unfortunately, there are two major problems with the use of incident reports—serious underreporting of assaults[18] and a lack of accurate measurement of *rates* of assaultive behavior. Studies using incident reports have produced differing rates of assault and conflicting patterns of patient characteristics.

Ekblom, in Sweden, found only 34 inpatients involved in reported assaultive incidents in a very large retrospective survey of a 10-year period.[10] Kalogerakis found only nine serious assaults in six years at a municipal hospital, and few assaultive incidents were reported by five directors of state hospitals.[16] Albee examined all accident and incident reports for a two-year period at a large psychiatric institute and found only 78 patients who injured others during that time.[2] He found an increased likelihood of assault by patients diagnosed as schizophrenic. Evenson and colleagues found 5128 incidents, not only assaultive, involving 1004 patients in a two-year period at a state hospital.[11] Using the hospital census figures they calculated an assault rate of 99/1000 patient years. Schizophrenics were at low risk for all types of incidents while neurotic patients and those with organic brain syndromes (OBS) and personality disorders all had an increased risk of assaultive behavior. Male and nonwhite patients had increased risk of assaultive behavior compared to female and white patients.

Fottrell examined incident reports at two large psychiatric hospitals and a psychiatric unit in a general hospital.[13] Although he used incident reports, he felt that there was not underreporting of assault since senior nursing and administrative personnel assured him that all assaults had been reported. Rates of assault in his survey cannot be calculated; however, he states that there were very few serious incidents. There was a preponderance of young and female assailants. Schizophrenia was the most common diagnosis and the most common victims were staff. Baseline data on age, sex or diagnosis were not reported.

One concludes that previous studies of assaultive behavior in hospitals have not been broad enough or have not relied on direct assessment. The survey, which is discussed below, directly assessed the frequency of assault, the characteristics of assaultive patients, techniques used to manage such behavior, and patients' eventual suitability for community placement.

SURVEY OF ASSAULTIVE PSYCHIATRIC INPATIENTS

Survey Methods

The following findings are from a series of studies by the author based on a two-month survey in 1979 of 5164 inpatients of two large state hospitals.[27,28,35] Patients who had been in these hospitals for less than one month were excluded since the author had previously assessed patterns of assault by patients around the time of admission to hospitals.[32-34] Patients in special treatment units for alcoholism or mental retardation and those less than 17 years old were also excluded.

The surveyors were experienced staff, predominantly nurses of the hospitals, but they did not assess patients on the wards where they worked. Surveyors participated in training workshops to familiarize them with the vocabulary of the survey instrument. Assault assessment included interviews of the patient and relevant staff and review of the medical record.

The survey instrument was a revised version of one used previously in an inpatient survey of the psychological and physical status of mental patients.[29] The instrument included a clear definition of assault—an aggressive act physically directed toward persons—and considered only those patients who had assaulted at least once within the hospital during the three months preceding the survey.

The survey instrument also contained data on demographic and clinical characteristics of patients, and an assessment of the likelihood of their release into the community. Treatment information included the type of psychotropic medications received by patients on a routine basis and the current daily dose. Emergency control measures such as seclusion or restraint, emergency medication, or constant observation in the preceding 30 days also were noted. Clinical characteristics included primary psychiatric diagnosis and information adapted from the Nurses' Observation Scale for Inpatient Evaluation (NOSIE).[14]

Our use of diagnosis merits special attention. The category "other nonpsychotic disorders" is comprised mostly of personality disorders. The data on patients diagnosed with paranoid schizophrenia, paranoid states, and manic episodes were grouped together under paranoid schizophrenia, because evidence suggests that these categories are more closely related to each other than they are to other types of schizophrenia.[36] The low frequency of manic episodes and paranoid states (1 percent) allays statistical concern about this combination of data.

Results

The basic demographic and clinical characteristics of the patients residing in the hospitals and included in the survey are presented in Table 1-1.

Table 1-2 compares patients who were assaultive in the hospital during the three months preceding the survey with those who were not assaultive during the same period. In addition, Table 1-2 presents the analysis of four variables, stratified by sex, which were associated with an increased likelihood of assaultive behavior. Race is not included because there was no statistically significant difference between white and nonwhite in assaultive behavior. There were 186 (7.8 percent) male patients and 198 (7.1 percent) female patients who physically assaulted other persons at least once in the preceding three months. Thus there was no significant difference between men and women in terms of the proportion of patients who were assaultive in the hospital. Approximately two-thirds of the assaults occurred within one month preceding the survey. Assaultive patients were more likely than nonassaultive patients to be younger than 44 years old and were especially overrepresented among patients 17–34 years old. Male patients from 17 to 34 years of age had a frequency of assault five times greater than that of the general patient population. Assaultive patients were more likely to have been in the hospital for a shortr period of time than nonassaultive patients, although both are often hospitalized for several years. Diagnoses of nonparanoid schizophrenia, psychotic OBS, other nonpsychotic disorders, and mental retardation were overrepresented in the assaultive population, and paranoid schizophrenia was surprisingly underrepresented. Assaultive patients were twice as likely to have a seizure disorder. Further analysis showed that only primary psychiatric diagnosis was a factor in differentiating assaultive patients with seizures from those without seizures. As shown in Table 1-3, assaultive patients with seizures were more likely to be diagnosed with psychotic OBS, mental retardation, or other nonpsychotic disorders. Only one-fourth of patients with seizures were diagnosed with psychotic OBS with epilepsy.

The NOSIE ratings showed assaultive patients to be more severely impaired than nonassaultive patients with regard to psychotic symptomatology such as delusions, hallucinations, inappropriate affect, and bizarre habits,

Table 1-1

Characteristics of All Patients

Characteristics	Percentage of Male (N = 2382)	Percentage of Female (N = 2781)
Age		
17–34 yrs	11	7
35–44 yrs	10	6
45–54 yrs	16	13
55–64 yrs	28	28
65+ yrs	35	46
	100	100
Duration of hospitalization		
1 mo–2 yrs	11	11
2 yrs–10 yrs	18	15
10 yrs–20 yrs	18	15
20 yrs–30 yrs	16	18
30 yrs–40 yrs	16	18
> 40 yrs	21	23
	100	100
Primary Diagnosis (DMS-II)		
Paranoid schizophrenia	28	34
Other nonparanoid schizophrenia	41	33
Depressions	3	6
Psychotic OBS	20	21
Mental retardation	5	4
Other nonpsychotic disorders	3	2
	100	100
Race		
White	79	85
Nonwhite (predominantly black)	21	15
	100	100

rituals, or behavior. Assaultive patients displayed more agitation, negativistic behavior, and antisocial behavior. Interestingly, assaultive patients were more likely than nonassaultive patients to cry and express feelings of depression. Assaultive patients of both sexes were three to four times more likely than nonassaultive patients to have attempted suicide at least once in the past.

Table 1-2

Characteristics of Psychiatric Inpatients by Presence of Assaultive Behavior and Sex

| Characteristics | Percentage of Male | | Percentage of Female | |
	Assaultive (N = 186)	Not Assaultive (N = 2196)	Assaultive (N = 198)	Not Assaultive (N = 2584)
Age				
17–34 yrs	34	9	17	5
35–44 yrs	16	9	15	6
45–54 yrs	19	16	12	13
55–64 yrs	17	29	29	28
65+ yrs	14	37	27	48
	100	100	100	100
	($\chi^2 = 121.72$, $df = 4$, $p < .00005$)		($\chi^2 = 62.73$, $df = 4$, $p < .00005$)	
Duration of Hospitalization				
1–3 mos	7	2	6	3
3 mos–2 yrs	18	8	15	9
2 yrs–10 yrs	28	17	26	15
10+ yrs	47	73	47	73
	100	100	100	100
	($\chi^2 = 84.45$, $df = 6$, $p < .00005$)		($\chi^2 = 56.09$, $df = 6$, $p < .00005$)	
Primary Diagnosis				
Paranoid schizophrenia	14	29	23	35
Nonparanoid schizophrenia	46	41	38	33 .
Depression	1	3	5	6
Psychotic OBS	11	5	7	4
Other non-psychotic disorders	3	2	3	2
	100	100	100	100
	($\chi^2 = 31.52$, $df = 5$, $p < .00005$)		($\chi^2 = 17.57$, $df = 5$, $p < .00005$)	
Seizure Disorder				
Present	23	9	19	9
Absent	77	91	81	91
	100	100	100	100
	($\chi^2 = 31.11$, $df = 1$, $p < .00005$)		($\chi^2 = 22.07$, $df = 1$, $p < .00005$)	

Table 1-3

Presence of Seizure Disorders in Assaultive Patients by Primary Psychiatric Diagnosis

Diagnosis	Percentage of Assaultive with Seizures (N = 81)	Percentage of Assaultive without Seizures (N = 303)
Paranoid schizophrenia	4	23
Nonparanoid schizophrenia	25	46
Depression	0	4
Psychotic OBS	45	19
Mental retardation	21	6
Other nonpsychotic disorders	5	2
	100	100
	$(\chi^2 = 59.49, df = 5, p < .00005)$	

Table 1-4

Comparison of Major Trends in Occurrence of Assault in Hospitals with Assault just Before or During Admission

Parameter	Current Study of Assault in Hospital	Previous Study of Assault just Before or During Admission
Sex	No difference between sexes in regard to assault	Men more assaultive than women
Age	Patients under 45 yrs more assaultive	Patients < 24 yrs and > 65 yrs more assaultive
Primary psychiatric diagnosis	For both sexes, nonparanoid schizophrenia, psychotic OBS, and mental retardation associated with increased assault. Paranoid schizophrenia associated with decreased assault	For both sexes, paranoid schizophrenia and psychotic OBS associated with increased assault. For men only, nonparanoid schizophrenia associated with increased assault
Presence of seizure disorder	Assaultive patients have greater likelihood of seizure disorders	No difference between assaultive and non-assaultive patients regarding seizure disorders
Presence of suicidal problems	For both sexes, assaultive patients have greater likelihood of suicidal problems	For men only, assaultive patients have greater likelihood of suicidal problems

Table 1-5
Percentages, by Age and Diagnosis, of Assaultive Patients Requiring Controls in the Preceding Month

All Assaultive Patients	Percentage Receiving Emergency Medication (N = 384)	Percentage Receiving Physical Restraints (N = 384)	Percentage Receiving One-to-One Supervision (N = 384)
	40	17	27
Age			
17–24 yrs	67	35	47
25–34 yrs	63	28	31
35–44 yrs	40	9	28
45–64 yrs	25	10	21
65+ yrs	14	4	8
Statistic	$(\chi^2 = 64.54, df = 4, p < .00005)$	$(\chi^2 = 37.70, df = 4, p < .00005)$	$(\chi^2 = 29.51, df = 4, p < .00005)$
Diagnosis			
Paranoid schizophrenia	41	18	26
Nonparanoid schizophrenia	44	17	32
Depressions	36	9	18
Psychotic OBS	25	8	16
Mental retardation	59	32	38
Other nonpsychotic disorders	46	36	46
Statistic	$(\chi^2 = 14.93, df = 5, p < .0107)$	$(\chi^2 = 14.31, df = 5, p < .0138)$	$(\chi^2 = 12.52, df = 4, p < .0282)$

Comparison of Results of the Chronic Inpatient Survey and
Preadmission Study

In Table 1-4, the major findings of the survey of chronic inpatients are compared to the findings of an earlier study of assault just before or at the time of admission to hospitals.[33] The rate of seizure disorders for assaultive inpatients was four times that of the patients who were assaultive just before or at the time of admission.

Emergency Management of Assaultive Behavior in Hospitals

The survey of inpatients assessed the emergency control methods used in the month preceding the survey. As expected, assaultive patients were more likely than nonassaultive patients to have received emergency medication, to have had some physical restraint or to have received special observation to control dangerous behavior. The data for assaultive patients are summarized in Table 1-5. Assaultive patients in the youngest age groups were more likely to have received all types of control measures. Assaultive patients in the diagnostic categories of mental retardation and other nonpsychotic disorders had a greater likelihood of receiving all three control measures, while nonparanoid schizophrenics were more likely to have received only emergency medication and one-to-one supervision. Although the control measures for the other diagnostic groups were not increased proportionately, the absolute numbers of assaultive patients receiving these measures, particularly emergency medication and one-to-one supervision, were substantial and no doubt represent considerable staff effort and time spent in managing dangerous behavior on the wards.

Routine Medication Used for Assaultive Inpatients

The type and dose of medications taken by the 384 inpatients with a history of in-hospital assault are described in Table 1-6. Drug combinations were infrequent and predominantly involved anticonvulsants and neuroleptics. As is seen in Table 1-6, approximately three-fourths of the patients were being given neuroleptics routinely, usually as the only drug or in combination with anticonvulsants. The most frequently used anticonvulsant was diphenylhydantoin, either alone or in a combination with sedatives or minor tranquilizers. Two patients were on lithium carbonate with neuroleptics and were placed in the "neuroleptic" category.

Two patient characteristics—age and diagnosis—were significantly related to the type of medication prescribed. Younger patients, especially those 17–34 years old (90 percent), were more likely than other patients to be on neuroleptic drugs, while patients 65 years old or older (26 percent), were more likely to receive no daily psychiatric medication. As expected, schizophrenics were

Table 1-6
Frequency of Medication Prescribed Daily for Assaultive Patients

Medication	Number of Patients	Percentage
No psychoactive medication	53	13.8
Chlorpromazine alone	52	13.5
Thioridazine alone	51	13.3
Haloperidol alone	57	14.8
Other neuroleptics alone*	76	19.8
Minor tranquilizers or sedatives alone	13	3.4
Anticonvulsants	49	12.8
Multiple neuroleptics	15	3.9
Tricyclic Antidepressants†	18	4.7
Total:	384	100.0

*Predominantly: thiothixene, mesoridazine or chlorprothixene.
†Most patients were on concurrent neuroleptics.

treated with neuroleptics; however, patients with diagnoses of mental retardation and other nonpsychotic disorders also were more likely than other patients to be treated with daily neuroleptics. Sixty-five percent of patients with psychotic OBS were on neuroleptics, either alone or with other medications.

Length of hospital stay, sex and race were not significantly associated with type of routine medication.

Patients taking routine neuroleptics, except chlorpromazine, were associated with a greater need for emergency medication, physical restraint, or seclusion, and one-to-one supervision during the 30 days before the survey.

Patients were classified as receiving "high," "regular," or "low" daily doses of medication as determined by comparison with the suggested daily dose range ("regular" dose) in *AMA Drug Evaluations*.[4] In patients taking combinations of anticonvulsants and neuroleptics, the dose of the neuroleptic was used for classification. Seven cases were excluded from this portion of the analysis because they could not be classified.

Of the assaultive patients on medication, 64 percent were on daily doses within the ranges suggested by the 1980 *AMA Drug Evaluations*,[4] while 20 percent were on higher and 16 percent were on lower doses than the suggested ranges. Chlorpromazine and thioridazine were more likely to be given in the low dose ranges, and haloperidol and the multiple neuroleptics were more likely to be given in the high dose ranges. Younger patients were on higher doses, and those 65 years old and older were on lower doses. Men were given higher doses than women. Nonparanoid schizophrenics were on high doses while patients with psychotic OBSs or depression were given low daily doses. In the 21 percent of the assaultive patients who had seizure disorders, daily doses of neuroleptics were not lower than those for other patients, despite evidence that neuroleptics can lower the seizure threshold.[15] Assaultive patients on "high" doses of medications were more likely than assaultive patients on lower doses to have received emergency medication, seclusion or physical restraint, and one-to-one supervision to control dangerous behavior during the month preceding the survey.

Level of in-Hospital Treatment Versus Community Placement

The surveyors placed each patient at one of four levels in terms of mental status and treatment needed (Table 1-7). Only patients who had been hospitalized for more than three months were included in these data, in order to be more certain that their illness generally had stabilized. The necessary levels of care ranged from "1" (most restrictive and intense) to "4" (patient stable and appropriate for community placement). As expected, male and female patients with a history of at least one in-hospital assaultive episode were more likely than nonassaultive patients to be seen as still dangerous to others and/or to require intensive psychiatric services (care level 1 or 2) at the time of the survey. Patients without a history of assault were twice as likely to be appropriate for community placement.

Of all variables analyzed, only age and diagnosis were significantly related to levels of supervision necessary. Those assaultive patients requiring a secure environment for current behavior dangerous to others were more likely to be less than 34 years old and to have a primary psychiatric diagnosis of mental retardation. Assaultive patients needing intensive supervision for severe psychotic symptoms but not currently dangerous to others were more likely to be less than 34 years old and to be diagnosed as having nonparanoid schizophrenia. Assaultive patients whose symptoms had stabilized but who were not appropriate for community placement, were more likely to be more than 65 years old and were overrepresented in the psychotic OBS and nonpsychotic diagnostic categories. Assaultive patients assigned to level 4, (i.e., appropriate for community placement) were more likely to be in 34–64 years old and in the diagnostic categories of paranoid schizophrenia and depression.

Age and Diagnosis of Assaultive Patients

In the population of chronic inpatients surveyed, 7 percent had assaulted persons in the hospital at least once in the three months preceding the survey.

Table 1-7

Current Mental Status and Level of Treatment Needed by History of Assault
in Past Three Months

Mental Status and Level of Treatment Needed	Percentage of Male		Percentage of Female	
	Assault (N = 173)	No Assault (N = 2155)	Assault (N = 186)	No Assault (N = 2516)
Level 1 Currently dangerous to others so as to require a highly secure psychiatric environment	7	<1	4	<1
Level 2 Currently showing severe psychotic symptoms so as to require intensive psychiatric services	31	11	32	10
Level 3 Psychiatric symptoms stabilized but still requires 24 hour behavioral supervision and *not* appropriate for community placement	49	59	52	66
Level 4 Psychiatric symptoms stabilized and is appropriate for community placement	13	30	12	24
	100	100	100	100
Statistics	(χ^2 = 156.80, df = 3, $p<.00005$)		(χ^2 = 120.91, df = 3, $p<.00005$)	

Often the last assault had occurred in the preceding month. The occurrence of
assaultive behavior was even more common in younger patients and those in
certain diagnostic categories. This reflects the seriousness of the problem faced
by staff and patients, even in chronic units where it has been thought that active
psychopathology and violent behavior are infrequent.

It is difficult to compare the assault rates in this survey to those in studies
using incident reports.[10,11,16] The rate in this survey, however, apparently
exceeds the rate in studies that relied on incident reports. Lion has speculated

that the studies of incident reports may suffer underreporting due to assaulted staffs' fears that they will be characterized as provocative or otherwise blamed.[19] Another possible explanation is that staff tend to report only those assaults of a serious or repetitive nature.

This author stresses the need for the complete reporting of all assaultive incidents, both minor and major, and possibly for periodic review of charts and other checks to assure complete reporting. Reports should include data concerning time, location, participants, and other circumstances. Assaultive incidents should be reviewed, as suicide attempts commonly are reviewed, at a staff conference intended to educate staff and preventing future occurrences. Minor incidents often escalate on the wards, either in the same patient or in contagion to other patients. One should not wait for staff and patients to be seriously injured before studying the problem in one's own hospital. Surveys of assaultive behavior at other hospitals may reveal different quantities and patterns of assaultive behavior, because of different patient characteristics, policies, and environmental factors.

Certain types of inpatients are more likely to be assaultive. The finding of increased risk among younger patients raises the question as to whether they should be segregated from other, especially older, patients. Evidence from Depp that young assaultive patients often direct their aggression toward older patients would support such policy.[8] On the other hand, the experience that assault breeds assault, would support the prediction that units for young assaultive inpatients might be counterproductive unless extensive resources could be used.

In contrast to this author's preadmission study, female inpatients were just as assaultive as male inpatients. As Maccoby and Jacklin have stated, physical aggression is considered more appropriate for males in our society.[20] The absence of sex differences in the hospital may suggest a blurring of sex role differences once a person becomes a chronic patient in a state hospital. Mental status and age may be more important than sex in determining whether a patient is likely to be physically aggressive.

Diagnosis is an important factor associated with the occurrence of assault and prospects for community placement. Patients with primary diagnoses of mental retardation, nonparanoid schizophrenia, and psychotic OBS were more likely to be assaultive and to be poor candidates for community placement, although it must be recalled that most patients in *all* diagnostic groups were not assaultive. Mentally retarded patients were more likely to require a secure environment because of continued dangerousness at the time of the survey. Furthermore, they were more likely than other diagnostic groups to have received emergency control measures such as seclusion, restraint, and emergency medication. Many of the mentally retarded assaultive patients were receiving routine neuroleptic medication. One must weigh the risk of long-term side effects such as tardive dyskinesia against the necessity of drug control of dangerous behavior in hospital. Nonbiological intervention often effectively prevents violence toward others.

Although nonparanoid schizophrenics with a history of assault were not quite as likely as mentally retarded patients to be currently dangerous, they were more likely than other assaultive patients to manifest severe psychopathology and to require intensive treatment. The nonparanoid schizophrenics were receiving high doses of neuroleptics and needed both emergency medication and constant observation more than other diagnostic groups. One is impressed with their lack of response to treatment even after long periods of hospitalization. Attention to the interpersonal and environmental factors associated with violence may assist in preventing assault in these patients as well.

Hospitalized paranoid schizophrenics were less likely than other patients to be assaultive, while paranoid schizophrenics assessed at the time of admission were more likely than many other types of patients to be assaultive. This suggests that paranoid schizophrenics may be more amenable to treatment with neuroleptics in the acute phase of hospitalization following admission. Those paranoid schizophrenic patients continuing to reside in hospitals may be more able to control their actions even though delusions or other psychopathology continue to exist. This is in distinction to nonparanoid schizophrenics, who are more disorganized, and those patients with mental retardation or psychotic OBSs who are less amenable to treatment. Paranoid schizophrenic patients with a history of assaultive behavior in hospital were more likely than other patients to be seen as no longer dangerous and appropriate for community placement at the time of the survey. However, it should be considered whether schizophrenics are prone to discontinue medication after discharge. This would result in reemergence of delusional thinking, loss of control, and subsequent increased likelihood of assaultive behavior. Perhaps consideration should be given to a policy, analogous to parole, and compulsory compliance with aftercare, use of depot neuroleptics, or even refusal to discharge paranoid schizophrenics with histories of assault who fail to comply. further cohort study is needed before contemplating such broad policy or legislation.

The fact that 21 percent of the assaultive patients had seizure disorders, more than twice the frequency for nonassaultive patients, is very interesting. The association of assault with epilepsy, particularly temporal lobe epilepsy is well documented,[6,22] yet temporal lobe epilepsy accounted for few cases in the current survey. Most of the problems with assault and seizures in this survey appeared to be associated with arteriosclerosis, senility, alcohol abuse, mental retardation, or other organic factors. Thus, seizures probably reflected gross brain damage which in turn resulted in loss of control, impulsivity, and violence. Association of mental retardation and serious ictal violence has been reported by Delgado-Escuta and his colleagues,[9] who reviewed videotapes of patients demonstrating violent and aggressive behavior during seizures. It should be noted, however, that the persons in the author's study do not represent the typical epileptic; stigmatization of epileptics should be avoided.

CONCLUSION

In the inpatient setting there are many factors associated with violence. Overcrowding and understaffing are observable, while subtle conflicts between staff or low ward morale are not as apparent but are transmitted to patients. Staff should give all patients, even agitated schizophrenics, the opportunity to talk rather than act.

The need for staff to analyze their reactions to violent patients is described vividly in two articles which should be required reading for such professionals: "Countertransference reactions to violent patients"[18] and "Impact of the threatening patient on ward communications."[7] At times, the violent behavior of one patient spreads to others and heightens tension on the ward. This may be compounded by an authoritarian approach by the staff. The importance of reacting to threatening patients in a nonprovocative manner has led Levy and Hartocollis to recommend that female aides work with assaultive patients.[17] There is some question about whether this method is as appropriate in the state hospital setting as it was in their private psychiatric hospital. Further, the potential need for rapid, overwhelming forces to physically contain a violent patient must be planned for in every hospital. (The complex topic of seclusion and restraint is discussed in Chapter 17. This topic will also be addressed by an American Psychiatric Association Task Force, which may submit model guidelines for Association approval.)

In the author's survey, assault was a problem even among chronic inpatients, and certain types of patients were more likely to be assaultive. The findings reported should alert all hospitals to the need for developing knowledge and expertise in the evaluation and management of assaultive behavior.

REFERENCES

1. Addad M, Benezech M, Bourgeois M, Yesavage J: Criminal acts among schizophrenics in French mental hospitals. J Nerv Ment Dis 169:289–293, 1981
2. Albee GW: Patterns of aggression in psychopathology. J Consult Psychol 14: 465–468, 1950
3. Bach-Y-Rita G, Veno A: Habitual violence: A profile of 62 men. Am J Psychiatry 131:1015–1017, 1974
4. American Medical Association Department of Drugs: AMA Drug Evaluations, 4th Edition, Chicago, AMA, 1980

5. Blackburn R: Emotionality, extraversion and aggression of paranoid and non paranoid schizophrenic offenders. Br J Psychiatry 115:1301–1302, 1968

6. Blumer D: Epilepsy and violence, in Madden D and Lion J (ed): Rage, Hate, Assault and other Forms of Violence. New York, Spectrum publications, 1976

7. Cornfield RB, Fielding SD: Impact of the threatening patient on ward communications. Am J Psychiatry 137:616–619, 1980

8. Depp FC: Violent behavior patterns in psychiatric wards. Aggressive Beh 2:295–306, 1976

9. Delgado-Escueta AU et al: The nature of aggression during epileptic seizures. N Eng J Med 305:711–716, 1981

10. Ekblom B: Acts of Violence by Patients in Mental Hospitals. Stockholm, Scandinavian University Press, 1970

11. Evenson RC, Altman H, Sletten IW, et al: Disturbing behavior: A study of incident reports. Psychiatr Q 48:266–275, 1974

12. Fareta G: A profile of aggression from adolescence to adulthood: An 18 year follow-up of psychiatrically disturbed and violent adolescents. Am J Orthopsychiatry 51:439–453, 1981

13. Fottrell E: A study of violent behavior among patients in psychiatric hospitals. Br J Psychiatry 136:216–221, 1980

14. Honigfeld G, Gillis RD, Klett JC: NOSIE-30: A treatment-sensitive ward behavior scale, Psychol Rep 19:180–182, 1966

15. Jonas AD: Ictal and Subictal Neurosis Diagnosis and Treatment, Springfield, Illinois, 1965

16. Kalogerakis MG: The assaultive psychiatric patient. Psychiatr Q 45:372–381, 1971

17. Levy P, Hartocollis P: Nursing aids and patient violence. Am J Psychiatry 133:429–431, 1976

18. Lion JR, Pasternak SA: Countertransference reactions to violent patients. Am J Psychiatry. 130:207–210, 1973

19. Lion JR, Synder W, Merrill GL: Underreporting of assaults on staff in state hospitals. Hosp Community Psychiatry 32:497–498, 1981

20. Maccoby EM, Jacklin CN: The Psychology of Sex Differences. Stanford, California, Stanford University Press, 1974

21. Madden DJ, Lion JR, Penna MW: Assault on psychiatrists by patients. Am J Psychiatry 133:422–425, 1976

22. Mark VH: Sociobiological theories of abnormal aggression, in Kutash SB, Schlesinger LB et al. (eds): Violence, San Francisco, Jossey-Bass, 1978

23. Planansky K, Johnston R: Homicidal aggression in schizophrenic men. Acta Psychiatr Scand 55:65–73, 1977

24. Ruben I, Wolkon G, Yamamoto J: Physical attacks on psychiatric residents of patients. J Nerv Ment Dis 168:243–245, 1980

25. Shader RI, Jackson AH, Harmatz JS, Appelbaum PS: Patterns of violent behavior among schizophrenic inpatients. Dis Nerv System 38:13–16, 1977

26. Tardiff K: Assault in hospitals and placement in the community. Bull Am Acad Psychiatry Law 9:33–39, 1981

27. Tardiff K: Emergency control measures for psychiatric inpatients. J Nerv Ment Dis 169:614–618, 1981

28. Tardiff: The use of medication for assaultive patients. Hosp Community Psychiatry 33:307–308, 1982
29. Tardiff K, Deane K: The psychological and physical status of chronic psychiatric inpatients. Compr Psychiatry 21:91–97, 1980
30. Tardiff K, Maurice W: The care of violent patients by psychiatrists: A tale of two cities. Can Psychiat Assoc J 22:83–86, 1977
31. Tardiff K, Sweillam A: Characteristics of violent patients admitted to public hospitals. Bull Am Acad Psychiatry Law 7:11–17, 1979
32. Tardiff K, Sweillam A: Age and assaultive behavior in mental patients. Hosp Community Psychiatry 30:709–711, 1979
33. Tardiff K, Sweillam A: Assault, suicide and mental illness, Arch Gen Psychiatry 37:164–169, 1980
34. Tardiff K, Sweillam A: Factors related to increased risk of assaultive behavior in suicidal patients. Acta Psychiat Scand 62:63–68, 1980
35. Tardiff K, Sweillam A: The occurrence of assaultive behavior among chronic psychiatric inpatients. Am J Psychiatry 139:212–215, 1982
36. Taylor M, Abrams R: Manic-depressive illness and paranoid schizophrenia: a phenomenological, family, and treatment-response study. Arch Gen Psychiatry 31:640–642, 1974
37. Whitman RM, Armao BB, Dent OB: Assault on the therapist. Am J Psychiatry 133:426–431, 1976

Frederick C. Depp

2
Assaults in a Public Mental Hospital

Adequate staffing, competent leadership, and an organization of therapeutic strategies that patients find coherent and assuring are prerequisites to attaining treatment objectives in the large public mental hospital. According to organizational theory, significant defects in the therapeutic enterprise may result in deficits in the attainment of goals and the maintenance of means. In the case of the large mental hospital, a variety of common-sense postulates have been formulated about the causes and consequences of these deficits. For example, inadequate staffing of wards often contributes to inadequate treatment programs for patients and to the demoralization and turnover of staff.

Since the mental hospital is committed to societally ascribed objectives for "people processing,"[21] which focus either on control (custodialism) or change (therapeutics), the success of its goals and means can be measured by the state of its patients. For example, a prison riot presumably indicates dysfunction in the correctional setting, and spouse abuse indicates dysfunction in the family. The administrator of the large public mental hospital therefore must be sensitive to press reports of dramatic episodes of patient violence; such episodes reflect managerial style and competence.

The assumed cause-and-effect linkages between organizational process and patient behavior are, however, highly complex and typically defy ready answers, even with careful clinical assessment of indicators such as those listed in Figure 2-1. The first set of indicators represent flight reactions of staff or patients. Staff are late or absent or leave or distance themselves from patients or decide to terminate therapies. In like fashion, patients overstay community visits, take unauthorized leave or leave against medical advice or stay and withdraw apathetically from ward process.

Fight reactions represent the alternative set of indicators. Staff chronically disagree and are hostile and at loggerheads, especially in treatment planning, while patients are self-destructive, destroy property, assault staff or other patients, or sabotage treatment plans.

This chapter will focus on only one of these dysfunctions in the large public mental hospital—physical violence between patients. This violence will be examined in relation to differences in socioenvironmental backgrounds among patients and to differences among patients that reflect social life on the wards. Assessing these factors will permit a tentative ordering of issues which may affect the problem of patient violence.

At this time our empirically grounded knowledge base does not allow us to confirm or deny with confidence most speculated relationships drawn between socioenvironmental factors in the large psychiatric treatment setting and dysfunctional flight or fight reactions of staff and patients of which patient violence is but one. Not only has there been insufficient direct examination of these relationships but additionally, there has not been any simultaneous control of extraneous factors likely to predict patient violence.

The data which will be presented here have been developed from a series of studies conducted at St. Elizabeths Hospital over the past several years. The report will emphasize characteristics of the violent patient dyad, which consists of the patient who strikes and the patient who is struck. The analysis of the patient pair in ward context was stimulated by Toch's study of police–citizen encounters[27] and Wolfgang's important analysis of Philadelphia homicides, especially those in the family setting.[31] Both studies reflect the growing realization that those who are assaulted need to be considered as potentially significant contributors to these encounters within an interactional study frame.

Causal implications will not be addressed. In this author's view the present level of systematic understanding requires rather that efforts be devoted to finding and comparing the strength and nature of associations between physical violence and a range of suspected precipitants. For example, James enumerates more than twenty of the "... commoner causes of aggressive behavior" among the subnormal which range from premenstrual tension and constipation to an unpleasant letter from home and jealousy of attention paid to another patient.[11]

Figure 2-1. Socio-environmental model to problematic hospital behaviors among staff and patients.

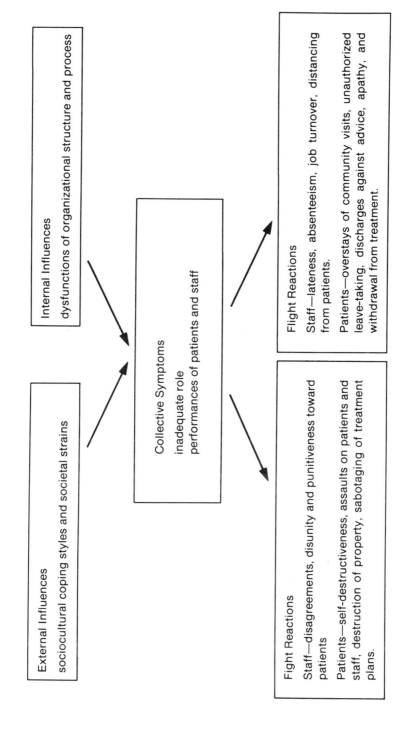

External Influences
sociocultural coping styles and societal strains

Internal Influences
dysfunctions of organizational structure and process

Collective Symptoms
inadequate role
performances of patients and staff

Flight Reactions

Staff—lateness, absenteeism, job turnover, distancing from patients.

Patients—overstays of community visits, unauthorized leave-taking, discharges against advice, apathy, and withdrawal from treatment.

Fight Reactions

Staff—disagreements, disunity and punitiveness toward patients

Patients—self-destructiveness, assaults on patients and staff, destruction of property, sabotaging of treatment plans.

Such lists tend to endless variety and description, usually without any rank ordering of relative importance. This chapter will provide comparative data on physical assault and will introduce possible significant predictors of institutional violence. Precipitating factors represent either an aspect of the ward's physical, social, or temporal structure; an aspect of the relationship between ward staff and patients in the incident; or an aspect of the relationship between patients involved in the incident.

STUDIES OF PATIENT VIOLENCE

Our initial effort[4] (hereafter called Study One) used 379 consecutively reported incidents of physical violence between patients, 238 of which (63 percent) occurred on the wards between pairs of patients whose identities were known. These 238 incidents were also similar in that only one patient was physically violent and medical attention was rendered in some form. Analysis focused on this largest subset of cases and ignored the remaining 86 incidents in which there was retaliation, staff involvement, off-ward occurrence, an unknown assailant, or more than two participants.

Study Two[3] retrospectively assessed 60 violent incidents using an orientation previously applied effectively to study suicides[14] and prison disturbances.[29] Interviews were conducted with those staff most closely involved with these incidents on 23 closed general psychiatric wards, using a structured questionnaire of 143 items. Those wards housing patients under criminal proceedings were excluded as were those treating special populations, e.g., drug addicts, alcoholics, children, or geriatric patients.

A violent incident qualified for study if both patients were identified, the injury sustained required medical attention and was not self-inflicted, and the incident occurred on a weekday on the first or second shift—between 7:30 A.M. and 11:30 P.M. This time limit was established to reduce variability in incident type and increase the likelihood of obtaining usable data.

Ward Context

Temporal Variations

Ward violence has shown to vary by hour of the day and day of the week (Study One). From 6:00 A.M. to 10:00 P.M. there were three periods of observed increase. Most significant among these is the 6:00 to 8:00 A.M. period, which showed 72 assaults while there were only 4 from 4:00 to 6:00 A.M. and only 34 from 8:00 to 10:00 A.M. Thus, 30 percent of all incidents (72 of 238) during the 24-hour day occurred in the 2-hour period between 6:00 and 8:00 A.M. This high proportion of violence in the morning is consistent with

Fottrells' reporting of a 30 percent rate of violence between 7:00 and 9:00 A.M. also in a 24-hour observation period.[7] The remaining two smaller increases during the day occurred between 12:00 noon and 2:00 P.M. and from 4:00–6:00 P.M. By day of week the highest assault rate is on Monday, the next highest is on Thursday, and the remaining days are unremarkable in rate variation.

Considering assault rates by time of day and day of week together raises the question of whether increases in demanded activity affect patient assault rates. Both Monday's weekly high and the 6:00–8:00 A.M. daily high represent periods of increase in demanded activity following periods of inactivity. This situation essentially corresponds with Melbin's finding of ward disturbance decreases during periods of staff reduction and fewer scheduled activities.[18]

Ward Organization

The demanded-activity hypothesis also is consistent with our finding (Study One) that sex-integrated, "mixed," wards have an adjusted annual rate of reported assault of 0.114/patient, which is slightly higher than the rate on male wards (0.101/patient), and is much higher than the rate on female wards (0.043/patient). One hypothesis offered to explain these data is that mixed wards present a more complex demand pattern for patients. While most observers believe this ward type gives substantial pressure for the normalization of behavior, it may have adverse consequences of heightened anxiety and inadequate information processing due to stimuli overload among very disturbed patients, especially those with organic deficits. Assaults in such an explanatory scheme could be seen as primitive means of coping by a disorganized individual unable to understand or function in his or her environment.

Architectural Blind Spots

One of the preconditions for violence on hospital wards is believed to be opportunity for nonobservation determined in part by architectural arrangements that produce blind spots in staff monitoring of patients. Although in many instances staff identified certain places in which it was difficult to observe patients (Study Two), only 13 cases of the 60 (22 percent) violent incidents occurred out of sight of staff. Table 2-1 shows the relative frequency of cases in which Study Two characteristics were found present. Narrative detail indicated that in 2 of these 13 instances, the setting for the violent incident was accidental and was determined primarily by a struggle over a record player, rather than by the deliberate selection of a blind spot. Thus, there were only 11 cases in which lack of observation appears to have been a possible contributing factor.

Table 2-1

Situations and Characteristics that Precede, Accompany, or Follow Violence
(Study Two, N = 60)

Situations and Characteristics	Frequency	Percentage
Either or both patients require relatively more supervision and observation and/or compete more than most for staff attention and favors.	55	92
The striker is physically stronger than struck patient.	47	78
Striker is more impaired or equal in psychiatric functioning.	43	72
Informal or formal staff discussion took place after the incident to reassess management of either or both patients.	41	68
One or both patients require more supervision and observation than does the remainder of the patient group.	40	67
One or both patients are more competitive for staff attention than is the remainder of the patient group.	40	67
Explicit restrictions or sanctions were placed on the striker following the incident.	34	57
The striker has an unusual problem in having others near or touching him or her, or the assaulted patient is unusually intrusive and meddlesome compared to other ward patients.	33	55
One of the pair is unusually concerned with the issue of justice and equity.	31	52
The ward indicates between zero and two reportable incidents of violence in the prior 30 days.	29	48
Staff are pessimistic about striker ever leaving the hospital or believe treatment is at an impasse or deadened.	29	48
There is a defined patient hierarchy on the ward.	27	45
Situational frustration or agitated behavior by the striker was evident just before incident.	25	42
The struck patient is either retarded, senile, blind, or has a substantial physical handicap.	24	40

(continued)

Table 2-1 (continued)

The striker is more impaired in psychiatric functioning in comparison to struck patient.	23	38
Either or both patients had a privilege request refused or were being actively considered for a privilege change.	23	38
The struck patient is unusually intrusive and meddlesome.	22	37
The struck patient is at least 40 percent older in age than the striker.	21	35
Striking patient has a primary diagnosis which importantly implicates organicity.	21	35
Defense of territory or possession was considered implicated in the incident's occurrence.	20	33
The striker has unusual difficulty with having others near or touching him or her.	17	28
Violence occurred out of sight of staff in ward space difficult to monitor.	13	22
Staff anticipated trouble between these two patients.	10	17
The striker was considered to be actively hallucinating just before the incident with evidence of psychotic transference to the struck patient in the incident.	9	15
There were marked ward changes in the seven days preceding the incident concerning important policies or rules, medications for either patient, staffing or patient group composition.	—	—

Patient Hierarchy

In the hospital surveyed staff speculated that violence often is initiated by patients who are in the middle positions of the ward's hierarchy of dominance against those at the lowest level in order to maintain status and influence. In Study Two staff were asked whether they could affirm the existence of fairly clear pecking orders or ranking structures among patients in terms of rights, privileges, and status (See Table 2-2). A well-defined pecking order or hierarchy was reported to be present in 27 instances of assault (45 percent of cases). In three other assaults, staff did not believe a generalized status hierarchy was present, yet were able to evaluate the status positions of both patients relative to one another and to most patients on the ward. For this reason that data also was used.

Table 2-2
Ward Hierarchy Position and Frequency of Violence (Study Two)

	Striking Patient	Struck Patient	Frequency	Percentage	
	Upper	Upper	—	—	
		Middle	6	20	50
		Lower	9	30	
Ward		Upper	4	13	
Position	Middle	Middle	3	10	26
		Lower	1	3	
	Lower	Upper	3	10	
		Middle	2	7	24
		Lower	2	7	
	Total		30	100	

When informants were asked to place patients from these incidents in the upper, middle, or lower part of these defined social structures, an interesting pattern emerged (Table 2-2). In 16 instances, the striking patient was perceived as having a higher position in the hierarchy compared to the struck patient; in 9 instances the struck patient was perceived as dominant; while in only 5 instances both patients were perceived to have equal status. This pattern suggests that violent acts may have importance for maintaining or challenging social status or position when a hierarchy is present, especially since only 5 cases show violence between equals, while 25 cases involve unequals. This view is also supported by the fact that one half the striking patients are located in the upper third of their ward's status hierarchies, while only 7 of those struck (23 percent) are in the upper third. When a hierarchy is reported present on a ward (see Table 2-3) the struck patient tends not to be intrusive ($r = -0.35$); staff do not place restrictions on the assaultive patient ($r = -0.25$), the striker is not concerned with justice and equity issues ($r = -0.28$); and staff can describe predictors or behavioral signs of the striking patient which tend to precede violence ($r = 0.31$). Each of these relationships suggests that an established dominance hierarchy importantly affects the character of violence in the ward environment. Further study of more cases using these typings (violent acts by dominants, subordinates, or peers) is necessary to determine how the ward hierarchy and patient positions in it may be useful to prevent violence.

Table 2-3

Associations Between Violence Factors (Study Two)

Violence Factor		1	2	3	4	5	6	7	8	9	10	11	12	13	14	15	16	17	18	19	20	21	22
Ward context— physical, social,	Blind spot	1		10	05	-19	00	16	10	-08	06	03	05	07	02	-19	-18	17	-12	-04	-04	-22	21	02
	social hierarchy	2			-22	-21	09	04	-25	03	-07	-26	-28	-01	-35	11	-17	-20	02	-04	-04	-22	21	02
	prior violence	3				01	12	-03	-09	-26	10	11	-12	-18	08	01	03	08	05	08	-08	12	08	-08
Staff Relations and actions	pessimism	4					19	02	-17	-26	-17	00	05	-26	11	-15	17	-10	09	-12	12	32	-20	-17
	privilege change	5						02	-11	02	02	03	-01	15	04	20	-01	03	03	-12	29	05	29	-02
	supervision, observation	6							19	30	03	-09	-08	-09	-03	03	-17	-04	-01	05	-05	-02	03	06
	restrictions	7								14	05	-09	21	23	07	17	08	26	-21	-07	15	08	01	-03
	reassessment	8									25	18	-06	-03	-08	15	-19	-06	14	03	-12	-12	05	18
Violent patient pair	territory, possessions	9										27	02	07	12	-06	-15	-18	-10	00	-22	-10	27	-06
	touch, closeness	10											02	02	00	-07	-10	01	22	-05	-10	17	04	-22
	justice, equity	11												07	-16	-14	25	01	-01	-17	-06	-14	24	-14
	retarded, senile, handicap	12													08	-12	09	00	00	07	-19	-15	-06	-09
	psychiatric intrusiveness	13														-24	14	17	06	03	12	26	-04	-12
	impairment	14															-02	00	-16	-15	05	21	-04	17
	physical strength	15																12	15	02	-03	05	-10	-11
	victimization	16																	-19	02	-09	04	-06	07
	frustration, agitation	17																		08	05	12	-05	-35
	chronicity	18																			-37	-26	00	11
	Organicity	19																				11	18	-14
	transference	20																					-24	-06
	competition	21																						09
	preincident signs	22																						

Violence Contagion and Preincident Signs

Effort also was made to determine whether there was evidence to support a social contagion theory of violence (Study Two, see Table 2-1) such as Stanton and Schwartz refer to as being a consequence of unaddressed staff conflict.[25] In such a model it could be expected that most observed incidents were preceded by a series of like incidents occurring in the recent past. We were interested in determining how frequently a "high" ward, with evident tension and previous violence, would be reported to us. Respondents were asked:

In the last 30 days, how many assaultive incidents, which involve physical attack (including fights), would you estimate have occurred here on the ward? (Not just incidents where there is an injury which results in a reportable occurrence.)

Sixteen wards reported no other incidents, 13 wards indicated 1 or 2, 17 had 3–6 incidents, 3 reported 9 and 10 each, while 10 others estimated between twelve and fifty incidents. Contagion is certainly subject to differing operational definitions and requires a formal comparison between adjacent time periods to argue persuasively for its presence or absence. Yet 29 of 60 wards presenting between 0 and 2 incidents does not strongly support this kind of explanation. In only 10 of 60 instances, staff said they had a basis for predicting trouble between these specific patients. There was no knowledge of any exchange of strong words or prior exchanges; although histories of recent conflict expressed with either verbal or physical assault is often frequent for certain kinds of intact resident populations, as for example in Berkowitz and Macauley's study of a correctional setting.[1]

Object Defense and Territoriality

The defense of physical objects and space defined as one's own territory also are often cited as contributors to patient violence. Questions were asked (Study Two, see Table 2-1) to determine whether either or both patients associated themselves strongly with specific places or with particular objects or possessions such as a book, a piece of clothing, or a pipe. There were 17 instances (28 percent of cases) in which objects or possessions appeared implicated in these acts, suggesting this factor merits more detailed study.

Significant Changes in Policies, Staffing, and Patient Group

Recent social change involving the ward community's policies, staffing, and patient composition also was evaluated to test the assumption that such alterations are elements frequently associated with violent acts. No marked changes were found for any of these ward level factors in the seven days preceding any acts of physical violence.

We believe these ward level factors do contribute to patient violence. However, changes in ward social organization such as departures of significant staff members, likely do not occur with sufficient frequency to explain the physical violence observed daily in the hospital milieu. For example, a prior analysis of 31 violent incidents on 4 general admission wards specifically addressed the extent of staffing coverage and incident occurrence.[5] Average staffing levels for the shift and day of the incident were compared with staffing levels for the same periods over the three previous days. Staffing coverage was examined for all nursing personnel assigned and male nursing personnel assigned. No significant differences in staffing were noted. However, there was some tendency for higher staffing levels on the shift or day a violent incident occurred.

The direct relation between staffing and frequency of violence is consistent with our daily and day-of-week patterns and Melbin's data reported above. It may also be consistent with Levy and Hartocollis' finding that a ward with female nursing personnel produced fewer violent incidents than did a control ward with male and female staff,[16] since our demanded activity hypothesis assumes the presence of a staff authority, backed up by physical coercion.

Kalogerakis' finding of an inverse relation between ward census and rates of assault[13] belies the popular belief about density or overcrowding and may tie in with our finding of a direct relation between staffing and violence. In both cases the proportion of staff to patients increases. In Kalogerakis' case due to a decrease in ward census while in ours due to an increase in staffing.

Staff–Patient Relations

Patient Privileges

One continuing index of the state of the authority relation between staff and patients is found in the privilege granting process. Because privilege requests and consequent denial or granting can be stressful and frustrating for patients, staff tend to implicate granting of privileges in the problem of ward violence. We found specific evidence of immediate situational frustration and unusually high levels of agitated behavior for 25 of 60 strikers (42 percent) just before their physical attacks (Study Two, see Table 2-1). Exploring the sources of prior frustration and unusually agitated behavior, we noted a denial by staff of a privilege request (in 10 of 60 cases) or found that the striking patient was actively under consideration for increased privileges involving more personal autonomy. These privileges had not been requested by the patient in 15 of 60 cases. Although some consider recently granted privileges for patients a source of stress and a possible explanation of assault, there was almost no evidence in our data to support that speculation (only 4 of 60 cases). These data therefore suggest that both the period following a patient's denied request and the period during with an additional privilege is under consideration may contribute to patient violence, while the period following actual receipt of a new privilege does not. These linkages between restrictions on privileges and violence are consistent with Quinsey's study in a forensic setting where patients and staff agreed that a restriction for patient misbehavior was one of the two major causes of assault.[22]

Staff Expectations

Hopelessness among these inpatients was indirectly assessed by obtaining staff expectations concerning the patient's probability of ever leaving the hospital and living again in the community. The staff were asked, "In your opinion do you expect patient (name) will probably never leave the hospital?"

This question was not asked in isolation, but followed other questions designed to determine whether the patient was believed likely to be living out of the hospital within the next six months and, if so, whether it was believed better for the patient to remain in the hospital longer than six months. In another phase of the interview, ward staff members were asked whether they believed effective treatment of the patient was currently at an impasse, or a "dead end." Responses reflecting either staff pessimism concerning the patient's release to community living or an opinion that effective treatment was at an impasse were combined to construct an index reflective of staff pessimism about positive change for the patient or as Guirguis puts it, a failure " . . . to communicate positive expectations to the patient."[9] Of the 60 striking patients, 29 (48 percent) were rated as persons about whom ward staff were pessimistic concerning any substantial change; in 10 instances (16 percent) an uncertain assessment was given; while in only 21 cases (35 percent) were staff hopeful for change.

When staff evidenced pessimism about a striking patient, they tended not to reassess management following the violence ($r = -0.21$). Further, staff tended to believe the striker was hallucinating at the time of violence with transference involving the struck patient ($r = 0.32$). Staff's tendency not to reassess management appears consistent with viewing the patient as hopeless and unchangeable, while absence of hierarchy may reflect the disorganized nature of those wards where no treatment program is operating to maintain staff morale and give hope for patient change.

Staff definitions of patient hopelessness and the frequent absence of reassessment after violence both may have a hostile component thus making these actions akin to more overt forms of staff provocativeness addressed by Quinsey[22] and Madden, Lion, and Penna.[17]

Competition for Staff Attention

Pursuing the dominance hypothesis, we also wanted to determine if status instability in the patient group might be evidenced by greater competitiveness for staff attention and favors among those patients implicated in violent acts. In 40 incidents (67 percent) one or both patients were identified as more competitive than most ward patients for staff attention and favors, with 20 striking and struck patients each so specified. Staff attention as an inadvertent social reinforcement for violence was indirectly assessed by asking whether

Table 2-4
Mean Differences Between Striking and Struck Patients (Study One)

Patient Characteristic	Patient Pairs (N = 238)	
	Striking	Struck
Age	37.00	53.01
Weight	156.01	142.38
Height (in)	66.88	65.20
Prior hospitalization (yrs)	9.84	13.99
Seclusion (hr/mo this admission)	22.04	5.79
Involvement in unusual occurrences (monthly rate)	0.23	0.25

Reprinted with permission from Depp FC: Aggressive Behavior, Volume 2:295-306, 1976.

either patient required relatively more supervision and observation than other ward patients. In two-thirds of all incidents (40 of 60, or 67 percent), either or both patients were so identified. In contrast to the competitive dimension however, staff reported 23 percent of struck patients (14 of 60) and 43 percent of striking patients (26 of 60) require relatively more supervision and observation. Noteworthy in these data is the large number of struck patients who often tend to be ignored in analyses of violence and the suggestions offered for its prevention.

Coupling this response pattern with prior data about competitiveness shows that in 55 of these 60 violent incidents (92 percent) either or both patients were considered a prominent part of the ward patient collective because they required continuing, extensive staff effort and supervision and/or had a marked tendency to compete more than most for staff attention. Thus, violent behavior for many of these patients as strikers or victim is related to substantial, ongoing relations with ward staff.

The prominance of both striking and struck patients also is evident by frequent reports of unusual occurrence. Although striking patients tend to receive a highly variable response following violent behavior, it is nevertheless true that they are more heavily secluded compared to struck patients. For example, in Study One strikers averaged 22.0 hours of seclusion time each month of their hospitalization while struck patients averaged 5.8 hours/month (Table 2-4). The greater ward control strikers suggests that their behavior is evaluated as substantially more dangerous to self or others or destructive of property—the three primary justifications for seclusion. Since destructiveness and dangerousness to self are comparatively infrequent, seclusion differences provide a useful index of the greater staff concern for aggression that strikers present. Whether staff concern contributes to a self-fulfilling pattern of assault-preventing seclusion that produces anger and resentment in patients and precipitates further assaults is uncertain.

Staff Reactions After Violence

While there was no evidence of intentional positive reinforcement by patients or staff for violent behavior, neither was there very much evidence of negative sanctioning (Study Two). In 2 cases, the striker voluntarily spent several hours in seclusion, in 32 cases the striking patient was involuntarily placed in seclusion while in the remaining 25 instances no seclusion was ordered. Involuntary seclusions were maintained for highly variable time periods. In some instances seclusion was ordered for only 1 hour, while at the other extreme seclusions were ordered for 60, 72, and 96 hours. Although a violence severity ranking was not formally developed, we believe these incidents would tend to be considered roughly equivalent acts on that dimension— neither trivial nor terribly serious and life endangering, as is true for example in the smaller incidence of cases Ekblom discusses.[6] Given this approximate equality, it is difficult to interpret the extremes in staff response or the absence of sanctions evident in many instances. Further, ward reporters indicated in about one-third of these cases (19 of 60) the incident did not result in any discussion, either informal or formal, by two or more staff members. Treating these incidents as nonincidents directly contradicts the prevailing wisdom expressed by Penningroth: "After a violent incident it is important to reassure other patients and encourage discussion of their feelings and reactions. It is equally important for staff to review the incident together, for they also have feelings and reactions."[20] Rada gives a third reason for a review after violence.[23] The patients' mental status needs to be assessed to help understand whether the behavior is situational, organic, or functional in nature.

Study Two also showed that striking patients are less likely to be restricted when there is a social hierarchy ($r = -0.25$) and when staff are pessimistic about change ($r = -0.17$). When a hierarchy is present there is a defined code of ward values which is likely to sanction physical violence. The association with pessimism may mean that when staff give up on a patient they relax restrictions on his or her behavioral excesses unless these threaten survival of the ward community. One could then see how pessimism and relaxed constraints would form a vicious cycle with each contributing negatively to the caregiving process and positively to the generation of violence.

The Violent Patient Pair

Age, Physical Dominance, and Chronicity

Our initial interest in the 238 incidents of Study One focused on the marked differences in age between striking and struck patients. Strikers were an average of 30 percent younger than those struck, with a mean age of 37. The assaulted patients averaged 53 years old (see Table 2-4).

Using hospital statistics for inpatient age groups, we found that struck patients were represented in approximate proportion to their numbers in the inpatient population while younger age groups tended to be overrepresented among strikers. This suggests that those assaulted are not selected for assault by age or age-linked behavior per se and may, to a large extent, be assaulted for reasons unrelated to age. However, age may be a contributory factor in assault by young patients due to the age variation now found among patients who are not segregated by their histories of assaultive behavior and assault potentials.

Study controls for the age relation between patients and evaluation of strength differences by physical weight showed that there was a tendency for striking patients to be heavier than those struck (see Table 2-4) whether strikers were younger, of the same age or older (the relative age percentages of strikers who were heavier were 59, 60, and 42 respectively). If physical strength were the primary factor overriding the age variable, one would expect to see proportionately more strikers of greater weight advantage in those cases where patients were of the same age or the striker was older. This was not found to be the case, suggesting that both a physical strength advantage and age difference represent contributing factors, and both merit further attention.

Most strikers in Study Two (47 of 60, or 78 percent) were assessed as stronger than those struck or equal in strength (20 of 60, or 17 percent). In only 3 instances of 60 was the striker believed to be physically weaker than the patient struck. By contrast, strikers tended to be assessed as sicker and more out of contact than struck patients. In almost 40 percent of cases, strikers were described as more mentally impaired (23 of 60 instances); as equally impaired in one-third of cases (20 of 60); and as functioning at higher levels in only 16 instances (27 percent of cases). Those patients with lower levels of internal control for coping with ward pressures tend to be identified in violent encounters as being physically stronger than those they strike.

Given the relative lower level of mental functioning among strikers, information was sought on the potential prevalence of psychotic transference in these incidents. In only 9 instances (15 percent) did staff believe striking patients were probably responding to either auditory or visual hallucinations during the violence.

Because patient age and length of hospitalization are positively associated, a question was raised also concerning the role of the latter factor in assault incidents. It was found that younger striking patients (average age 37 years) had been hospitalized the same proportion of their lives as had older struck patients (average age 53.01 years). Struck patients averaged just 42 percent more prior hospitalization time with a mean of 13.99 years while striking patients averaged 9.84 years, thus demonstrating the struck patients, although older, were not in fact more "chronic" (see Table 2-4).

The lack of difference in prior inpatient time between strikers and those struck, after adjusting for mean differences in age, may parallel a previously reported lack of difference between assaultive and nonassaultive patients using first admission status versus readmission status as the index of chronicity reported by Tardiff and Sweillam.[26] These findings suggest that length of hospitalization does not affect role selection in violence or the adoption of a violent or nonviolent coping style in the ward.

Patients admitted within six months tend to be overrepresented in these incidents on both sides of the assaultive relationship. As one examines categories reflecting longer hospitalization, assaultive patients are decreasingly represented in these incidents.

At the other extreme of hospitalization, only 10 percent of the striking patients and 22 percent of those struck[2] were among the 30 percent of inpatients with more than 25 years in residence. This finding contradicts the prevailing belief that patients hospitalized the longest bear the brunt of assault by those younger. It appears that length of hospitalization does not affect the age differences in the violent pair. For example, among the 33 incidents in which both patients had been hospitalized for less than 6 months, struck patients (average age 36 years) are still 30 percent older than are strikers (average age 28 years).

In Study Two chronicity was defined as two or more years of cumulative inpatient hospitalization time. Using this definition chronicity was found to be associated with organicity ($r = 0.37$) and inversely with both transference ($r = -0.26$) and concern with justice and equity issues ($r = -0.17$). Interestingly, no relation was noted between chronicity and physical strength differences, victimization, defense of territory or possessions, or intrusiveness by the struck patient.

Effects of Gender and Race on Assaultive Behavior

Not only is age linked to assault but gender and race are as well (Table 2-5—Study One). Assault with a physical injury tends to be found pre-dominantly among male patients. Although there are almost equal numbers of male and female inpatients, 63 percent of strikers and 62 percent of those struck are male (Table 2-5). Our data further show that there is significantly less assault across gender lines than predictable by chance (only 27 percent involved a male and female when exactly 50 percent were expected). It should be noted that 90 percent of those cross-gender assaults (54 of 60) were initiated by black patients with males initiating only a few more assaults than females (29 versus 24). Males tend to assault males and females strike females. This part of our analysis was of course directed specifically to those 30 or so hospital wards in which patients of both sexes reside. Whether this pattern results from a cultural constraint, from patients' associations on the wards, or from peer competition or rivalry remains unclear.

Black patients are overrepresented in the striking role (73 percent of strikers are black while 58 percent of inpatients are black), and whites are

Table 2-5
Comparison Between Striking, Struck, and All Patients (Study One)

Patient Characteristics		Patients Percentage of all assaults		
		Striking	Struck	All Inpatients
Race and gender	White male	17	33	19
	White female	10	21	23
	Black male	46	29	29
	Black female	27	17	29
Age group	Under 63 yr	91	58	61
	63+	9	42	39
Primary diagnosis	Functional psychoses*	54	50	51
	OBS†	20	31	26
	Mental retardation‡	15	6	5
	Other	11	13	18
One or more major and visible physical handicaps		34	28	§

Reprinted with permission from Depp FC: Aggressive Behavior, Volume 2:295-306, 1976.
*Diagnostic and Statistical Manual (DSMII) Codes 295 through 298.
†DSM Codes 290 through 294 and 309.
‡DSM Codes 310 through 315.
§Percent unknown.

overrepresented in the struck role (54 percent of those struck are white while 42 percent of inpatients white). In the striking role males of each race exceed females, while white patients of each sex are underrepresented in this role. While the gender and racial data are limited, it is interesting to note that in-hospital overrepresentation of male and black patients in violent incidents appears to be substantially lower than is true for community rates reported by Webster,[28] Wolfgang,[30] and Hindelang.[10]

White males take the striking role in proportion to their numbers in hospital. In contrast, the situation among those struck is somewhat different. Black females are heavily underrepresented among struck patients, black males and white females are struck in approximate proportion to their numbers in the hospital, and white males are prominently overrepresented among struck patients.

Diagnostic Combinations

Considering assaultive incidents as dyadic interactions also produced an interest in determining whether differences in patient behavior patterns were reflected by marked diagnostic patterns in violent dyads (Study One). We were interested not only in assessing the proportionate representation of hospital patients by diagnosis in both assault roles, but also in the possibility that specific diagnostic combinations might repeatedly be evident.

Using diagnostic data for inpatients we found those with functional psychoses proportionately represented in the roles of striking and struck patients (see Table 2-5), although there is a widespread belief in hospital settings that these patients are substantially overrepresented in assaultive incidents.

Patients with organic brain syndrome (BOS) are underrepresented as strikers, probably because those patients tend to be older and physically less able. That tendency also likely explains the overrepresentation of these patients among those struck in assault (see Table 2-5).

Patients with a primary diagnosis of mental retardation, by contrast are overrepresented in the striking role relative to their numbers in hospital (see Table 2-5). These patients deserve additional special attention as a subgroup in such settings, particularly with respect to their means of expressing tension and interpersonal conflict.

In Study Two striking patients with a primary diagnosis of OBS or mental retardation were defined for analytic purposes as an organic deficit subgroup to determine whether differences in the character of their violence could be observed. Twenty one of the 60 striking patients (35 percent) had an organic deficit relfected in a primary diagnosis such as alcohol-related deterioration, profound or severe mental retardation, or psychosis with brain trauma.

Goldstein characterizes these organically deficient patients' reactions as "catastrophic" when cognitive demands made on them exceed a level which can be internally processed.[8] One catastrophic reaction is physical violence toward others. Goldstein hypothesizes that the organic patients' physical violence tends to be characterizable as an explosive outburst which is relatively undirected. The notion that organic patients exhibit violent behavior distinct from that of nonorganics was confirmed in some ways and not in others in these data. For example, following the assumption that the violence of organic patients is less directed and organized, one would not expect to find organics selectively striking those weaker than themselves while such behavior would be found among those without these deficits. There was almost no association, however, between organicity and victimization ($r = -0.09$). On the other hand, we did find staff reported less predictability of violence for organic patients by way of prior behavioral indications ($r = .14$) and the privilege changes were more frequently implicated in the violence of these patients ($r = .29$). Beginnings of an empirical pattern of differences in violent behavior for these patients may be seen, although several contradictory tendencies are also found.

In summarizing diagnostic data from both studies, although there were not any diagnostic combinations particularly evident in patient assault, we did note that certain diagnoses were linked to either the role of striker or struck patient. Some caution must be exercised since the frequencies are small but in these data there also was some tendency for patients with personality disorders, transient situational disturbances, and behavioral disorders to be overrepresented in the striker's role. In contrast, patients with neuroses, major affective psychoses, psychoses with intracranial infection, alcoholic psychoses, and senile psychoses were overrepresented in the struck role. As indicated, age plays a part in certain of these apparent linkages between specific diagnoses and assault roles. Due to insufficient data, however, an analysis of the age-variables' effect upon these relations is not feasible at this time.

Equity Concerns and Physical Proximity

In Study Two staff considered 17 of the assaultive patients and 19 of those struck to be unusually concerned with the issue of justice, with "people being taken advantage of" and not getting a "fair shake." These patients are found in more than half of the incidents sampled (31 of 60) and this pattern is consistent with the repeated concern about perceived encroachments by others on possessions or privileges. In many instances, patients appear to quickly interpret these encroachments or intrusions as significant moral issues and threats to self worth.

Additionally, 17 of 60 striking patients and 11 of 60 struck patients have an unusual and persisting difficulty, compared to most ward patients, with having other people near them or touching them. This assessment corresponds to other work or anxiety and proximity among the institutionalized.[15] We did not find that specific ward places or territories are strongly associated with these personal approach sensitivities $(r = 0.13)$. This finding suggests that sensitivity to personal approach operates independently of specific place in the ward environment.

Victimization

In 24 instances of 60 (40 percent) assaults, the struck patient was noted to be either retarded, senile, or to have a substantial physical handicap. Such a patient was therefore less likely or able than other patients to assess risk and use discretionary strategies to avoid conflict (Study Two).

Struck patients are often visibly incapacitated. Not only were 11 either retarded or senile, but another 3 were restricted to wheelchairs. Whether these incapacities contribute to violence because they indicate weakness and a lower risk of retaliation or whether they trigger status anxiety and issues of self-definition among striking patients or both is unclear.

The age factor (which is positively correlated with physical strength) was used to construct an overall index of victimization. If a patient struck another patient 40 percent older than him or herself, this was defined as a substantial level of victimization. If the struck patient was older than the striker by less than a forty percent age difference, this was defined as a mild level of victimization. In more than one-third of the incidents studied (21 of 60) there was substantial victimization using this operational definition.

These data also reflect the price paid for mixing patients without regard to differences in age, disability, and behavioral characteristics. While there are advantages to mixing, in recent years the disadvantages have been increasingly stressed. Danger of serious injury and even death by ward violence due to extreme patient differences is certainly one important factor in recent growing staff concern in many hospitals.

Role Consistency

Concerned with the issue of multiple involvement in assault, we found 87 patients reported in an assault more than once. Of the 324 incidents involving one-way assault or reciprocal striking each with 2 roles—striker and struck patient—for a total of 648 role positions, these 87 patients accounted for 38 percent or 249 role positions. Of the 486 patients in these incidents, 87 patients accounted for more than one-third of all role positions.

Staff usually are surprised to find that in any careful enumeration of violent incidents a small number of patients are responsible for a large proportion of violent incidents. For example, Quinsey found that 13 percent of the patient grouping accounted for 61 percent of the assaults in a forensic setting studied.[22] Fottrell also highlights the focused nature of violent behavior as an institutional problem in his study of three large English hsopitals. He found that of the total number receiving inpatient treatment, 3 percent were involved in 70 percent of incidents in the first hospital, 1 percent produced 41 percent in the second and 4 percent produced 59 percent of incidents in the third.[7]

Our data also show a high degree of role consistency; those patients in more than one assault tended to take the same role. Defining these roles— striker, struck, or participant in reciprocal striking—we observed that of the 249 roles taken by patients more than once, in 173 instances or about 70 percent of the time, patients took the same assaultive role. When a patient was involved in an assault more than once, there was about a seven in ten likelihood that he or she would appear again in the same role. Further, there was not one instance in which a patient repeatedly involved in assault took the roles of both striker and struck patient except one patient who was found in all three role positions in five assaults. Patients involved in more than one assault were most often found taking the striker's role (45 percent of these 249 role positions) with the nonstriker patient role next most in evidence.

CONCLUSION

These data indicate that violent behavior is frequent and occurs pre-dominantly between pairs of patients. Violence is usually unilateral, i.e., without retaliation by the struck patient.

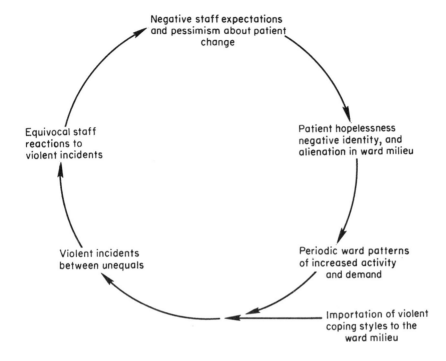

Figure 2-2. Conceptualizing socioenvironmental factors in hospital violence.

While these separate findings contribute to an emerging objective view of hospital violence and therefore have value for those responsible for ward management, they also need to be considered in our ongoing, collective effort to understand hospital violence through systematic study. Three major organizing concepts suggest themselves in the data and may allow us to better focus our thinking about socioenvironmental factors. These are the demanded activity concept of the ward milieu; staff expectations for patient change or inability to change that are communicated to the patients; and the dominance-submission features in the violent dyad.

Figure 2-2 exemplifies different ways these three concepts might operate together in the ward milieu. Other modes of action and reaction are not ruled out.

Staff expectations of no change for certain patients are communicated to them, especially by withdrawal of significant personal involvement and concern. Hopelessness about change becomes an important part of the patients' self-definition, precipitating alienation and depersonalization. When ward activity demands are increased, they are experienced as external requirements unrelated to the patients' interests. Ward demands are perceived as being useful for meeting the needs of others but of no significance for the patients' fate. As reflections of the custodial demand system, orders to rise, bathe, eat, or leave the dormitory may evoke resistance which serves to confirm the continued operation of the self and the vaguely autonomous sense of choice and decision remaining within. Resistance to staff's demands results in anger, which is displaced to expressed as violence toward one's other patients as physical assault. Striking weaker, more helpless patients is a dramatic violation of societal norms and undermines staff expectations for order and cooperation. The data indicate substantial competition for staff attention. That most violent dyads are comprised of patients with differing social statuses on the ward also implies that the staff–patient authority difference may be implicated. To the extent that the striker identifies himself as an actual or potential victim, may his violence communicate both a protest to staff and a punishment to encroaching patients.

Violence may also represent a response consistent within a patient subculture with its own normative code for weighing right and wrong actions and administering primitive forms of retributive justice. The data on object defense, equity concerns, patient hierarchy and extreme variability in staff responses are all suggestive of a patient-based normative code governing peer relationships. We are aware that the withdrawal or breakdown of formal authority in a collective will stimulate member development of an informal set of replacement mores. Levy and Hartocollis' data on patient surrogates exercising peer control functions on a female staffed ward exemplifies this pattern.[16]

Finally, in order to provide an assessment of the predictive usefulness of these data, eight statistical efforts were made to identify our violence cases along selected dimensions of clinical importance. For example, a discriminant function analysis was used to identify cases of violence initiated by patients with an organic deficit from those without such a deficit.[19] The same procedural approach was used for seven other dimensions of clinical interest seeking to identify their presence or absence in these incidents (Table 2-6).

As shown in Table 2-6, the procedure failed to successfully classify violence cases based on the pair of statistical models applied to these data. Accuracy levels ranged between 42 and 63 percent using the stringent split half method and between 68 and 87 percent for the whole sample technique. Interestingly, the two sample prediction levels closely approximate estimates of predictive accuracy of between 40 and 46 percent given for assessing dangerousness.[12]

Our inability to more accurately predict the presence or absence of an organic deficit in the striking patient, using information about the nature of the violent incident, suggests that we do not yet have a usable approach for modelling this problem behavior. Alternatively, one may argue there is no objective data to substantiate that the organic patient's violent behavior is substantially different in kind from that of other patients. Similar statements

Table 2-6
Predicting Characteristics in Violent Incidents (Study Two)

Characteristic	Number of Cases		Percentage of Classification Prediction Accuracy		
	Present	Absent	Method 1: Split Half		Method 2: Whole Sample
			Equation	Balance of Cases	All Cases
Ward Hierarchy	27	33	100	63	87
Ward assault rate	31 (high)	29 (low)	80	44	68
Legitimacy of incident*	26	34	92	53	74
Staff pessimism	29	31	100	52	68
Striker—organicity	21	39	97	59	83
Striker–chronicity	48	12	85	62	85
Intrusiveness of target	22	38	94	46	80
Victimization of target	21	39	89	42	73

*An incident was called legitimated violence if no sanctions or restrictions were placed on the assaultive patient following its occurrence.

apply to other violence features; for example, the victimization of older patients or the presence of absence of a patient hierarchy. Application of such concepts as explanatory factors after violence occurs must be done with an awareness that good objective and systematic evidence is inadequate.

We need to exercise caution when easily assigning functional responsibility to hospital leadership for violence and other fight or flight reactions among both patients and staff. Smith argues that the mental hospital is a type of "front line" organization with significant power decentralized to its peripheral units.[24] Our data reflect extreme variability between wards while also describing certain structural inter-relations between patient violence and ward process. There is no systematic data, however, to support causal linkages between administrative decision making and patient behavior. Almost all of the hard work of objective assessment remains to be done to make more specific those common causal sequences which determine violent or nonviolent response patterns among inpatients.

REFERENCES

1. Berkowitz L, Macauley J: The contagion of criminal violence. Sociometry 34:238–260, 1971
2. Depp FC: Preventing injuries inflicted on elderly psychiatric patients. Issues in Mental Health Nursing 3:353–363, 1981
3. Depp FC: Socio-environmental Factors in Hospital violence. Final Report. The Hoffman Division of Research, St. Elizabeths Hospital, Washington, D.C., 180
4. Depp FC: Violent behavior patterns on psychiatric wards. Aggress Behav 2:295–306, 1976
5. Depp FC: Ward Violence and Nursing Personnel Staffing Levels. Unpublished report. St. Elizabeths Hospital, Washington, D.C., 1973
6. Ekblom B: Acts of Violence by Patients in Mental Hospitals. Transl by Helen Frey, Svenska Bokforlaget, Uppsala, 1970
7. Fottrell E: A study of violent behavior among patients in psychiatric hospitals. Br J Psychiatry 136:216–221, 1980
8. Goldstein K: Functional disturbances in brain damage, in Arieti S (ed): American Handbook of Psychiatry. Second Edition Vol 4: Organic Disorders and Psychosomatic Medicine. Basic Books, New York, 1971, pp. 182–207
9. Guirguis E: Management of disturbed patients, an alternative to the use of mechanical restraints. J Clin Psychiatry 39:295–299, 1978
10. Hindelang M: Race and involvement in crimes. Am Sociol Rev 43:93–109, 1978
11. James J: Practical care of the aggressive patient. Nurs Times 68:1352–1353, 1972
12. Kahle L, Sales B: Due process of law and the attitudes of professionals toward involuntary civil commitment, in Lipsett P, Sales B (eds): New Directions in Psychological Research. Van Nostrand, Reinhold, New York, 1980
13. Kalogerakis M: The Assaultive Psychiatric Patient. Psychiatr Q 45:372–381, 1971

14. Kastenbaum R: Psychological Autoposy: A case commentary. Bull Suicidology 1:15-24, 1967
15. Kinzel AF: Body buffer zones in violent prisoners. Am J Psychiatry 127:59-65, 1970
16. Levy P, Hartocollis P: Nursing aides and patient violence. Am J Psychiatry 133:429-431, 1976
17. Madden D, Lion J, Penna M: Assaults on psychiatrists by patients. Am J Psychiatry 133:422-425, 1976
18. Melbin M: Behavior rhythms in mental hospitals. Am J Sociol 74:650-655, 1969
19. Nie NH, Hull CH, Jenkins JG, Steinbrenner K, Brent DH: Statistical Package for the Social Sciences. McGraw-Hill, New York, 1975
20. Penningroth PE: Control of violence in a mental health setting. Am J Nurs 75:606-609, 1975
21. Perrow C: Hospitals, technology, structure and goals, in March JG (ed): Handbook of Organizations. Rand-McNally, Chicago, 1965 pp 910-971
22. Quinsey VL: Studies in the reduction of assaults in a maximum security psychiatric institution. Can Ment Health 25:21-23, 1977
23. Rada R: The Violent Patient: Rapid Assessment and Management. Psychosomatics 22:101-109, 1981
24. Smith D: Front-line organization of the state mental hospital. Adm Sci Q 10:381-399, 1965
25. Stanton A, Schwartz M: The Mental Hospital. Basic Books, New York, 1954
26. Tardiff K, Sweillam A: Assault, suicide and mental illness. Arch Gen Psychiatry 37:164-169, 1980
27. Toch H: Violent Men: An Inquiry into the Psychology of Violence. Aldine, Chicago, 1969
28. Webster W: Crime in the United States—1977 F.B.I. Supt. of Docs., U.S. G.P.O. Washington, D.C., 1978
29. Wilsnack R, Ohlin L: Preconditions for Major Prison Disturbances. Paper presented to the American Sociological Association. New York, N.Y., August 1973
30. Wolfgang M: From Boy to Man—From Delinquency to Crime. National Symposium on the Serious Juvenile Offender. Minneapolis, 1977
31. Wolfgang M: Patterns in Criminal Homicide. Wiley, New York, 1966

Park Elliott Dietz
Richard T. Rada

3

Interpersonal Violence in Forensic Facilities

Forensic facilities as a class span a range that resembles psychiatric units at one extreme and the worst prisons at the other. Their patients and inmates, mostly men, are typically described as violent and psychotic, though one or both of these features is absent more often than is generally assumed. Moreover, the relationship between a history of violence and a psychotic mental disorder is highly complex. Both the outcome of legal proceedings, which often determine admission, release, and disposition of these men, and the very designation of the facilities as "forensic" are directly related to presumptions and debate about the relationship between violence and mental disorder.

A major nationwide study of forensic facilities has recently been completed by Steadman et al.[13] They identified 256 facilities providing care to mentally disordered offenders. In 1978 only 32 of these were specialized *primary facilities* devoted solely to forensic activities. The other 224 (88 percent) were *secondary facilities*, mostly specialized, secure units within larger psychiatric institutions, such as forensic units within state mental hospitals. Of the 32 primary facilities,

20 (63 percent) were run by departments of mental health; the other 12 were run by correctional agencies. Departments of mental health ran 201 (90 percent) of the secondary facilities. Not including pretrial evaluation cases, the average daily census of these forensic facilities in 1978 was 14,140 persons. Admissions during 1978, again excluding pretrial evaluation cases, totalled 20,143 persons, a figure not dissimilar from that reported a decade earlier.[12] Given that these data do not include pretrial evaluation cases, which often comprise half of the institutional census at any given time, the total number of individuals institutionalized in forensic facilities on any given day in the United States may be closer to 30,000.

Researchers who have attempted to study episodes of interpersonal violence in forensic facilities have anticipated considerable resistance from the staff. The shared experience seems to be that research of any kind is viewed skeptically and unenthusastically. To some extent, the skepticism is justified in that the treatment resources of many such settings are so sparse that deployment of manpower for the long-term goals that research might promote seems inappropriate in the context of immediate suffering and a bottomless pit of needs for basic services. Staff members and administrators of these institutions have been embarrassed[9,11,14] and even indicted on criminal charges[9] following exposure in the media and are understandably suspicious of anyone who might write about what goes on within their walls. As in any bureaucracy, recordkeeping is designed—to the extent that it is designed at all—for purposes of day-to-day administrative needs, not for science or history, and certainly not to document failures or outright abuses. These difficulties are only a part of the challenge facing one who would study interpersonal violence in forensic facilities.

These difficulties can be overcome; studies of interpersonal violence in at least five forensic facilities have been published during the past five years. These include Quinsey and Varney's[7] study of a unit at Penetanguishene in Ontario, Thornberry and Jacoby's[15] study of Fairview State Hospital, Rogers and colleagues's[10] study of a unit at Chester Mental Health Center in Illinois, Stokman and Heiber's[14] study of Mid-Hudson Psychiatric Center in New York, and our own studies of a maximum security hospital (MSH), which the administrators preferred not to identify.[1,2,3]

In this chapter, we highlight findings from these various studies, and share our view of the clinical and policy implications of these findings.

LIMITATIONS OF AVAILABLE QUANTITATIVE STUDIES

The validity and generalizability of published studies is severely comprised by two problems: the unknown extent of underreporting and underdetection and the "apples and oranges" phenomenon.

Lion, et al. documented a remarkable degree of underreporting of incidents of all types in a state hospital.[6] Elsewhere, we interpreted data on the rates of reported incidents under low- and high-census conditions at MSH as suggesting that underdetection of incidents must be taken into account along with underreporting.[3] Particularly under high-census conditions, staff may be unaware that certain incidents have occurred. Thus, even complete reporting of incidents known to staff may fail to disclose those kept secret by patients. Official incident reports are therefore analogous to police arrest records in that they exclude cases handled informally[5] or never detected.[4]

Of the published studies conducted in forensic facilities, only that by Quinsey and Varney seems to have overcome the problem of potentially large reporting biases.[7] They did so by limiting their study to a single unit with a mean census of approximately 138, by conducting their study prospectively, and by interviewing both staff members and patients about the reported incidents. The other studies have relied on institutional incident reports, with varying degrees of confidence in the completeness of those reports.

The "apples and oranges" phenomenon, i.e., the fact that various authors have studied dissimilar events, was overcome by Quinsey and Varney by limiting their study to events involving "physical contact of a forceful nature between two or more persons."[7] Our studies began with the delineation and pretesting of descriptive criteria for classifying incidents as batteries (involving physical contact), assaults (threats of various kinds without physical contact), parasuicides (self-destructive actions or threats), and disorderly conduct episodes. The incident classification scheme is shown in Table 3-1. In contrast, Thornberry and Jacoby did not disaggregate their data according to whether physical contact had occurred, since their analyses were not focused on violence within the institution.[16] Rogers et al. lumped together assaultive behavior, self-destructive behavior, and behavior resulting in property damage as "aggressive behavior," and compared this class of incidents with socially disruptive behaviors such as verbal abuse, theft, and persistent rule-breaking.[10] Stokman and Heiber lumped together incidents of all types in their analyses.[14]

Dietz compared assaults with batteries in our data base and found multiple significant differences which suggest that threats and blows should be differentiated from one another in the study of violence within institutions.[1] Threats differed from blows in location of occurrence, social role of the participants, religion of the assailant, preadmission criminal charge of the assailant, and legal status of the assailant. In addition, although people were injured in both assaults and batteries (since many injuries occur as the staff respond to incidents, the probability and severity of injury differ between assaults and batteries. In our study of battery incidents and batterers, we found many differences when these were compared to all nonbattery incidents and the patients involved in them.[2] Studies of incidents within institutions therefore must be interpreted with attention to the exact type of incidents

Table 3-1

Criteria for Classifying Nonfatal Intrainstitutional Incidents

Incident Class		Behaviors coded for inclusion
Battery	A.	At least one of the following: Assaultive impact with weapon Assaultive impact with body* Forcible sexual contact Matter† set in motion striking another
	B.	No parasuicide behavior more serious than the battery behavior
Assault	A.	At least one of the following: Threatening another with weapon (action) Threatening another with body (action) Threatening another with weapon (verbal) Threatening another with body (verbal) Threatening talk Matter† thrown at another without striking another Provocative talk‡
	B.	No battery behavior and no parasuicide behavior more serious than the assault behavior
Parasuicide	A.	At least one of the following: Suicide attempt Self-mutilization Other self-harm Suicide threat (action) Self-mutilization threat (action) Other self-harm threat (action) Suicide threat (verbal) Self-mutilation threat (verbal) Suicide talk Self-mutilation talk Other self-harm talk
	B.	No battery or assault behavior more serious than the parasuicide behavior
Disorderly Conduct	A.	At least one of the following: Destruction of property§ *Striking inanimate object* *Matter*† set in motion without human target Escape attempt Stealing Possession of contraband Bizarre or psychotic conduct Disobedience Walking beyond designated area Making noise
	B.	No battery, assault, or parasuicide behavior

*Includes striking, hitting, tackling, grabbing, and body blocking.

†Thrown food and drink are included here for the sake of conceptual clarity and conformity to common legal definitions.[1]

‡Provocative behavior is included here because it is extremely difficult to differentiate from threatening behavior. Efforts to separate these two classes decrease the reliability of classification.

§Firesetting may be included here or, depending on intent and consequences, under any of the other incident classes.

studied, for some are studies of apples, some of oranges, and some of fruit in general.

When the limitations discussed above are taken into account, our established knowledge of interpersonal violence within forensic facilities seems meager. In the following sections, we highlight the state of corrent knowledge.

INTERPERSONAL VIOLENCE AMONG PATIENTS AND CORRECTIONAL OFFICERS

Timing and Location

The month of the year and day of the week are not significantly related to the occurrence of interpersonal violence,[1,7] and popular beliefs regarding phases of the moon are not borne out.[7]

We noted that the highest frequency of batteries at MSH was on Thursdays, the day that patients from most units assemble for movies, and suggested that it would be worthwhile to determine whether the type of film shown is related to the frequency and type of subsequent incidents.[2] Dr. Bruce Harry recently conducted the proposed study and found that the types of films shown did indeed relate to changes in postviewing frequencies of incidents of specific types, classified according to our incident typology, shown in Table 3-1.* He found that batteries increased significantly after patients had viewed adventure films (though none of these were graphically violent), and did not increase following comedies, romances, or mixed-genre films, though other types of incidents increased significantly after patients had viewed comedies and romances.

In contrast to month and day, hour of the day has a dramatic association with the occurrence of interpersonal violence.[1] Figure 3-1 shows the distribution of assaults (i.e., threats) and batteries (i.e., blows) from our data at a forensic facility, MSH. The doors to patients' rooms are unlocked at 7:00 A.M. and the frequency of both assault and battery immediately rises above that observed during the night. Assaults and batteries tend to peak from 8:00 A.M. to 9:00 A.M., 11:00 A.M. to noon, and 4:00 P.M. to 5:00 P.M.; these are the time intervals when patients go to the dining room for meals. The violence drops after 6:00 P.M., the hour at which the first wave of patients retires to their rooms for the night, and decrease again after 10:00 P.M., when the remaining patients retire.

Two differences in the hourly distributions should be noted. The first is that from 2:00 P.M. to 3:00 P.M. batteries decrease but assaults do not.

---

*Harry B: Movies and behavior among hospitalized mentally disordered offenders. Unpublished data. (Manuscript available from Dr. Dietz.)

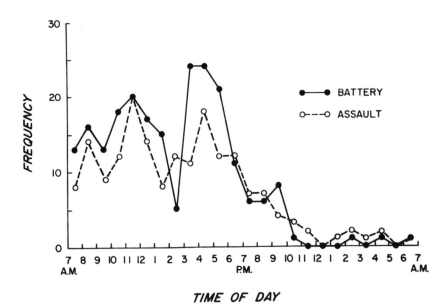

Figure 3-1. Distribution of reported assaults and batteries in a forensic facility by hour of occurrence. From Dietz, PE: Threats or blow? *Int J Law and Psychiatry, 4* p.406, 1981. ©1982 Pergamon Press. With permission.

Batteries may decrease at this time because patients are assembled under correctional officer supervision and are counted in preparation for the officers' change of shift. At MSH this process involves patients exiting to the yard and returning single-file. This activity apparently is associated with little change in the frequency of reported assaults and a clear decrease in the frequency of reported batteries.

The second noteworthy difference is in the relative frequencies of assault and battery at night. Approximately two-thirds of the patients are locked in single rooms for the night. Although assaults are possible from these rooms, batteries are not, accounting for the higher frequency of assault than battery from 10:00 P.M. to 7:00 A.M. One-third of the patients are selected by the officers to sleep in four-man dormitories. These are the patients whom the officers typically describe as "no trouble" and cooperative." These dormitories are supposed to remain unlocked so that patients retain access to a common bathroom in the hall, and it is among these patients that batteries occasionally occur during the night.

Quinsey and Varney also found dramatic variation by hour of day,[7] but the specific variation was quite different from that we observed. In the institution they studied, the first sharp rise in frequency occurred at 8:00 A.M., after breakfast but before patients went to work areas or to organized activity. This was a time when patients mopped the corridor or engaged in unstructured activity. At lunchtime the frequency declined, but rose again between lunch and dinner. At their institution the highest rates occurred in the evening when patients were watching television, shaving and showering, or talking in the yard or in the corridor.

The observed differences between these two institutions and the timing of batteries becomes understandable when considered in relationship to the location of incidents. At MSH batteries were particularly likely to occur in the dining room and in the ward dayrooms. These two locations accounted for a statistically significant association between the density of patients at certain locations and the proportion of incidents at these locations that were batteries.[2] The same observation held true when batteries were compared with assaults, i.e., batteries were disproportionately likely to have occurred in the dining room or in dayrooms.[1]

In contrast, Quinsey and Varney found that two-thirds of the batteries occurred in the corridor and in patients' rooms, with few if any occurring in the dining room.[7] They noted that locations, such as the dining room, to which patients gained access only if they had demonstrated sustained stable behavior were rarely the locations for batteries.

Thus, we found high frequencies of battery in the dining room because at the institution we studied, all patients except those in seclusion went to the dining room, where many different wards simultaneously mingled in one large room. At Penetanguishene battery rarely occurred in the dining room; patients earned the privilege of going to the dining room and fewer patients were assembled there at any one time. Conversely, the patients at Penetanguishene frequently battered in their own rooms.[7] At MSH, since patients had individual rooms unless they had proved themselves to be "no trouble," patient rooms were rare sites for battery not only at night, but also during the evening when many patients began to retire to their rooms. Timing and location therefore are closely interrelated. The distribution of batteries in time and space varies between institutions, but in comprehensible ways. In both institutions, batteries occurred with greatest frequency at those times and places with the highest levels of interaction among patients.

These observations provide one of the most important practical implications of the published studies. The evidence strongly suggests that the goal of reducing the frequency of batteries could be furthered by changing patterns of interaction through environmental design and institutional policy. At MSH the observed frequency of batteries in dayrooms suggests such options as structural enlargement of these areas, or diversion of some patients to other areas at times of peak use. The frequency of dining room incidents might be reduced by staggering the arrival of different units in the dining room to a greater degree, by seating fewer patients at each table, or by exercising a greater degree of selection over which patients may go to the dining room. At Penetanguishene, the frequency of batteries might be reduced by structural changes leading to a higher proportion of single rooms or by policy changes restricting patients' unsupervised access to corridors.

Whether such changes are measurably beneficial will be known only if naturally occurring changes are properly studied or if experiments are properly conducted with such changes. In any case the potential benefits must be weighed against the costs of such structural and policy changes. These costs include not only the financing of architectural changes or personnel shifts, but also the impact on the overall treatment program. If all patients were confined to individual rooms 24 hours a day, there would be no batteries, no treatment, and no opportunity for the patients to prove themselves able to live with others. Nonetheless, institutions concerned about levels of interpersonal violence can further their conceptualization of the extent and nature of the problem by studying the frequency of incidents in relationship to specific locations and time of day.

Characteristics of Patients in Relation to Interpersonal Violence

Although the age variation among patients in forensic facilities is not great, some evidence suggests that in these facilities, as in the population at large, younger patients have higher rates of interpersonal violence than older patients. Quinsey and Varney found that batterers were significantly younger than nonbatterers.[7] Thornberry and Jacoby provide evidence that the rate of incidents of all types combined (mostly violent) decreases with increasing patient age.[16]

Differential rates of interpersonal violence between the sexes are unknown and likely to remain unknown since 95 percent of patients in forensic facilities are men[13] and the patients in most of the larger institutions are exclusively men. Correctional institution folklore has it that mentally disordered women prisoners are impossible to manage and require male guards. Those who promote this belief, however, are often male correctional officers who believe they might lose their jobs to women officers or fear they might be jeopardized during violent confrontations if their partners were women. In one study, the rate of all incidents combined was higher for women than for men, but the rate of injury associated with these incidents was lower for incidents involving women patients than for those involving men patients.[14]

The only study to have addressed race was our own, but with inconclusive results. Although nonwhites were disproportionately involved in batteries, this might be because nonwhites were disproportionately prison transfer cases who were housed on a unit with a small dayroom and the highest rate of batteries of any of the nine residential units.[2]

Targeted data have not been gathered on diagnosis in relation to interpersonal violence within forensic facilities (in our case, because chart diagnoses were too unreliable). Looking at incidents of all types combined, Stokman and Heiber found no strong relationship with diagnosis.[14] Since there is a widely shared assumption that paranoid schizophrenic patients are disproportionately violent even within institutional settings, it may be worth looking at the available clues as to associations with diagnosis, meager as these are. Stokman and Heiber found a slight tendency for patients with diagnoses of schizophrenia, personality disorder, or drug dependence to have fewer incidents than expected, and for those with mental retardation or organic brain syndrome (OBS) to have more incidents than expected.[14] Quinsey and Varney reported the diagnoses of the 18 patients with the highest frequency of batteries. Diagnoses among these were schizophrenia (10), mental retardation (5), epilepsy (1), psychosis associated with encephalitis (1), and transient situational disturbance (1), though the diagnostic distribution for other patients was not reported.[7] Thus, correct data do not support the assumption that any specific diagnostic category is disproportionately associated with interpersonal violence within forensic facilities.

No association is known between the types of charges brought against patients before admission to their involvement in violent incidents within forensic facilities. We found no association between preadmission criminal charge and involvement in batteries, once we had controlled for duration of hospitalization.[2] Batterers did, however, differ from assaultists in preadmission criminal charges; the most common preadmission criminal charge among batterers was battery, and the most common preadmission criminal charge among assaultists was assault. In addition, batterers were more likely to have had no preadmission criminal charges, indicating that they had been transferred from a state mental hospital as being unmanageably violent.[1] Despite these minor differences between patients committing battery and patients committing assault within the institution, administrators and clinicians should not assume that preadmission criminal charges are predictive in any meaningful way of patients' propensity toward violence within the institution.

Quinsey and Varney found that batterers were more likely than other patients to have a history of previous admissions to psychiatric hospitals or retardation facilities and were more likely to have been referred to the forensic facility from a psychiatric or retardation facility.[7] Batterers were less likely to have a criminal offense as the reason for their admission and were less likely to have been adjudicated unfit to stand trial or not guilty by reason of insanity. We found that batterers were disproportionately individuals who had been transferred from prison to the forensic facility and were somewhat more likely to have been transferred from a mental hospital.[2] A reciprocal interpretation of our data would be that patients undergoing pretrial or presentencing evaluations are somewhat less likely to become involved in batteries than other patients.

Quinsey and Varney noted that approximately 13 percent of the patients accounted for 61 percent of the batteries.[7] This is analogous to the observation, widely replicated in studies of crime within the community, that a small number of offenders are responsible for a large share of the offenses. This observation requires critical analysis in terms of probability theory in order to determine the extent to which it is a statistical artifact.

The relationship between violent incidents and duration of hospitalization is difficult to determine because violent incidents are routinely used to justify continued hospitalization. Evidence from Quinsey and Varney[7] and from Thornberry and Jacoby[16] is consistent with a hypothesis that violent incidents are particularly likely to occur soon after admission or among patients with particularly prolonged hospitalization.

The most important generalization that can be made about existing knowledge of the relationship between patient characteristics and violence within forensic facilities is that no strong associations are known. The variable with the greatest impact, although still not a particularly strong association, appears to be legal status. We think that the most useful predictors of intrainstitutional violence will ultimately be shown to be history of intrainstitutional violence, mental status, legal status, and age. Charges and diagnosis are less likely to prove useful.

The Process of Interpersonal Violence

In interviewing participants in violent incidents, Quinsey and Varney found that staff members and assaultive patients connected with incidents gave very different accounts of the motivations for the event.[7] Staff most frequently reported that there was "no reason" for a battery, while patients most often reported that they had been teased by other patients or provoked by the staff.

Although our data from MSH are limited to the content of official incident reports, they permit us to examine the correctional officers' accounts of the events in some detail. The most prevalent accounts given indicate that a battery in progress or already completed received the attention of officers. From the standpoint of the officers, the battery itself marked the initiation of the incident. This was the case in 170 (76.9 percent) of 221 batteries, none of which was anticipated by the officers. The other 51 battery incidents were recorded as having begun with some other disruptive or assaultive conduct that was followed by a battery. The particular behaviors noted as preludes to battery were all such commonly occurring events that they had little or no predictive value.[2]

We found that the patients who initiated batteries, either through their provocative behaviors or by striking the first blow, were themselves likely to be hit by the time the incident was completed. In some instances, a provocateur was struck in return by another patient, in others a batterer was struck in return by another patient, and in many a batterer was forceably subdued by officers. The patient who initiated the incident was hit in 153 (69.2 percent) of 221 batteries. This proportion is significantly greater than the proportion of provoking patients ultimately hit in assault incidents[1] or in all nonbattery incidents combined.[2]

Of 221 batteries, 30 resulted in serious injury, 59 in minor injury, and 132 in no injury. Many of the injuries associated with batteries (and all of the injuries associated with assaults) occurred in the course of officers' efforts to subdue patients. Some incidents resulted in more than one injury. The 221 batteries resulted in 32 injuries requiring treatment (such as lacerations, bite wounds, and fractures), and 89 minor injuries not requiring medical treatment (such as bruises, small cuts, and scratches). Including violence associated with subduing activities, patients were hit 317 times, officers 91 times, and other staff members 5 times. Of these, 181 occurred while patients were being subdued by officers, accounting for 45.7 percent of the bodily impact to patients and 39.6 percent of the bodily impact to officers.[2]

Preliminary analysis of other MSA data—incident reports, census, and staff—suggests that while the frequency of injury was greater for patients than for officers, the injury rate per waking hour in the institution was substantially higher for officers than for patients. For other staff members, both frequency and rate were low.

An unwritten MSH rule requires that all noncorrectional staff members immediately leave the scene when an incident is occurring. This rule is said to reflect concern about the safety of the noncorrectional staff member. Compliance with this rule has led to a secondary effect, whether intended or not, that incidents in progress are rarely observed by clinicians. Officers' formal accounts of subduing, almost without exception, use the phrases, "the patient had to be forcibly subdued," or "a violent struggle ensued." Patients' accounts of subduing suggest that most often there is an uncoordinated descent of all available officers on the individual perceived as the aggressor.

Regardless of the validity of these divergent accounts, it is clear that noninjurious techniques for subduing patients might have enormous impact on the rate of injury to both patients and officers. This is an area for intervention in which it is not necessary to await the results of observational studies of subduing practices before attempting to change those practices. The effects of such changes can be reasonably evaluated by monitoring injury rates and injury severity before and after implementing the change.

"Soft" Observations

In the absence of hard data and in an area with few empirical studies, we may perhaps be allowed to mention some unsystematic observations. The first of these is the extraordinary difference we have observed between traditional forensic facilities and specialized forensic units in teaching hospitals. The forensic units at the Royal Ottawa Hospital and at the Clarke Institute of the University of Toronto, for example, receive patients for the same purposes as the large forensic facilities in the United States. Patients are screened for admission to these units, no doubt making it possible to provide a very different sort of care than is provided in the large forensic facilities. The units are operated like the inpatient units of most teaching hospitals, with both men and women patients on the same unit, regular attendance by nurses, physicians, and other clinical staff, and a conspicuous absence of the symbols of police power (such as barbed wire, metal detectors, armed officers, and correctional uniforms). Such units are so vastly preferable to the usual sort that the visitor cannot escape recognition of the extent to which we have elsewhere isolated our forensic populations from good and humane care. We are told that the incident rates on these forensic units are similar to or even lower than those on the other units of the same hospitals. Likewise, the forensic unit at the Augusta Mental Health Center in Maine operates much like the other units of that hospital without any discernible difference in incident rates. In that instance, the patients are not specially screened for admission but are told upon arrival that they are entering a hospital, not a prison, and are expected to behave accordingly.

The issue of patient expectations has received insufficient attention. We suspect that much of the violent and disruptive behavior within forensic facilities reflects the success with which the institutional physical and social structures and the initial interaction with newly admitted patients convey the message that they are expected to be violent and psychotic. A wealth of experimental and survey data over the past decades documents the power of expectations and self-fulfilling prophesy in determining human behavior. We think that forensic facilities could be vastly different from what they are today and that major changes in the expectations held out to patients would be critical in implementing needed improvement.

CONCLUSION

Several investigators have examined interpersonal violence within forensic facilities. These investigations are in a relatively early stage of development. We do not yet know, for example, whether the rates of battery and resulting injury are different in forensic facilities from other psychiatric institutions, in part due to inconsistencies among studies in the selection of units of analysis and in the definitions of assaultive acts. Comparisons between institutions will become possible only when some consensus has been reached about definitions, and would be best achieved through collaborative prospective studies.

Although we recognize that intrapsychic and interpersonal factors must be assessed when the clinician evaluates individual acts of violence,[8] we believe that the strategies offering the greatest hope for reducing injury rate and severity from interpersonal violence within forensic facilities are changes in environmental design, institutional policy, and techniques for subduing patients whose behavior is considered unacceptable. The false assumption that forensic patients are all violent and psychotic even if true would not justify the conditions under which so many of them live, the abuses to which so many are subject, or fatalism toward the occurrence of interpersonal violence within these institutions.

REFERENCES

1. Dietz PE: Threats or blows? Observations on the distinction between assault and battery. Int. J Law Psychiatry 4:401–416, 1981
2. Dietz PE, Rada RT: Battery incidents and batterers in a maximum security hospital. Arch Gen Psychiatry 39:31–34, 1982
3. Dietz PE, Rada RT: Seclusion rates and patient census in a maximum security hospital. Behav Sci Law (in press)
4. Gold M: Undetected delinquent behavior. J Research in Crime and Delinquency 3:27–46, 1966
5. Goldstein J: Police discretion not to invoke the criminal process: Low-visibility decisions in the administration of justice. Yale Law J 69:543–589, 1960
6. Lion JR, Snyder W, Merrill GL: Underreporting of assaults on staff in a state hospital. Hosp Community Psychiatry 32:497–498, 1981
7. Quinsey VL, Varney GW: Characteristics of assaults and assaulters in a maximum security psychiatric unit. Crime and Justice 5:212–220, 177.
8. Rada RT: The violent patient: Rapid assessment and management. Psychosomatics 22:101–109, 1981
9. Rawls, W., Jr.: *Cold Storage.* New York: Simon and Schuster, 1980.
10. Rogers R, Ciula B, Cavanaugh JL, Jr: Aggressive and socially disruptive behavior among maximum security psychiatric patients. Psychological Reports 46:291–294, 1980
11. Ryan T, Casey B: Screw: A Guard's View of Bridgewater State Hospital. Boston, South End Press, 1981
12. Scheidmandel PL, Kanno CK: The Mentally Ill Offender: A Survey of Treatment Programs. Washington, D.C., American Psychiatric Association, 1969
13. Steadman HJ, Monahan J, Hartstone E, et al: Mentally disordered offenders: A national survey of patients and facilities. Law Hum Behav 6:31–38, 1982
14. Stokman CLJ, Heiber P: Incidents in hospitalized forensic patients. Victimology (in press) 5:175–192, 1980
15. Thomas, B & Stebel, S.L.: *The Shoe Leather Treatment.* Los Angeles, J.P. Tarcher, Inc., 1980.
16. Thornberry TP, Jacoby JE: The Criminally Insane: A Community Follow-up of Mentally Ill Offenders. Chicago, University of Chicago Press, 1979

Lois M. Conn
John R. Lion

4

Assaults in a University Hospital

This chapter examines assaults that occurred in the psychiatric unit of a large, urban, university teaching hospital during the 18-month period of July 1979 through December 1980. Ours is a 54-bed psychiatric facility in an 800-bed general hospital. Forty-four beds are reserved for adults and 10 are for children. Admissions are, for the most part, elective and scheduled. Patients are also admitted on an emergency basis through the emergency room and by way of community mental health centers. All admissions are voluntary; certified and court-ordered patients are not accepted. Psychiatric residents have primary responsibility for all admissions.

The data in this chapter were obtained primarily by reviewing formal incident reports which are required to be filed with the Office of the Hospital Director for any assault or other out-of-the-ordinary incident occurring on any ward. During the 18-month study period, reports were filed on a total of 2165 incidents that occurred throughout the general hospital; 61 were identified as involving some degree of physical violence, determined by key phrases such as

Table 4-1

Distribution of Assaults over an 18-month Study Period

Service	Number of Assaults	Percentage of Total Assaults
Psychiatry	25	41
Emergency Rooms (Adults and Pediatric)	11	18
Medicine	8	13
Surgery	5	8
Pediatrics and Adolescent Medicine	4	7
Shock-Trauma Unit (A critical care service) and other Intensive Care Units	4	7
Prison Ward	2	3
Obstetrics/Gynecology	1	1.5
Location not listed on incident report	1	1.5
TOTAL	61	100

"hit," struck," "assaulted," and so on. In cases of ambiguous incident reports, personnel were interviewed to determine whether the incident was an accident or the result of willful behavior.

Of the 61 assaultive incidents, 25 (41 percent) occurred within psychiatric units. This high percentage becomes even more significant in view of the fact that the psychiatric service at our hospital comprises only about 7 percent of total hospital beds. Eleven assaults (18 percent) occurred in the emergency room. The remainder were distributed throughout the general hospital. Table 4-1 gives a breakdown of the number of assaults occurring on various hospital services during the study period.

We found that 9 of the 36 assaultive patients in the general hospital (25 percent), regardless of the service on which they had been hospitalized, had been identified previously as having some form of psychiatric history such as prior antisocial behavior or evidence of severe agitation or assaultiveness, a history of psychiatric hospitalization, or mental retardation. Table 4-2 gives a breakdown of this phenomenon. Because of incomplete documentation on incident reports, the percentage of general hospital patients with a psychiatric history is probably underestimated. Interestingly, a number of patients who assaulted staff in the general hospital had already been subjectively perceived by nursing personnel on their wards as being potentially volatile and had therefore been provided with a full-time "sitter" to keep them under constant surveillance.

Assaults during the study period ranged in seriousness from the infliction

Table 4-2
Evidence of Psychiatric History in Nine Assaultive Patients in the General
Hospital

Hospital Location	Patient History
Emergency Room (ER)	Prisoner from area penitentiary.
ER	Patient presented to ER in "hysterical" state.
ER	Patient from area penitentiary.
ER	Patient recently discharged from psychiatric hospital.
Prison Ward	Prisoner from area penitentiary.
Medicine	Previously violent on the ward—had been provided with a full-time sitter.
Surgery	Previously agitated on the ward—had been provided with a full time sitter.
Surgery	Mentally retarded patient.
Surgery	Previously agitated on the ward—had been provided with a full-time sitter.

of minor cuts and bruises to several broken teeth and a lacerated lip when a
nurse on the psychiatric unit was struck in the mouth by a psychotic patient.

Information concerning the diagnoses and backgrounds of the offenders
as well as the circumstances under which an assault occurred was obtained with
difficulty. A formal diagnosis was usually given on psychiatric incident reports,
but was commonly overlooked on reports filed from the emergency room and
other areas of the general hospital. Delineation of assault profiles could, therefore, only be carried out by review of the attacks occurring on the psychiatric
ward.

Table 4-3 lists general categories of assaults occurring on the psychiatric
wards. As shown, most injuries (32 percent) occurred during seclusion procedures. Unfortunately, formal training for staff in restraint and seclusion techniques is lacking at most facilities (including ours until very recently). The high
percentage of injuries occurring during seclusion of a patient points to the need
for such staff training on a routine basis at any institution that admits
dangerous patients.

It is also noteworthy that roughly only one-fourth of assaults were felt, in
retrospect, to be unprovoked or unanticipated. These were in general committed by psychotic patients whose distortions of reality led them suddenly to
act out aggressively against those around them. For example, on one of these
cases, a psychotic patient who previously had been docile on the ward
unexpectedly struck a nurse when he incorporated her into a delusional system
in which he thought she intended to harm him.

Table 4-3

Types of Assaults Occurring on the Psychiatric Service

Type of Assault	Percentage of Total
Unprovoked	
Unanticipated; no warning even when viewed retrospectively	28
Provoked	
Injury of staff or patient during a seclusion procedure	32
Assault by a patient on another patient following a verbal argument, or by a patient on a staff member attempting to break up the argument	20
Assault by a patient on a staff member following the verbal denial of a privilege such as smoking or leaving the ward	16
Miscellaneous	4
Total	100

Escalation of a verbal argument accounted for 20 percent of assaults. This clearly demonstrates the need for rapid staff intervention when such a situation arises.

Excluding injuries that occurred during a seclusion procedure, the offenders were patients in all of the assault incident reports examined, with one exception. In that case a physician grabbed a hospital visitor around the neck and chest following a verbal dispute. Unfortunately, the details of this incident could not be elucidated as the physician involved was unavailable at the time of this writing.

METHODOLOGICAL PROBLEMS

We would like to acknowledge some difficulties we encountered in gathering this data which are inherent in this kind of research at present.

Although a formal incident report is required to be filed for any assault at our institution, in our experience on the wards, there is significant underreporting of such episodes. Staff members shared several reasons for this with us. Primary among these was that minor assaults occurred with such frequency in psychiatric settings that they tended to be taken for granted and only the more serious assaults were reported. As one psychiatric aide commented: "If I wrote up a report every time a patient took a swing at me, I'd be doing nothing but writing all day." A second reason was a feeling among the staff that filing a report did not result in improved security on the ward and they thus experienced reporting an incident as futile. Further, staff often worried that an assault by a patient represented an instance of negligence or poor job performance on their part and they were therefore not eager to draw attention to the event. Perhaps another reason for underreporting is that our hospital's policy is unclear regarding what constitutes a reportable "incident"; the reporting is left up to the discretion of each ward.

The incident reports which do exist are generally quite vague, e.g. "acting-out patient kicked psychiatric aide following dispute over ward rules" may be all that is written. In reviewing the charts of patients who assaulted others, we were amazed to find that often there was no mention whatsoever in the progress notes tht the assault had even occurred. This absence of both detailed documentation and uniform reporting made it difficult to draw hard conclusions from the reports regarding the incidence of assaults, the circumstances under which they occur, the effects on the victim and on the milieu, and interventions which might have prevented the attack. To supplement the data, therefore, and to reconstruct episodes in order to make such conclusions, we relied on interviews with staff and patients and personal experience working on the wards in addition to reviewing incident reports and studying charts in those cases where detailed documentation existed. While this approach is anecdotal to be sure, it provided us with much valuable information from which we were able to delineate assault profiles and offer recommendations for prevention.

REACTIONS OF VICTIMS AND EFFECTS ON THE MILIEU

Little has been written about the reaction of staff members to having been assaulted. This issue was explored in several interviews with individuals at our hospital who were seriously injured when attacked by patients under their care.

Following the assault victims typically suffered from the psychological sequelae that have come to be regarded as the "Posttraumatic Stress Disorder" including insomnia, eating disturbances, anxiety, an exaggerated startle-response, depression, trouble concentrating, and "flashbacks" in which the attack would be vividly relived. Staff members who had been attacked often developed fear of working with unpredictable or dangerous patients, particularly a hesitancy to confront them or to set limits. One staff member reported that after she was assaulted, feelings of helplessness and vulnerability when she was at work persisted for several months.

Staff members reported experiencing considerable anger at the patient who assaulted them, coupled with anger at the hospital's administration for allowing the patient to remain on the ward; these emotions came into sharp conflict with the individual's sense of professional responsibility toward the patient and his or her desire to continue to provide the patient with appropriate care. This conflict—anger versus a wish to provide the patient with appropriate care—is typically experienced by the entire staff on a ward following an assault, which may result in staff splitting over the question of whether or not the patient should remain on the ward and may considerably delay resolving such a question. In some cases, assaulted individuals felt that the patient's care had been given priority over the staff member's physical protection, leaving the victim with feelings of having been abandoned and unsupported.

Following the assault, staff often reported feeling that administrators minimized the seriousness of the incident and were slow to correct the factors which might have contributed to it. Such factors included staffing shortages (particularly the shortage of male staff), poor physical design of the wards—staff working in enclosed areas with no ready route of escape if threatened by a patient—and a laissez-faire attitude toward simultaneously admitting several potentially dangerous patients despite the fact that there was no adequate way of managing them. It is particularly noteworthy that in several cases which came to our attention, a patient had in fact assaulted several individuals before any action was taken. We speculate that this might have grown out of a need on the part of the hospital administration to deny that unsafe conditions existed within their facility.

Several concerns in addition to personal safety may plague assaulted staff members. Primary among these is self-doubt regarding professional competency and worry about how colleagues and supervisors will view them. Even in cases in which the attack appeared clearly unprovoked and unpredictable, staff members sometimes found their clinical abilities questioned; others assumed that the assaulted individual had necessarily in some way "brought it upon himself." We wonder whether this stance is used defensively in order to allow colleagues to feel assured that they are personally immune to being attacked.

The staff we interviewed differed with respect to whether they received emotional support from other staff and administrators following the incident. A nurse who was punched in the jaw by a psychotic patient told us that the daily phone calls she received from co-workers provided a great deal of support in working through the episode. Others told us that staff tended to avoid them and to refuse to discuss the attack with them. Almost unanimously, the victims of assault agreed that the emotional impact of having been attacked far exceeded the impact of physical injury, and that the need for emotional support following the assault was enormous. Victims reported that they needed time to ventilate their feelings about the incident, an opportunity to learn from what had happened in a nonjudgemental environment, and to discuss the dynamic issues of the patient who had contributed to the attack.

A resident who was seriously injured when an adolescent patient suddenly assaulted her pointed out to us that nowhere in her training program—neither in supervision nor in formal lectures—had the topic of how to assess or manage dangerous patients had been discussed until *after* she was attacked. In retrospect, the resident felt that she might have unwittingly contributed to the assault because of her naiveté about dealing with potentially volatile patients. We recommend that this essential area of training be routinely incorporated into the first year of psychiatric residency programs as a preventative measure.

Patients witnessing an assault on the ward often have profound reactions. A physical attack represents such a serious transgression of boundaries that important questions arise regarding authority and limit-setting in the milieu. Other patients with aggressive urges may be confronted with their own fears about losing control of these impulses. Patients usually welcome the restoration of ward stability that occurs when the assaultive patient is contained. Alternatively, a forcible seclusion of the assaultive patient may create additional tension on the ward. If the patient is precipitously transferred to another facility, particularly if patients feel that the attack was provoked, an adversarial relationship may be established between staff and patients. For these reasons, we suggest holding a meeting of everyone in the milieu community after an assault has occurred; at this time, facts can be clarified, rumors can be dispelled, and patients can ventilate their feelings about the incident.

Profile of an Assault

Prevention of assaults largely depends on the identification of potentially violent patients, so that steps can be taken to minimize the likelihood of assault. This case illustrates several points which we noted repeatedly in our series of assaults and which appear to have value as predictors of patient dangerousness in hospital settings:

Case Study 4-1

Allen B. was 26 years old, unemployed, had a history of heroine abuse and wife beating, and had been admitted for detoxification. He was medicated with gradually diminishing doses of methadone hydrochloride; this went smoothly from a medical standpoint, although Allen continually complained of "nervousness" and insomnia and made repeated demands for tranquilizers. He was not given such medication because the resident managing the case felt it was ill-advised to give this patient an addicting drug; instead, small doses of hydroxyzine (Vistaril) were prescribed. The rationale for this was explained to him briefly, but because the resident was feeling irritated with the patient's "dependency," she did not take the time to learn from him that he felt tranquilizers were being withheld in order to punish him for his drug habit. Allen stated on a number of occasions that the staff was "out to get him" because of several restrictions designed by the staff to minimize the chance of illicit drug use on the ward.

The morning of the assault, Allen asked to depart early for a planned leave from the hospital and was told by a nurse on duty that he could not do so. Allen became quite annoyed, pounded his fist on the counter at the nurses' station, and shouted that if he wanted to leave early he would—he was fed up with all of the "ridiculous rules" that the staff imposed. The nurse responded that her word was final and instructed

Allen to leave the nurses' station. At this point, Allen picked up a glass ashtray from the countertop and hurled it at the nurse, hitting her on the forehead.

This case is typical in a number of respects that will be useful to discuss.

The patient gave warning signs that he was becoming stressed beyond his ability to control himself. Few assaults occur without some warning. If one observes carefully, patients usually do give some indication that they are likely to behave violently; the staff may miss these signals however, generally because of their own countertransference feelings. The latter point will be discussed below.

In Allen's case, the warning signs that could have alerted the staff to the fact that Allen was a potentially dangerous patient began soon after admission. For example, he revealed that he was incapable of tolerating discomfort when he repeatedly sought tranquilizing medication to relieve his internal tension. Allen also expressed his feeling that he was in an adversarial relationship with the staff, stating that they were "out to get him," rather than viewing the ward rules as simply routine procedure.

Just before he threw the ashtray, Allen gave several additional clues that he was losing control. He raised his voice, pounded his fist on the countertop, and again indicated that the staff was antagonistic toward him, stating that he was "fed up with all the ridiculous rules."

Assaultive patients have difficulties with rules and authority, and tend to view virtually any restriction as a threat to their autonomy. In our series we repeatedly observed that these patients acted out violently in response to staff denial of even minor privileges. Useful tactics for dealing with these unusually volatile patients include maintaining clear, *realistic* expectations, the rationale for which are discussed with the patient. Such patients are highly sensitive to arbitrary, contradicting, or overly restrictive rules; a frank, nonjudgemental explanation of the reasons for various ward policies can go far in enlisting the individual's cooperation and thus in preventing violent outbursts. Whenever feasible, these patients should be given choices in matters concerning their own treatment to encourage a feeling of participation in the therapeutic program.

Countertransference feelings may have interfered with staff's ability to recognize a potentially volatile patient. Countertransference feelings must be explored constantly, as potentially violent patients characteristically behave in ways which provoke anger in staff members. We have found staff meetings useful for discussing countertransference feelings and for exploring how such feelings relate to patient management issues.

Like many patients who have problems tolerating frustration, Allen made repeated demands on others to relieve his internal discomfort. The resident became angry and annoyed with this "dependent" behavior and responded by withdrawing from the patient, a situation which served to frustrate him still further. Had the resident recognized Allen's "dependency" as part of his pathology rather than responding to countertransference feelings, she would have spent some time with him discussing in depth the rationale for his treatment. Such a therapeutic maneuver might have resulted in improved cooperation with treatment, in diminishing feelings of alienation toward the staff, and thus in helping to prevent Allen from acting violently on the ward.

The nurse who was assaulted also acted on countertransference feelings and thus in some ways provoked the attack. She responded to the patient's demands as a threat to her authority and engaged him in a power struggle over who was in charge. A more prudent tact might have been simply to restate the hospital's policy regarding leaves of absence in a nonjudgemental tone. Her countertransference feelings toward Allen in this situation prevented her from recognizing the clues that Allen had tenuous control over his anger and was about to assault her.

The patient had a history of assault and other impulsive behaviors. A patient who has acted impulsively or aggressively under stress in the past is at increased risk to respond similarly when frustrated again. In Allen's case the patient was an immature individual with a low tolerance for frustration and tenuous impulsive control as evidenced by his history of physically abusing his wife, his poor work record, and his history of drug abuse. Other historical factors which we have found useful for alerting us to a patient's difficulties with impulse control and therefore the patient's increased propensity toward assaulting others include: arrest record (including traffic violations), dishonorable military discharge, unstable personal relationships, suicide attempts or gestures, alcoholism, gambling, accident-proneness, and a history of truancy, expulsion from school, or dropping out. Such patients usually blame others for their difficulties rather than assuming responsibility themselves, leading to an increased likelihood of acting aggressively toward others.

SUMMARY

In our survey an attack by a patient was most likely to occur (1) during a seclusion procedure, (2) following a verbal argument, and (3) following the denial of a privilege. Prevention largely depends on recognizing not only these predisposing circumstances, but also on identifying potentially dangerous patients. The latter can be accomplished by screening patients for a history of impulsive behaviors and by paying attention to behavioral warning signs on the ward, which are usually present before a patient loses control.

Interventions that are likely to reduce the risk of assault include setting unambiguous, realistic expectations for patient behavior; enlisting the individual's cooperation in the treatment plan; giving the patient choices whenever feasible; and constant attention to countertransference feelings.

Joseph A. Ionno

5

A Prospective Study of Assaultive Behavior in Female Psychiatric Inpatients

Violent behavior is not unexpected in the psychiatric hospital, nor is concern for potential injuries.[1,5,6,8,10] Efforts to reliably and consistently predict violence as an aspect of human response have been of considerable concern to both the medical and legal professions.[12] Our degree of accuracy is less than optimal, particularly when long-range prediction is involved.[9,12,13] Perhaps related or causal factors preceding acts of violence could be identified in a "controlled environment." If so, perhaps more effective methods of intervention and/or prevention could be developed.

A selected review of the literature regarding violent behavior in hospital settings revealed discussion of a variety of topics. Management techniques were often emphasized, but data regarding psychopathology, demography, method of assessment, prevention, or feasibility or effectiveness of different interventions were limited.

This author's interest in the subject was stimulated by what appeared to be an increase in assaultive activity by a group of severely disturbed inpatients at the Institute of Living in Hartford, Connecticut. (This facility is a 417-bed, nonprofit, long-term psychiatric treatment hospital.) An early attempt to collect available data was confined to incident reports which primarily focused on injuries, their management, and their sequelae. There was limited and variable commentary about the events preceding the assaults, as well as about management of patients during the acute phase of the incidents. Although some demographic features could be extracted, the information was often inconsistent, incomplete, and of limited teaching value.

The foregoing prompted the initiation of a prospective study which would permit us to evaluate our own experience in regard to frequency and extent of injury to both patients and staff from patient assaults. Of additional concern were the characteristics of assaultive behaviors and the identification of any associated and/or precipitating events which might have been related to a particular patient's psychopathology. Management techniques used to deal with specific situations were the topic of a parallel investigation.

SURVEY OF FEMALE INPATIENTS

A unit which housed our most severely disturbed female patients was selected for this study. Clinical data indicated that this group of patients, who exhibited varying psychopathology, were responsible for a major portion of the assaultive incidents in our facility.* Patients' ages varied from 15–41 years. The major diagnostic categories represented were schizophrenia, paranoid type, chronic; borderline personality organization; antisocial personality with severe impairment of impulse control, and on rare occasion, organic brain syndrome (OBS) with disordered behavior.

The unit is capable of housing 23 patients, and only rarely was the census below capacity. The ward's physical configuration permitted maximum observation of both a west and a south corridor from the nursing station, with a large day room directly in front of the station. In addition, a group room (eight-patient capacity) was also in direct view at the end of the south corridor. Patients housed in the group room were those with self-destructive behavior requiring constant observation and/or recent demonstration of marked potential for such behavior. Patients who are placed on constant observation are in direct view and close contiguity with a psychiatric technician 24 hours each day.

Staffing consisted of a mixture of senior and less experienced technicians, recent graduates of a three-month training program, and individuals in training. The registered nurses assigned had varying levels of experience and training. The unit staff maintained communication with individual therapists

---

*A similar unit for all male patients underwent a comparable study; the results are not included in this report.

regarding their patients. The frequency of interaction between staff and therapists varied from once to many times during the daily work period, depending on the patient's clinical condition. It should be noted that unit staff might be required to contact over 20 separate therapists. An additional management resource for the unit staff was the availability of a nursing supervisor and a unit administrator. The latter was available for consultations regarding maintenance of appropriate unit milieu and aid in identifying unit issues (such as problems with patient–staff interaction). Unit meetings with staff and patients were held twice weekly, during which individual and group issues were defined and explored.

A form for reporting assaults was devised and tested. It included a simple definition of assaultive behavior and required a brief written comment by the staff member completing the post-assault assessment. A specific individual was assigned the task of completing the form and submitting it to the unit administrator no more than 24 hours after an incident. Both self-destructive and verbally assaultive activity was to be excluded. The report was to focus on not only the individuals involved, but also on the means of assault and the extent and location of injury, if any. An attempt was made to identify the factors which might be related to the incident, such as patient psychopathy or self-defense. Characteristics of the preassault phase which might lead to some degree of future predictability were also elicited. Finally, the management of each incident, varying from verbal intervention to some form of physical restraint, was evaluated.

Data were collected during a six-month interval from July 1, 1980 to December 31, 1980. The individuals recording and reporting the information were members of the unit staff. The forms were collected daily and reviewed Monday through Friday of each week. Reports obtained during weekends or holidays were reviewed immediately following the weekend or holiday period, thus ensuring as complete and accurate a report as possible. One individual was responsible for collecting and collating the data. Postassessment review was not feasible due to time constraints.

Study Results

The number of assaults each month and the day of the week on which each occurred are shown graphically in Figure 5-1. The majority of assaults (40–65 percent) took place during the evening shift (3:00–11:00 P.M.). Table 5–1 compares the frequency of assaults that involved unit staff with those that involved patients or damage to property.

The most frequent means of physical contact were with hands and feet, with occasional biting (seven instances out of 87 assaults). The extremities and trunk were the body areas most frequently contacted. The injuries described were primarily abrasions, with occasional contusions of an extremity. There

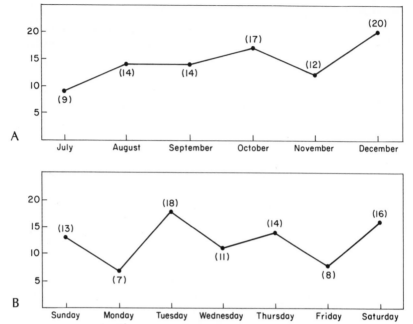

Figure 5-1. Number of assaults by month (A) and by day of the week (B). Data for day-of-the-week assaults are the total number of assaults occurring on that day during all of the months surveyed.

was one incident of a traumatic myositis. There were no lacerations which required suturing, no fractures of the skeletal system or loss of consciousness, and there was no necessity for hospitalization for either observation or additional medical treatment. There was rarely staff absence related to trauma sustained as a result of assault.

Table 5-2 presents various information collected for each recorded

Table 5-1
Receipt of Assaultive Behavior

Month	Staff	Other Patients	Property
July	5	3	1
August	11	3	0
September	11	2	1
October	13	3	1
November	7	5	0
December	20	1	0
Total	67	17	3

Table 5-2
Six-Month Survey of Assaultive Behavior

Month	Number of Assaults	No. of Individuals Responsible for No. of Assaults	Diagnostic Factors Related to Assaults	Management	Assaults During Evening Shift	Time within which Assaults Occurred
July	9	1 for 3 assaults 1 for 2 assaults 4 for 1 assault each	4 character disorder 5 psychotic state	PRN medications (3) Seclusion (4) Verbal intervention (not recorded in 2) CWP (3)	6 (67%)	2 in 3 h 2 in 1 h
August	14	1 for 5 assaults 1 for 4 assaults 5 for 1 assault each	6 character disorder 8 psychotic state	PRN medications (4) Verbal intervention (not recorded in 11) Seclusion (11) CWP (1)	9 (64%)	3 in 5 h 2 in 1 h 3 in 6 h
September	14	2 for 2 assaults 1 for 3 assaults 7 for 1 assault each	8 character disorder 6 psychotic state	PRN Medications (5) Verbal intervention (not recorded in 6) Seclusion (8) CWP (4)	6 (43%)	4 in 8 h
October	17	1 for 5 assaults 3 for 3 assaults 3 for 1 assault each	14 character disorder 3 psychotic state	PRN medications (10) Verbal intervention (not recorded in 6) Seclusion (4) CWP (7)	9 (53%)	3 in 7 h 2 in 2 h 2 in 2 h 2 in 1 h
November	12	1 for 3 assaults 2 for 2 assaults 5 for 1 assault each	9 character disorder 3 psychotic state	PRN medications (2) Verbal intervention (not recorded in 6) Seclusion (4) CWP (5)	7 (58%)	5 in 4 h 4 in 3 h
December	21	1 for 5 assaults 2 for 4 assaults 1 for 3 assaults 1 for 2 assaults 3 for 1 assault each	10 character disorder 11 psychotic state	PRN medications (13) Verbal intervention (not recorded in 4) Seclusion (9) CWP (8)	9 (43%)	3 in 6 h 2 in 7 h 3 in 3 h

Total Assaults = 87

CWP = Cold wet pack

instance of assault. In Table 5-2 it appears that particular individuals were responsible for the majority of the incidents (over 50 percent). The diagnostic category (e.g., psychotic state and/or character disorder) did not appear to be a dominant feature. One might only speculate about a trend toward a higher frequency of assault when the patient population contained more persons diagnosed as having a character disorder.

Analysis of Study Data

It is apparent that certain individuals are responsible for the majority of instances of assaultive behavior in this study. Those individuals are more likely to be hospitalized with a severe personality disorder (e.g., antisocial or borderline or conduct disorder) than with an active psychotic process. What remains unclear are the precipitating events which may be related to these violent expressions. One might speculate that disturbing communications or visits could lead to assault; however, the bases for occurrence of agitated/ assault behavior in the absence of these remains elusive. One major hypothesis suggests that the patient replicates significant pathologic intrafamilial events with others on the unit (patients and staff), and that this can culminate in a behavioral reenactment of the patient's pain or rage.

There was approximately a 1.4:1 ratio of patients with severe personality disorders to those having a psychotic process involved in the assaults. There may have been a population skew of the unit from month to month; however, in evaluating those individuals most frequently involved, those with severe personality disorders predominated. It is my impression that when there is a preponderance of either diagnostic group—i.e., active psychotic process or severe personality/conduct disorder—a polarization can occur in the quality of patient interaction with may lead to (unit-wide) stimulation and subsequent agitated and assaultive behaviors. In this scenario, a major mode of interaction involves those with a severe personality disorder using the psychotic patient as a scapegoat.

Exposure to the chaotic, regressed, delusionally-distorted cognitive state of the psychotic patient is quite threatening to maintenance of psychological integrity by patients with severe borderline personality organization. This seems particularly true for those with antisocial personality and related conduct disorders. Thus, one might perceive scapegoating and clique formation as an active, defensive process which attempts to maintain psychological integrity in the nonpsychotic patient. Conversely, the psychotic patient's experience of rejection and alienation as a consequence of significant misperception of the human and other environment confirms his need to continue the very delusional and/or hallucinatory precepts which perpetuate interpersonal and intrapsychic difficulty.

Whenever approximately three to five patients are admitted to such a unit environment within a 48–72- hour period, a pulse of increased tension appears. This provides an environment in which polarization can develop (e.g., the new patients versus the old), with exacerbation of tension states and enhanced propensity for agitated and assaultive activity. These in turn may be related to recrudescence of personal issues of acceptance, inclusion, control, and relatedness for the members of both "groups."

The time of the day and week was tabulated for purposes of detecting any overall pattern of occurrence. It is noteworthy that 50 percent or more of assaults took place during the evening shift (3:00–11:30 P.M.). There are fewer opportunities for involvement in off-unit programs during this part of the day, and thus a higher density of patients for a sustained period. As a result of this study, more on-unit activities are being provided, some in conjunction with the Department of Rehabilitation Services. In addition, the gymnasium is now used for team sports. These additions have been valuable in permitting unit staff to deal more effectively with periods of increased tension and/or escalating behaviors.

The number of assaults by day of the week is illustrated in Figure 5-1 combined for all months. When the frequencies for each day during a six-month period are tabulated, the results show that the highest number occur on Tuesday, Saturday, Thursday, and Sunday, in that order. Although the differences are not statistically significant, it is interesting that Tuesday, Saturday, and Sunday are visiting days on this ward (hours 2–4 P.M.), and that unit meetings take place on Tuesday and Thursday of each week. The latter often entail the development of significant individual and group issues.

It is noted that there was sporadic clustering of assaultive events, and some thought was given to the possibility of "assaultiveness inducing assaultiveness," i.e., whether a "communicability" factor existed. When there were three or more assaults in a day, they usually all occurred within a period of three to six hours. The individuals involved in the clustered events were usually different; the phenomenon was not due to repetitive behavior of one or two patients.

The management techniques available were verbal interventions, psychotropic medications, and containment procedures (*side room*, seclusion, and cold wet pack). When a side room was used, the patient was escorted to a sparsely furnished room in which she was to remain for a prescribed period of time. The door to the room remained open. In seclusion, the door was locked and could only be opened from the corridor. The patient was evaluated by a physician during the initiation of the procedure and periodically thereafter by a staff member (every 15 minutes). The duration of seclusion varied, up to a maximum of two hours. The cold wet pack management technique consisted of wrapping the patient in a series of bed sheets which had been soaked in tepid tap water and wrung dry. This permitted maximum control of the patient's behavioral responses in a setting in which a staff member was present throughout treatment. Vital signs and other information were recorded every 15 minutes.

The use of side rooms, seclusion, or cold wet pack varied in frequency, and the study does not indicate a discernible pattern of their use on a month-by-month basis. However, when the patients are considered in two categories, psychotic and nonpsychotic, seclusion is seen to have been utilized to a greater extent for the former, and cold wet packs for the latter.

It would appear from the data collected that verbal intervention is seen as having limited value. In many instances the use of verbal intervention was not recorded as a management technique. This study has highlighted a need to focus on verbal intervention. Although verbal interventions were not recorded as a means of intercession in slightly more than 50 percent of the incidents during the study period, it is likely that they were used throughout. The failure to indicate such interaction might more accurately reflect the value placed upon this modality of intervention.

It seems reasonable to assume that a clearer comprehension of psychopathology in general terms, as well as of the specific psychopathology of the patient concerned, would facilitate appreciation of behavior as an expression of affect. One hopes that this would enhance staffs' ability to interact more meaningfully and appropriately in their verbal interchange with patients. Thus, one would vary the approach to, say, a hostile, threatening patient based on the context of his or her behavior (e.g., psychotic state versus antisocial personality structure).[11]

The exploration by unit staff of their perceptions and attitudes regarding the use of containment and physical restraint and the management of patients is essential. The issue of touching another human being in order to restrain him or her is rarely discussed among mental health professionals. The impact of these restraining behaviors on unit staff and the requirement to impose a variety of containment measures is seldom commented on in the literature.[3,4,7,14] Hesitancy to set firm limits in a consistent manner may be related to staff anxiety. Reluctance to make use of physical containment techniques in order to restore homeostasis has significantly contributed to escalation of an evolving, conflictual situation in some institutions.[2] In the patient population a parallel process involving high levels of anxiety due to inadequate control measures and insufficient psychological structuring of the environment also contribute to escalation of agitation on the unit.

Hypothesis for Assault Clusters

The foregoing suggests a hypothesis for explaining the frequent clustering of assaultive behavior that was observed throughout the six-month period. It is important to emphasize that these observations apply to all levels of the treatment hierarchy and can be quite useful therapeutically once recognized and accepted.

The objective of identifying predictive factors leading to assaultive behavior was not accomplished. However, the study renewed our awareness of a of issues that need to be focused on in order to improve our understanding and management of patients who require a highly structured therapeutic milieu. The data thus far suggest that the following should be considered:

1. A program that would enhance unit staffs' understanding of the patient's behavior in light of his or her psychopathology.
2. Frequently repeated inservice training, as well as "mock exercises" in physical containment of the agitated and/or assaultive patient.
3. Exercises in modes of verbal intervention in conjunction with plans 1. and 2.
4. Elaboration of the principles and methods of restraint such as seclusion or cold wet pack.

The development of a cyclic program of inservice seminars would use case studies as a means of enhancing unit staffs' understanding of the patients' behavior in terms of their psychopathology. This would also encourage staff self-evaluation of their contributions to individual and unit dynamics. The stage would then be set for the development of recurring training exercises on physical containment of the agitated and/or assaultive patient. Ideally, this would permit the development of higher levels of confidence in one's ability to contain such an individual and enhance the quality and quantity of verbal interventions. The unit as a therapeutic instrument would move toward a higher level of functioning.

SUMMARY

This study has provided specific demographic data which permit a number of observations. There were no serious injuries during the study period. The individuals directly responsible for assaultive behavior comprised between 20 and 30 percent of the total population. The majority of assaults occurred during the evening shift (3:00–11:30 P.M.), and there was a tendency toward certain days of the week. The use of physical containment, seclusion and cold wet pack, occurred more frequently in the management of the nonpsychotic group. The results have enhanced our awareness of population skew related to diagnostic category. The arrival of three or more new patients within a 48-hour period has considerable impact on unit dynamics. All of the foregoing has facilitated more effective unit management in general.

It is important to emphasize the need for ongoing exploration of staff attitudes regarding treatment of the assaultive patient, and to perceive this as a process which is parallel to certain patient group dynamics and is related to the provision of an effective therapeutic milieu.

REFERENCES

1. Abbott A: Accident and its correlates in a psychiatric hospital. Acta Psychiatr Scand 57:36–48, 1978
2. Adler G, Shapiro L: Some difficulties in the treatment of the aggressive acting out patient. Am J Psychother 27:548–556, 1973
3. Bursten B: Using mechanical restraints on acutely disturbed psychiatric patients. Hosp Community Psychiatry 26:757–759, 1975
4. DiBella WGA: Educating staff to manage threatening paranoid patients. Am J Psychiatry 136:333–335, 1979
5. Evenson, RC, Altmanh, H, Sletten, IW, et al. Disturbing behavior: A study of incident reports. Psychiatr Q 48:266–275, 1974
6. Fottrelle E, Bewley T, Squizzoni M: A study of aggressive and violent behavior among group psychiatric inpatients. Med Sci Law 18:66–69, 1978
7. Gair DS: Limit setting and seclusion in psychiatric hospital. Psychiatric Opinion 17:15–19, 1980.
8. Greenland C: Evaluation of violent and dangerous behavior associated with mental illness. Semin Psychiatry 3:345–356, 1971
9. Guze S, Woodruff RA, Clayton P: Psychiatric disorders and criminality. JAMA 227:641–642, 1974
10. Kalogerakis M: The assaultive psychiatric patient. Psychiatr Q 45:372–381, 1971
11. Lion J, Pasternak S: Countertransference reactions to violent patients. Am J Psychiatry 130:207–210, 1973
12. Monahan J: The clinical prediction of violent behavior. U.S. Department of Health and Human Services, Rockville, Maryland, 1–124, 1980
13. Rubin R: Prediction of dangerousness in mentally ill criminals. Arch Gen Psychiatry 27:397–407, 1972
14. Soloff P: Behavioral precipitants of restraint in the modern milieu. Compr Psychiatry 19:179–184, 1978

Wolf N. Adler
Christopher Kreeger
Penelope Ziegler

6

Patient Violence in a Private Psychiatric Hospital

In a 312-bed privately endowed psychiatric facility, clinical staff and lay administrators became alarmed at what they perceived to be an escalating trend of patient assaultiveness and formed a committee to address the problem in the fall of 1981. At that time the annual incidence of violence-induced injuries to patients and staff had been rising for several years. This chapter reports the committee's findings and efforts to recognize, manage, and prevent violence among the inpatient population.

The authors gratefully acknowledge their indebtedness to the following members of the Committee to Study the Violent Patient: Mat Acuff, R.N., Donna Dittberner, R.N., Betty Lake, R.N., Barbara Molicki,R.N., Helen Wenzel, R.N., Pat Zeiser, R.N., Gordon Bush, M.H.W., Michael Maskovyak, M.H.W., Peter McGunigle, Michael Gerred, and Lynne Apostolides.

DESCRIPTION OF THE HOSPITAL

The hospital's 300-plus beds are organized into three major divisions. The largest of these, the General Adult Division, consists of eight patient units with a total capacity of 150 beds. These treat a heterogeneous adult population, emphasizing individual psychotherapy during often lengthy inpatient treatment. Its population is predominantly young adult, but ranges in age from 18 to 64. Median length of staff is approximately four months. Another division, the Adult Specialty Division, consists of four units, one each for the treatment of alcoholics, geriatric patients, substance abuse, and general patients needing short-term evaluation and treatment. A third division includes an 84-bed adolescent service and a 12-bed unit for children. The median length of staf for this division is approximately seven months.

Patients are predominantly well educated, from middle-class background. In recent years there has been a rise in the number of involuntary patients, from 5 percent five years ago to 12 percent in 1981. It is very uncommon for patients to be committed to the hospital by a court, and very few have any history of criminal behavior or legal problems. Many admissions are transfers from other psychiatric facilities, often because of management difficulties at the sending facility.

In fiscal 1981 the hospital admitted 871 patients. One-third of those admitted to the General Adult Division were from out of state, but most patients admitted to the hospital came from the local metropolitan area. Substance use disorders became the most common primary diagnosis (25 percent) for the first time in the hospital's history. Previously, this diagnostic category had accounted for only 5–15 percent of inpatients. This increase was probably related to the opening of a new substance abuse unit, a higher daily census on the alcoholism unit, and a change in diagnostic practices resulting from the implementation of the DSM-III. Schizophrenic disorders and major affective syndromes were equally prevalent (20 percent), followed by dysthymic disorder (15 percent).

Much emphasis is placed on milieu therapy. Community meetings occur almost daily on each unit, and smaller discussion groups and task-oriented gatherings are regular features of unit life. A strong effort is made to involve patients in structured activities off the unit as well. Patients participate in verbal, nonverbal, and physical and vocational therapies, most of which are conducted in a centralized location. A central dining room is used by both patients and staff. A patient government with representatives chosen from each unit organizes social events, examines issues of patients rights and responsibilities, discusses grievances, and provides patients with an opportunity to experience leadership roles.

In an effort to coordinate this complex multidisciplinary approach, interdisciplinary treatment team meetings are held three to four times each week. Smaller team conferences may be arranged to discuss a patient's treatment plan, areas of particular difficulty, and so on. In addition, an increasing awareness of the need for staff to discuss feelings which arise in working with severely disturbed patients and to work through interstaff conflicts has led to the development of stress management "rap" sessions, therapists' discussion groups, and so on. Time spent in these meetings, as well as the increasing demand for accountability and documentation, are often perceived as intrusions upon the time available for direct patient care.

Each inpatient is assigned a primary therapist, who might be a psychiatric resident, a staff psychiatrist, or a staff psychologist. Individual psychotherapy is offered universally in the General Adult Division, whereas more emphasis is placed on primary group therapy on the Specialized Adult Units. On the adolescent and child units, a combination of individual and group therapy is employed. With few exceptions, all therapists are salaried staff. Patients rarely have a change of therapist.

In general, patients remain on the same unit from admission to discharge. No single unit is designed to provide a higher level of security or staffing for more disturbed patients; patients are not segregated according to diagnosis. The size of units varies from 12 to 22 beds, and each may be locked or unlocked depending on the needs of the patient group. Each unit has one seclusion room available. The only means of physical restraint used are cold wet sheet packs and seclusion. The former is used infrequently and must be terminated after two hours. It is prescribed more often to sedate a distressed patient than to restrain one who is physically aggressive. Seclusion is used more frequently; it is uncommon for patients to remain in seclusion for longer than a few hours.

THE RECOGNITION OF VIOLENCE AS A PROBLEM

Given the obtrusive and anxiety-provoking nature of violence, it is more than a bit surprising that it took several years of escalating levels, before it came to be recognized as a serious problem. Several factors may have contributed to this selective inattention. The hospital's cherished psychodynamic tradition and its founders' legacy of Quaker pacifism gentility and idealism may have dulled the staff's perception of such a harsh reality, and thus inhibited their reactivity. Awareness of the problem must have been inhibited by denial of a more defensive nature, whereby those working in the midst of violence attempted to sustain a sense of security. The staff may have needed to deny the effect of violence in order to contain feelings of guilt for not having prevented it. Still another source of denial may have been a misplaced desire to avoid stigmatizing the mentally ill by attributing to them the opprobrious and criminal-like character of violent behavior.

The first stirrings of concern about the problem began appearing in early

Table 6-1

Incidence of Injuries Due to Patient Assaults

Calendar Year	Staff Injured	Patients Assaulted
1975	56	36
1976	21	44
1977	57	53
1978	79	64
1979	137	107
1980	289	85

1979. Previously, there had been an almost nonchalant acceptance of occasional patient assaultiveness. Indeed, there had been an uneasy recognition by many staff members of an occasional failure to maintain a consistent approach in responding to assaultive behavior. Some patients could get away with threatening or injurious behaviors which would not be tolerated in others.

As the data to be presented later in this chapter demonstrate, the incidence of staff and patient injuries gradually increased from 1975 through 1978. By 1979, the staff's previous sense of control and imperviousness to threats had noticeably declined. Along with this greater sense of vulnerability came an increase in interdisciplinary tension. Staff began to criticize the administration for seeming indifferent to the problem. Eventually, an analysis of data derived from the hospital's incidence reports supported the staff's impression that the incidence of violent episodes was rising rapidly.

The Data

Data on the number of staff and patients injured by assaultive patients from 1975 through 1980, as reflected in official incident reports, are shown in Table 6-1. In 1979 and 1980 the number of staff reported injured increased over 1975 by 145 percent and 316 percent, respectively. A similar, albeit not quite so dramatic, increase occurred in the number of patients injured: 197 percent in 1979 and 136 percent in 1980.

The number of staff who lost workdays due to injuries, and the number of workdays lost, are shown in Table 6-2. These data tend to confirm the growing nature of the problem. During the three years 1957–1977, there were only 62 workdays lost, in contrast to 422 workdays lost during 1978–1980.

Caution must be exercised in assessing the incident data. The study committee recognized that the reporting system was subject to artifactual fluctuations, including those related to the motivational level of the reporters. The nursing staff might have been encouraged to report incidents more

Table 6-2
Workdays Lost Due to Patient Assaults

Calendar Year	Number of Workdays	Number of Staff
1975	24	7
1976	0	0
1977	38	4
1978	118	3
1979	165	15
1980	139	10

rigorously, but we found no evidence that this was the case. The nursing staff never received feedback about their reporting efforts, and had little reason to believe that anybody, other than the hospital's insurance carrier, was paying any attention to these reports. Other efforts to discover artifactual causes for the increase in workdays lost were also unsuccessful.

The Committee to Study the Violent Patient

From an initial group of 17 volunteers (seven psychiatrists, six nurses, two mental health workers, and two administrative support staff), a smaller committee was eventually formed. Its primary mission was to reduce the incidence of injuries due to patient assaultiveness, with a goal of a 50 percent reduction by the following year.

It quickly became obvious that the hospital's crisis training program had been giving insufficient attention to teaching people about the nature of violence and techniques for preventing and managing assaultive behavior. However, the kind of training that would optimally meet staff needs had not yet been determined. Certainly, management had to make a stronger commitment to training and what was taught had to fit the hospital's clinical philosophy. In order to improve our crisis training, other hospitals and groups were contacted about their own programs; several committee members attended a workshop on the topic, and a consultant conducted a two-day workshop at the hospital. Very few of the hospitals contacted had training programs that seemed appropriate to our needs. An extensively revised and extended training program for aggression management was eventually developed. All new and old employees are now required to attend three hours of this new inservice training.

Discussions about staff training merged into discussions about the nature of violence, its causes, and approaches to preventing and containing it. A staff procedure manual was proposed in order to standradize responses to patient violence. It addressed immediate measures, rapid organization, and predetermined roles of staff in assaultive incidents. The "crisis" team approach was eschewed in favor of general but flexible guidelines applicable to many different assaultive settings.

Staff Attitudes and Responses

The committee found that a key element in the management of physical aggression is the staff's general attitude on this issue. In order to function effectively, the treatment team must share a common value system with regard to violence. Of crucial importance is the core belief that physical aggressiveness has no place in the hospital social system, as well as the recognition that individual autonomy does not require, nor is it consistent with, a permissive attitude toward violence. A unit staff in conflict about these basic assumptions will experience difficulty setting limits, making value judgments, confronting inappropriate conduct, or even establishing clear and consistent rules of behavior. The patient who is confused, or who lacks self control, needs the constraining influence of staff's refusal to permit or ignore physical aggressiveness. When staff fails to provide such influence in a firm and consistent manner, the patient may force staff to exert the control he or she needs.

Those staff members who are most successful in discouraging violent acting out often demonstrate qualities of toughness, fair-mindedness, and self-confidence, combined with a genuine concern for patients' needs and sensitivity to their levels of function. Such assets are rare in inexperienced staff. For example, one inexperienced nurse had obvious difficulty with limit setting during her initial months at the hospital. Her previous experience had focused on individual interviews with patients; her training had stressed the importance of empathy, understanding, and acceptance. The sense of responsibility for the safety of patients and staff had not yet become a part of her role identity, and she was unable to easily adopt an authoritative mode of behavior. When her patients' acting out behavior was confronted by other members of the treatment team, she responded with remarks like, "Well, I'm not sure how I feel about that yet . . . I think he [the patient] probably needs more time."

In contrast, an experienced nurse who is generally regarded as being especially effective in running her adolescent inpatient unit was interviewed about her approach toward patient assaultiveness: she said, "We do not allow physical violence. We do not allow verbal abuse; it usually escalates to physical violence. When it happens, patients are told they must go to the quiet room right now . . . we tell them, 'No drugs, no physical contact, no violence.' . . . We need a commitment from the patient. We do not play games about who is tougher."

This unapologetic, straightforward stance is accompanied by a reality-based concern and a genuine warmth. She added, "Staff too often make the mistake of thinking they can motivate patients by being overcontrolling. The characteristics I look for in staff are gentleness, warmth, relatedness, and absence of guilt feelings about setting limits."

These qualities are prerequisites for successful functioning as a member of the treatment team. New staff members who possess these attributes must be oriented to the team's value system and provided with the tools needed to implement that system, i.e., training and experience in both preventive verbal intervention and physical techniques of managing aggression.

Explaining the Increase in Violence

The simplest explanation for an increasing rate of violent behavior in an inpatient population is the admission of larger numbers of more aggressive patients. Although the percentage of patients admitted to this hospital with a previous history of violence had not changed during the six-year period studied, the total number of patients admitted increased substantially, while the average length of stay was decreasing. Thus, the absolute number of aggression-prone patients in the patient population did increase, and more patients, at any given time, were in an acute stage of decompensation.

A second explanation had to do with the growing concern about violent crime in our society. Heightened sensitivity to violent behavior could have led staff to perceive and report more occurrences of violence. It also could have generated a climate of fear on the units which in turn may have provided fertile soil for outbreaks of violence.

A third explanation stems from the Jaunary, 1979, New Jersey court case of *Rennie* v. *Klein*, which affirmed the right of involuntary psychiatric patients to refuse to take psychotropic medication.[1] This profoundly affected both attitudes and practices at the hospital. Previously, whenever a patient had been too psychotic or depressed to be accessible to psychosocial rehabilitation, or whenever a patient was thought to be too out of control to be managed safely, appropriate medication was routinely prescribed and dispensed. If the patient resisted taking medication, but was thought too ill to be deprived of this form of treatment, he or she was offered the choice of taking the medication by mouth or receiving an intramuscular injection. In almost all instances, the patient chose the oral medication, and there was no struggle.

After *Rennie* v. *Klein* the pattern of drug prescription changed dramatically at our hospital. Medication was no longer prescribed unless the patient consented to take it, or unless the patient had already become intolerably aggressive or combative. Paranoid and litigious patients were especially reluctant to take psychotropic medication. Many patients aggressively asserted their right to go unmedicated, and some flaunted their control over staff to the point of provoking other patients into aggressive reactions. A nine-month sampling of persistent medication refusers who were considered potentially dangerous showed that 40 percent eventually injured either themselves or someone else.

Finally, in 1980 a number of administrative changes spawned a series of factional disputes which led to many staff feeling disheartened and frustrated by the temporary instability that ensued. The resulting increase in staff tension could have lowered the patients' threshold for violence, although it is also very likely that staff began to register their discontent by reporting a greater percentage of potentially reportable incidents.

Patients Most at Risk

Common denominators notwithstanding, violence springs from certain types of patients more than others. The committee constructed two sets of profiles of patients who were found to be overly represented in the hospital's population of physically assaultive patients.

The first set of profiles is based on the traditional diagnostic classification system. For example, *manic* patients, especially during the early phase of their illness, are comparatively more prone to combative behavior. They often seem to function as sponges for other people's rage, and their treatment is often complicated by their being too "entertaining" to treat or to confront. Manic patients with a history of alcoholism are, in our experience, even more violence-prone. The aggressive threat posed by dysphoric manics is easy enough to spot, but even euphoric patients aggressive guard their euphoria, sometimes to the point of violence when staff press them with reality. It is usually easier, and safer, to distract acutely manic patients than to confront them with the inappropriateness of their behavior.

Regressed schizophrenic patients may become violent because of their need for distance in order to maintain their own sense of identity. The need to withdraw from stimulus-laden interpersonal reactions can impel them to aggressively fend off approaches by staff and other patients. Some become violent in the midst of a homosexual panic. Others respond to hallucinatory commands to attack imagined persecutors. Because some of the patients in this group are socially inept, they are often scapegoated by other patients; if their verbal skills are insufficient to adequately defend or assert themselves, they resort to the more primitive defense of physical retaliation. These patients are also frequently barometers of the tension level of the patient unit.

The *acting-out adolescent* often needs to engage in increasing levels of exciting activity in order to avoid feelings of depression. Sometimes adolescent violence results from peer competition, in which a patient wants to prove that he is the group leader or the most antisocial group member for reasons of prestige. For some adolescents, flouting the rules against physical aggressiveness is a way of saving face—avoiding the humiliation of being needy. Violence can also be a way of gaining attention; negative attention is better than little or none. Some adolescent patients follow others into violence in order to be recognized as members of their peer group. Finally, some adolescents are violent by remote control—they never become violent themselves, but their influence over others is so strong that other patients act for them.

Other types of patients who pose a significant risk of becoming assaultive include some substance abusers, especially those with a history of violence; patients with temporal lobe epilepsy; the agitated demented; a few of the mentally retarded; and those with an antisocial personality.

A second set of profiles was constructed along motivational lines.[2] For example, the *pressure remover* is the type of patient who is deficient in verbal skills and thus is unable to effectively negotiate with or defend himself against an environment that is perceived as being unyielding or menacing. These patients usually have organically-based cognitive deficits. sometimes they are unable to negotiate reasonably because of learned patterns of communication that are too provocative. The *irritable* patient is one whose threshold for violence is lowered because of organic problems or because of affective volatility, as in the manic patient. The *fear producer*, needs to master his own vulnerability to fear by demonstrating his power to produce it in others, as in the case of patients who behave sadistically or as bullies. Then, there are the *misperceivers*, who misinterpret, in a paranoid fashion, the intention of others.

CONCLUSION

Psychiatry can ill afford to view violent behavior as simply another symptom of emotional distress, nor can it pass off this phenomenon as a sociopolitical aberration, the responsibility for which belongs to some other profession. More often than we like to admit, violence occurs within psychiatric institutions. Its victims are not only the perpetrators themselves, but psychiatric staff, the patient's peers and the entire therapeutic environment. It is a human frailty which is becoming increasingly prevalent and for which our conventional mode of thinking does not prepare us well. We need to face the problem and design specific preventive as well as reactive methods of effective intervention.

REFERENCES

1.   Rennie v. Klein, 462F. SVPP. 131 (DCNJ, 1981)
2.   Toch H: Violent Men: An Inquiry Into the Psychology of Violence. Chicago, Aldine, 1969

Ernest A. Haffke
William H. Reid

7

7
Violence Against Mental Health
Personnel in Nebraska

Patient violence against psychiatrists and other mental health personnel is an infrequent occurrence. Fear of such acts, and occasionally actually experiencing them, are among the more anxiety provoking aspects of a clinical career. Among health care workers, not only mental health personnel are victims of serious assaults, including murders; emergency rooms and some other hospital locations are occasionally sites of patient violence. Nonetheless, publicity and lay stereotypes about the dangerousness or unpredictability of "mental patients" affect the clinician's perception of the mental health profession as being potentially hazardous.

When a psychiatric patient commits a violent crime, it is often highly publicized. This may be due in part to the bizarre nature of some such acts and in part to the frequent absence of apparent personal gain. For example, the mugging of a physician to obtain money or narcotics may be seen quite differently from a bizarre assault whose motivations might be considered "psychotic," or striking out by a confused patient whom one is trying to help.

Statistically speaking, reliable data indicate that arrest rates among psychiatric patients for all crimes are about the same as those for the general population: 7/1000 total pop. psychiatric patients versus 6/1000 total general pop.[16] Violence in general is less common among psychiatric patients than among the general population.[2] There is some indication that the number of violent incidents is increasing; however, the source of such trends is difficult to define because of shifting diagnostic classifications and blurred boundaries between populations of "criminals" and the "mentally ill."

The prediction of violence in psychiatric patients is a difficult matter. In one study psychiatrists overpredicted violent behavior in specific individuals by more than 800 percent.[15] To further complicate the search for reliable data on the topic, retrospective reviews of mental hospital records reveal considerable inaccuracy (usually underreporting) in official documents such as incident reports.[7]

In a 1976 survey of psychiatrists, Madden and co-workers found that 42 percent had been assaulted by a patient at least once, usually early in their psychiatric training.[8] A further survey supported that finding.[14] In another study, 48 percent of psychiatric residents said they had been attacked by a patient.[11]

In order to explore and attempt to replicate the above survey data and to prepare for prospective studies of some of the issues, two statewide surveys were conducted by investigators at the Nebraska Psychiatric Institute.

Definition of Violence

"Violence" and "dangerousness" have been defined in many ways.[9, 10] Violent behavior may be described as activity that uses force to inflict injury on another.[12] The concept can be extended to include overt threats and/or behavior that is likely to physically harm another person.[1]

In the Nebraska surveys, the investigators chose to use broad definitions such as those above when asking participants to report and describe their experiences. Although strict definitions and experimental controls are important to good research, we felt that the participants' personal perceptions of violence ("assault") were also important.

THE SURVEYS

Nebraska Demographics

The State of Nebraska has a population of just over 1.5 million (1981 census), and covers an area of 76,612 square miles. The economic base is largely agricultural. There are only two cities with over 100,000 inhabitants (Omaha and Lincoln). These are in the eastern portion of the state and contain almost half the total population.[3] In addition to agriculture-related industry, these larger population centers include and are significantly influenced by military installations, educational institutions, and business/financial centers. Omaha is located at a sort of midcontinent crossroads. Psychiatric patients in public institutions in the Omaha area are often non-Nebraska residents *enroute* to the east or west coast.

In July 1980 there were 88 psychiatrists in six mental health "regions" of the state. The three major Nebraska state mental hospitals ("regional centers") had a combined inpatient capacity of over 700 beds.[4]

Survey of Psychiatrists

A nine-page confidential questionnaire was mailed to every psychiatrist in the state in order to assess the frequency and quality of assaults on them by patients. Respondents were asked to complete demographic data and rate several kinds of incidents on six-point scales of severity. Written comments about assaults, related feelings, or other issues were also solicited. ·

Two-thirds of the psychiatrists responded (n=54). Of these, seventeen (32 percent) had been the victim of at least one assault during their careers; nine had been assaulted within the preceeding year.* Most episodes were minor; only one required medical attention.

Part of the survey requested information about violence against the psychiatrist's staff, and 26 respondents reported such assaults. One involved the stabbing to death of an aide on an inpatient unit. As might be expected, clinicians in large institutions reported the highest number of assaults, primarily against nursing staff.

Forty-three percent of the responding psychiatrists reported receiving noteworthy threats. Some respondents described being threatened several times a year. The most common responses to these were said to be frustration, fear, feelings of helplessness, and psychologic stress reactions. A few clinicians said that they responded to these potentially dangerous situations with detachment. Legal action was taken in only three instances.

Six psychiatrists reported aborted attacks which had been potentially dangerous, and in one case tragic. The most serious of these involved a paranoid patient who entered the wrong house and killed the neighbor of his intended victim—the psychiatrist's wife. (It is of interest that his intent to kill the psychiatrist's wife was not clarified until some time later, after the patient had committed suicide and other "revenge" murders were traced to him.)

---

*For purposes of this survey, "assault" was described in such a way as to include, but not be limited to, the legal concept of "battery."

Assaults tended to be by patients from lower socioeconomic groups, in large institutions. The significance of this trend is, however, unclear since the numbers involved were low and statistical manipulations necessary to eliminate other variables, such as demographic skew, are not reliable for this group. The assaulted psychiatrists tended not be be inolved in subspecialities that one might associate with violent behavior, for example substance abuse programs or forensic practice. There were indications of administrative underreporting of assaults and threats. Fear of adverse publicity for the facility appeared to be one reason for the noteworthy lack of legal sanctions against assaultive patients.

Survey of Community Mental Health Centers

Another perspective of violent behavior by patients was obtained in a survey of all psychiatric facilities in the state, including community mental health centers, Veterans Administration medical centers, other public facilities and private hospitals (see Appendix 7-1). A structured interview format was used. The format was mailed to appropriate representatives of the surveyed facilities along with a request that they review their records for violent incidents during 1979 and 1980. A telephone interview was then conducted by an experienced investigator.

Results from the hospitals, both public and private, were consistent with those of more comprehensive institutional studies,[8] many of which are reported elsewhere in this volume. Those data will not be reported here.

The findings for community mental health centers (CMHCs) were different. Thirty-four assaultive incidents were reported by eleven CMHCs over a two-year period; about 1.5/year in each center. Over 20 percent of the assaults were directed toward nonclinical personnel, especially secretaries and receptionists. The type of assault—which was not always violent—varied from extreme verbal abuse to threats of physical harm to displaced assaultive gestures (exhibitionism, property damage, theft) to actual physical contact. Only one victim received injuries leading to lost time at work. (See Tables 7-1 and 7-2.)

Actions taken by individual personnel or by the CMHC itself in response to assaultive behavior were varied. In one case nothing at all was done. A chart note was entered in 28 of the total of 34 cases. Although the policy in all agencies required an incident report, reports were completed in less than one-half of the assaults reported to us. Local police were notified on 12 occasions, and psychiatric commitment procedures were initiated as a result of seven of the incidents. Discharge of the patient from CMHC care was a fairly common response ("loss of patient status").

Many respondents indicated that they felt that the rural nature of the state decreased the incidence of patient violence in their clinics. There were a number of concerns expressed, however, such as the patients' ready access to firearms.

Table 7-1
CMHCs: Attacks Directed Against Staff

Staff Position	No. Attacks
"Therapist"*	13
Secretary/Receptionist	8
Nurse	6
Social Worker	4
Security Guard	2
Psychologist	1

*A generic term for clinical staff not described as "Nurse," "Psychologist" etc.

Another difficulty voiced was the frequent proximity of the mental health clinic to local bars, and the (apparently) resulting frequency of patients' being intoxicated during appointments. In addition, staff and their families in rural communities, where there is apparently less anonymity and more difficulty concealing one's address or telephone number, are often more accessible to patients outside the clinic environment. Nonclinical staff appear to be particularly vulnerable by virtue of their "front-line" setting and their frequent lack of training in handling emotional crises.

Although assault on staff appears to be an uncommon event, the numbers may be increasing. Anticipation of potential dangers, practice in the management of violent situations, and the existence of broad support systems for victims are all important. Some mental health centers have staff rehearsals in the management of the violent patient, much as they have fire drills.[6] Architectural measures such as elevated or otherwise protected reception desks,

Table 7-2
CMHCs: Types of Assault

Type	No. Assaults
Extreme verbal abuse	1
Verbal abuse with specific threat	8
Verbal abuse with show of weapon	2
Displaced assault (property damage, exposure theft)	3
Physical assault attempted	5
Physical assault completed	15

and therapy rooms with multiple exits[5] are being used, as are hidden call buttons and other electronic warning systems. The integration of staff and patient safety with modern warm, open therapeutic environments is a challenge which can be met in a number of ways.

Finally, it was apparent in the survey that the administrative policies of the responding centers were beginning to recognize the need for intrastaff communication and support. Group "rehash" sessions to discuss violent incidents were routine in some CMHCs, as was individual support of victims to combat guilt, lowered self-esteem, feelings of loss, and the like.

CONCLUSIONS

The experience of the authors and our colleagues indicates that assaults on staff are infrequent but, for a number of reasons, may be increasing. The sequelae—for staff, patients, and the mental health professions in general—of even a few violent incidents seem so important that our continued interest in the topic is imperative. It is important for staff to realize that lack of recognition of problems or improper handling of violent confrontations will only escalate potential danger.[13]

One priority at this time should be the training and support of mental health personnel with respect to the realistic, not sensationalized, vulnerability to which they are heir. A second area of concern, and one which must be addressed before broad policy issues can be discussed, is that of obtaining accurate information about the incidence and prevalence of assault in psychiatric facilities. A large prospective study, headed in part by one of the authors, is nearing completion.

REFERENCES

1. Andrew JM: Are left-handers less violent? J Youth & Adol 9:1-9, 1980
2. Assaults on doctors. Br Med J 62:1229-1230, 1978
3. Department of Commerce, Bureau of the Census: 1980 Census of the United States (for Nebraska). Washington D.C., US Government Printing Office, 1981
4. Department of Public Institutions State of Nebraska: Unpublished data, 1981
5. Edelman SE: Managing the violent patient in a community mental health center. Hosp Community Psychiatry 29:460-462, 1978
6. Gertz B: Training for prevention of assaultive behavior in a psychiatric setting. Hosp Community Psychiatry 31:628-630 1980
7. Lion JR, Snyder W, Merrill GL: Underreporting of assaults on staff in a state hospital. Hosp Community Psychiatry 32:497-498, 1981
8. Madden DS, Lion JR, Penna MW: Assaults on psychiatrists by patients. Am J. Psychiatry 133:422-425, 1976

9. Monahan J: The Clinical Prediction of Violent Behavior. Rockville, MD, NIMH, 1981, pp 3-5
10. Monahan J: The prevention of violence, in Monahan J (ed): Community Mental Health and the Criminal Justice System. New York, Pergamon, 1976, pp 13-34
11. Ruben I, Wolkon G, Yamamoto J: Physical attacks on psychiatric residents by patients. J Nerv Ment Disease, 168:243-245, 1980
12. Shah SA: Dangerousness: A paradigm for exploring some issues in law and psychology. Am Psychologist, 33:224-238, 1978
13. Symonds M: Violence and the mental patient—a two-sided phenomenon. Roche Report 11(12): 1, 1981
14. Tardiff K, Maurice WL: The care of violent patients by psychiatrists: A tale of two cities. Can Psychiatr Assoc J, 22:83-85, 1977
15. Wenk E, Robison J, Smith G: Can violence be predicted? Crime Delinq, 18:393-402, 1972
16. Zitrin A, Hardestry A, Burdock EI, Drossman AK: Crime and violence among mental patients. Am J Psychiatry 133:142-142, 1976

(*This chapter continues with Appendix 7-1, on page 98*)

APPENDIX 7-1

Client Violence in Community Mental Health Centers

Description	Against	Injury	Response Action	Diagnosis
Assault Male client, fist to gut of female staff	Therapist	Minor injury; stunned but not hurt	Incident Report, loss of patient status	Unknown, or not given
Property damage Female client, hammer to waiting area	Receptionist, and those in waiting area	No physical injury	Incident Report, reported to police and Board of Mental Health (BMH)	Psychotic chronic client at day treatment center
Stolen property Adolescent male client took purse of female staff	Therapist	No physical injury	Arrested, tried, sent to state inpatient facility	Unsocialized aggressive reaction of adolescence
Assault Female client had handgun in purse, showed to female staff and talked of using guns against others and self	Therapist	No physical injury	Chart Note, client referred to inpatient setting and BMH as "dangerous"	Antisocial personality
Assault Male client pulled hunting knife on female staff	Receptionist	No physical injury	Incident Report, reported to police (plus client given an immediate appointment)	Character disorder

Incident	Staff	Injury	Action	Diagnosis
Assault Adolescent client struck staff	Therapist (halfway house manager)	Slight injury to face drew blood	Incident Report, reported to police through parents, loss of privileges, consider inpatient treatment if another incident	Mentally Retarded
Assault Male client struck male staff	Therapist	Minor	Chart Note	Not given
Assault Client struck staff	Therapist	Minor	Chart Note	Not given
Assault Client struck staff	Therapist	No physical injury	Chart Note, reported to police, BMH Commitment recommended in staff "rehash"	Schizophrenia
Assault Client struck staff	Therapist	Medical attention considered	Chart Note, reported to police, BMH Commitment recommended in staff "rehash"	Unknown Alcohol abuse suspected at time of incident
Assault Male client struck female staff in head from rear	Nurse	Medical attention considered	Chart Note, Incident Report, medication and seclusion	Personality Disorder
Assault Husband of client struck female staff during therapy session	Social Worker	Minor injury	Incident Report, reported to police, escorted out by police	Domestic violence Alcohol involved

(*continued*)

Description	Against	Injury	Response Action	Diagnosis
Harassment Use of abusive language to female staff regarding policy of agency	Receptionist	No physical injury	Incident Report, reported to police, escorted out by police	Unknown
Threat Intoxicated client threatened female staff	Receptionist	No physical injury	Incident Report, reported to police, escorted out by police	Unknown Alcohol involved
Threat Client threatened assault to staff	Social Worker	No physical injury	Chart Note, no action taken	Not given
Harassment Male client verbally abused and threatened bodily harm to female staff	Receptionist	No physical injury	Chart Note, summoned therapy staff	Paranoid Schizophrenia
Assault Male client threatened bodily harm and swung at male staff	Therapist	Physical injury avoided	Chart Note, Incident Report, loss of client status, notified county attorney, asked for BMH hold	Paranoid Schizophrenia
Assault Client struck staff	Therapist	Minor	Chart Note, reported to police, loss of patient status	Chronic Schizophrenia

Type of incident	Staff member	Injury	Action/Documentation	Diagnosis
Assault Male client verbally threatened and grabbed at female staff	Receptionist	No physical injury	Chart Note, summoned other staff	Paranoid Schizophrenia
Threatened assault Male client to male staff	Therapist	No physical injury	Chart Note, reported to police, recommended BMH action	Paranoid Schizophrenia
Assault Client struck staff	Nurse	Medical attention given Loss of one work day	Chart Note, Incident Report, client transferred to more secure institution	Paranoid Schizophrenia
Assault client scratched and pulled staff	Nurse	No physical injury Medical attention required by policy	Chart Note	Not given
Assault Client struck staff	Security Guard	Minor Medical attention required by policy	Chart Note, Incident Report, seclusion	Not given Alcohol believed involved
Assault Client struck staff	Nurse	No physical injury Medical attention required by policy	Chart Note, Incident Report, loss of patient status	Not given
Assault Client scratched and bit staff	Security Guard	Minor Medical attention required by policy	Chart Note, Incident Report, seclusion	Not given Alcohol believed involved
Assault Client struck staff	Security Guard	Minor Medical attention required by policy	Chart Note, Incident Report, seclusion	Not given Alcohol believed involved

(continued)

Appendix 7-1 (continued)

Description	Against	Injury	Response Action	Diagnosis
Assault Adolescent client struck staff and broke glasses	Social Worker (manager of group home)	Broken nose and cut under eye Loss of many work days	Chart Note, Incident Report, civil suit against parents dropped when they agreed to seek BMH inpatient treatment	Unsocialized Aggressive
Male client exhibited himself to female staff	Receptionist	No physical injury	Chart Note, Incident Report, reported to police and BMH	Not given Alcohol believed involved
Threat Phone call at home; threatened family and staff	Psychologist	No physical injury	Incident Report, reported to police and local phone company	Not given Alcohol believed involved
Threat Phone call to home; threat to staff	Social Worker	No physical injury	Incident Report, reported to police and to phone company	Not given
Threat Phone call at home; threatened staff and family	Therapist	No physical injury	Incident Report, reported to police and phone company	Not given
Threat Phone call; threatened violence to staff and family	Therapist	No physical injury	Incident Report, reported to police and phone company	Not given Alcohol believed involved

Herbert N. Ochitill

8
Violence in a General Hospital

The growth of psychiatric units in the general hospital setting has been phenomenal. At the same time there has been an impressive expansion of psychiatric consultation and liaison activity in the general hospital. The influx of mental health professionals into this treatment setting has increased attention to identifying and caring for behavioral disturbances.

Violence in the general hospital presents the staff with a situation alien to their training, interest, or sometimes their sense of professional responsibility. While the medical professional understands that there is no guarantee of patient satisfaction, he or she hardly expects belligerent declarations or actions from the patient. Conversely, patients do not expect hostility or violence from the medical staff. Though such interactions seem unlikely and incompatible with the mission of the hospital, such incidents do occur. This chapter will consider the background, development, resolution, and prevention of these assaults.

In the medical treatment setting the predominant approach to patient care is often biological. Thus, when assaultive behavior occurs the mental health clinician is asked to bear a considerable burden of the assessment and resolution of the violent incident. This intervention occurs in the medical setting unless the patient represents an ongoing, significant risk of assault felt to be associated with a mental disorder. Then, if medical conditions permit, the patient is treated in a formal psychiatric setting.

Although there has been some exploration of aggression and hostility in general hospital patients, there has been little exploration of the occurrence of violent and assaultive behavior among these patients. The potential for assault in a general hospital varies with the community served, the self-defined mission of the institution, the physical and staff organization of the hospital, and the degree of recognition and resolution of assaults. Unfortunately, our under-standing of assaults in the general hospital is hampered by the lack of sufficient investigation. The extant literature can only provide suggestive leads for the investigation needed in this important area.

STUDIES OF VIOLENCE

The Problem of Documentation

The study of violence in a general hospital depends on available documen-tation procedures or on a prospective design. Documentation requirements vary among hospitals; the staff is often allowed wide discretion insofar as hospital chart documentation, and it is not unusual to find no specific institutional insistence on recording violent incidents. Thus the investigator must tolerate incomplete information or hope to implement a more effective data-collection system.

The case for adequate documentation requires a clear and substantial rationale. The professional and administrative staff of the hospital must see that assaultive behavior is a definable problem, an obstacle to the work of the hospital, and a difficulty whose characterization will permit preventive steps to be taken.

Defining Violence

It is a truism that people define violence differently. Differences in definition are particularly important for the large proportion of assaultive incidents which occur without a clear institutional definition. For one indi-vidual the loud and angry accusation by the patient is violent; another may brush off an attempted assault without further comment. The definition of assaultive behavior often says as much about the victim as the assailant. Provocation of and response to violent behavior are shaped by the individual's psychological and sociocultural background. These determinants strongly influence the person's propensity for violence and the particular meaning that she or he assigns to the incident. Additionally, the victim and the eyewitness can define events and the need for documentation differently.

Violent behavior that is unexpected, inexplicable, targeted against oneself, and bizarre in its form or expression often has a greater impact than otherwise on those involved with the incident. Such features partially determine its definition and the response of others.

The situational context also plays a role in the person's understanding and response to events. The circumstances in which the violence unfolds influence its meaning for the individual. The violent threat from a stranger being escorted off the hospital ward by the security police has a different meaning from the wild but inadvertent gesticulations of the delirious patient who is being restrained. The degree to which a person feels he or she has contributed to the violence can effect the individual's perspective. Those who feel thay may have contributed to the violence can exaggerate or minimize events.

Setting and Timing of Assaults

The modern general hospital is a complex, multifaceted institution. Three of the main components are the inpatient, ambulatory, and emergency services. Although no area is exempt from assaultive behavior, claims have been made that assaults occur more frequently in the emergency service than elsewhere.[9,19] Clearly, more has been written about violence in the emergency department than other areas of the general hospital. Nonetheless, there has been no definitive work on the relative incidence of assaults in various areas of the general hospital.

Many features of emergency care contribute to the potential for violence. The medical staff in the emergency department more frequently than other departments treats acutely intoxicated patients, some of whom have a greater likelihood of assaultive behavior. Violence-prone individuals with traumatic injuries often must be treated first in the emergency setting. In some emergency treatment settings the unwilling patient is frequently involved in an assaultive incident. The unwilling patient may be intoxicated, delirious, or so fearful that he or she is unwilling to acknowledge an obvious need for acute medical care. The staff feels obligated by the patient's condition to treat without delay and a confrontation ensues.

Frequently, patients and the staff are mutual strangers without a repository of trust to allay frustration and fear. Even in a private hospital the patient's personal physician is not always available to attend to the emergency care of his patient. Generally, patients are in great discomfort with an urgent need to be examined and treated. Staffing may be inadequate to the workload, resulting in long waits before and during the staff's often brief contact with the patient and his family. Staff morale and frustration tolerance drop concomitantly. The collection of difficulties for the patients, their families, and the staff provides generous tinder for an explosion of hostility and assault. For many of the same reasons, so-called walk-in clinics are likely to be relatively less safe.

Ochitill and Krieger investigated the occurrence of violent behavior over a two-year period at the San Francisco General Hospital.[13] Several sources of data were reviewed: 11 violent episodes occurred on a general medical ward, 17 on general surgery, and two in the emergency department. In terms of clinical activity, these figures dramatically underrepresent the emergency service. Some of the possible discrepancies in reporting practices have been discussed. Future investigation should explore the incidence of assault with a standardized case-finding system to avoid the questions raised about retrospective data.

The timing of an assault is strongly related to context and circumstances. The relationship of assaults to conventional time measures and periodic changes within the hospital is not well established. Ochitill and Krieger found that almost all violent incidents occurred within the first 10 days of hospitalization with the average on day seven. Incidents occurred throughout the day and night but were most frequent from 7 P.M. to 7 A.M. It is a time when patients are usually less distracted from the reality of their pain, the implications of their illness, and the persistent worries about other aspects of their life. The hospital wards tend to be less well staffed during these hours, reducing the availability of nurses.[13] There are no studies that relate assaults to other time periods in the general hospital, such as during nursing shift changes and medical rotations.

The Assailants

In the Ochitill and Krieger study, a majority of reported violence involved men less than 37 years old.[13] Female assailants had a mean age of 30 years. Women had a greater proportion of assaults against property or person than men, who were more often reported for threats of violence.

All the reported assailants were patients. Although such a reporting system would be unlikely to describe a staff contribution to violence, it would not necessarily exclude assaults by patients' visitors. However, no report of an assault by a visitor was filed.

Although little has been noted regarding family assaults on staff, such incidents are not unheard of. The following example, drawn from this author's clinical experience, emphasizes the need for effective communication between medical professionals and families, and indicates the potential for assault when adequate communication has not occurred.

Case Study 8-1

The patient, a 66-year-old woman, was admitted to the hospital to investigate the full extent of a cancerous lesion of the mouth that had been diagnosed several months before.

Her sons and daughters noted that she had consistently dismissed the idea of surgery before hospitalization and they understood the goals of admission to be limited to "testing." The patient, a highly respected member of the family, was honored in her intentions by the family. Before hospital admission she shared her reluctance about surgery with her physicians.

On admission, testing was conducted and the question of surgery raised anew. The patient softened her resistance and surgery was performed five days after admission.

Within hours of surgery while recuperating in the Intensive Care Unit, the patient was approached by her two daughters. Claiming they had difficulty locating her in the hospital, they professed ignorance of the surgery. Upon entering the unit they impatiently asked for their mother. The charge nurse asked that staff be allowed a few moments to prepare the patient. The sisters became agitated with this delay; they became angrier still when a benign comment by the nurse was misinterpreted as a slight against their mother. Without further warning, they attacked the nurse. Other staff members intervened before serious injury occurred.

The patient's family later confided their frustration and anger on several counts. They had thought surgery was no longer a consideration given the sentiments of the patient, and several of the patient's children felt she had been unduly coerced to accept the procedure. Her daughters were distressed that no persistent effort was made to contact them when the surgical decision was pending. Once aware that the patient had undergone surgery, they claimed to have difficulty locating the patient in the hospital. The assault was precipitated by a sense that they were being further excluded from their mother's care by a staff not appreciative of the patient or the family's perspective.

Though in this instance a staff nurse was assaulted, the situation implies hostility toward others on the professional staff. The example highlights the possible discontinuity between ambulatory and inpatient care and between the intent of the family and the staff. It also suggests the presence of unresolved disagreement among family members.

The Victims

Work in other settings suggests violence may be "diffused" or directed against a specific target, often the spouse of the patient.[8, 10] In alcohol-related violence, the victim often is both inebriated and the assailant's spouse.[18] Rada notes that when patients in a general hospital setting are angry with the staff they are less likely to express anger with the physicians but will redirect their feelings toward nurses, aides, and family.[14] He adds that patient violence against family members can be a continuation of prior familial conflict and not only a displacement of hostility from the hospital staff. Ochitill and Krieger's work suggests that most assaults of the staff involved nurses, with an appreciable number of assaults against other patients. A very small number of assaults were against visitors. Only a single incident included an attack on a physician.[13] In using nursing incident reports as a source of data, these findings may underrepresent assaults on nonnursing staff.

The Assailants

Medical Status

Certain medical conditions have been strongly associated with violence in many settings, while others can be present in violent patients but have no well-documented relationship. Within the emergency service, intoxication and withdrawal states involving alcohol and drugs, primary CNS injury, or illness such as epilepsy, and systemic conditions such as chronic renal disease have all been associated with assaultive behavior.[9, 14, 15] These conditions are thought to increase the risk of violence through their influence on brain function. Other medical conditions such as chronic pain syndromes are associated in some patients with hostility and violence without evidence of gross brain dysfunction.[2, 14] Among hospitalized patients, it has been noted that the majority of reported assaults were associated with relatively benign medical conditions.[13] In a substantial number of these assaults, contention over pain management was a vital issue. In six of 29 incidents, there was evidence of gross organic brain dysfunction.

Solomon and Kleeman indicate that certain characteristics of the violent episode imply important involvement of medical illness: no premeditation, minimal or absent provocation, bizarre quality of behavior, limited awareness by the patient of the behavior, and other findings of organic brain syndrome (OBS).[16]

In addition to the patient's medical condition per se, medication of many classes—e.g., antiinflammatory agents, cardioactive drugs—has been associated with disturbances of thought, mood, or behavior. Severe mood lability, agitation, perceptual disturbance, or delusional thinking increase the risk of assaultive behavior. These difficulties may occur in therapeutic dosages or herald the onset of a toxic reaction. The hospitalized patient often receives several medications at the same time, increasing the possibility of interactive drug effects.

Psychiatric Status

In the emergency service of a general hospital, clinical experience suggests that intoxication and withdrawal states, delirium, psychoses such as schizophrenia or manic-depressive disorder, paranoid states, acute anxiety, and personality disorders such as borderline or sociopathic are the conditions most likely to be associated with assaults.[3, 9, 14, 15]

Violent behavior among hospitalized patients is associated with a variety of psychiatric conditions. Chronic substance abuse was the most prevalent disorder associated with violent incidents in a large municipal hospital.[13] Acute OBS also was frequently noted. The functional psychoses did not account for a substantial number of incidents while there was little evidence of personality disorders. The latter could have been underrepresented, given the difficulties in obtaining comprehensive data in a retrospective study. Considering only actual assaults on others, the preponderance of substance abuse among assailants was unchanged. The substances abused were opiates or, less frequently, alcohol.

Although alcohol use has been related to violence,[5,8] there is some suggestion that violent behavior is less strongly associated with opiate abuse. Once hospitalized, the patient with a substance abuse history is generally not intoxicated but often experiences the special problems of withdrawal. Excluding withdrawal, many of these patients experience no direct effect of drugs or alcohol despite chronic patterns of abuse. Links between the patient's previous substance abuse and assaultive behavior in hospital might include the patient's continued psychological dependence on drugs and the dementia associated with alcoholism that impairs the patient's modulation of mood and behavior.

Authors such as Bender and Rada have noted the difficulties in staff-patient relations when patients present with pain. They have emphasized the potential for hostility and violence in the care of chronic pain and psychogenic pain patients.[4,9] In Ochitill and Krieger's report neither of these diagnoses was well established but pain assessment and management played a critical role in many cases.[13]

Another factor in assaults which should gain increasing attention is the use of psychotropic medication. With widespread use of minor tranquillizers and growing use of antipsychotic medications in the medical setting, the report of aggressive side effects[1,7] requires more vigorous investigation.

Clinical Context

Rada and others have commented on the situational aspects of assault. He reviews elements of the preassault, assault, and postassault phases and calls for review of provocative interaction between the staff and patient before the assault. Rada also emphasizes the degree to which the assault is goal-directed.[14]

Rada considers the patient's feelings about himself and the illness, his family, and the staff. Noting that hostility arises as a consequence of self-blame for the illness, he comments that certain patients may feel unworthy of the staff's care. Rada suggests that allowing this patient increased control of his care will be helpful. He notes that the fear and confusion generated by illness can contribute to the development of a violent episode.[14] The difficulties are compounded when there are problems in communication with the staff, indicating that patients and their families feel they are not obtaining clear, comprehensive information. The various stresses of illness and hospitalization for the patient have been amply considered in a chapter by Strain.[17]

Familial conflict is noted as a source of violence. However, it is unclear how often and in what fashion prior conflict prompts a hospital assault between family members or family and staff. After family disturbance results in injury and hospitalization, threats of violence sometimes continue among the nuclear or extended family. Family contribution to illness and the impact of illness on families have been relatively neglected areas of investigation that are gaining increasing interest.[11]

Several investigators have described the potential for hostility and violence in caring for pain patients. Bender describes the difficulties in the care of seven hospitalized patients with psychogenic pain.[2] The patients feel unsatisfied in their requirements for pain relief while the staff typifies patient's needs as "excessive". The patient's behavior can escalate from decorous requests to strident demands. These demands can evoke hostility, avoidance, or both from the staff. In this way a turbulent situation develops rapidly. Bender proposes that several possible dynamics underlie the patient's interaction: a powerful though ambivalent need for intimacy intensified by a stress-induced reduction of self-esteem and a need for punishment. The latter theme is well reviewed in a classic paper by Engel on the "Pain-prone Patient."[4]

Ochitill and Krieger documented the prevalence of pain management problems in their survey of hospital violence. Difficulties generally involved the care of patients who abused drugs and/or alcohol. For a few of these patients, there was disagreement over the indications for methadone and, if indicated, its dosage and duration. Another very small group attempted to satisfy their drug requirements illicitly while still in the hospital. The largest proportion of these patients was locked in contention with the staff about the frequency, dose, and duration of analgesia. Those who habitually used drugs to reduce tension and frustration felt ineffectively treated with analgesics and grew more tense and even more desirous of the anxiolytic effect of the medication regimen.[13] The dispute can become most difficult when the patient has significantly improved in all respects except pain. This discrepancy raises questions for the staff about the determinants of the pain. In the context of troublesome issues of pain management, the assault may be immediately preceeded by events not directly related to these difficulties.

Case Study 8-2

One young female patient with a seven-year history of drug abuse was admitted with the diagnosis of bacterial endocarditis. On the morning of her 17th hospital day, the patient frequently requested pain medication, often "screaming for the nurse." That evening, in the context of continued dispute with the staff regarding pain management, the patient was visited by a friend. The staff called the hospital security when the friend refused to honor visiting hours. The patient became enraged and threw a pot at the nurse who had summoned security.

Another group of substance abusers struggled with the staff over the control exercised over their activities in hospital. They felt the staff was unnecessarily interfering with their desire to leave hospital briefly and return, or to change the discharge date. These patients also balked at the regulation of visiting hours.

Case Study 8-3

One patient, chronically abusive of heroin and alcohol, was admitted for multiple abscesses. Six days after admission, in transgression of hospital rules, she refused to leave the room of a male patient. The nursing staff thought the patient was interfering with staff duties, and so called the security guard. The patient left the male patient's room but returned to her room yelling and later threw an ashtray at her roommate. She was transferred to another ward but chose to leave the hospital, refusing to sign the "against medical advice" form.

Patients with OBS were most likely to become violent when their symptoms were most severe. These incidents seemed unpredictable and unprovoked.

Case Study 8-4

A chronic alcoholic was admitted with a diagnosis of right knee arthropathy. During the first several days of his hospitalization, he remained disoriented to time and place, muttered continually to himself, and showed considerable agitation and insomnia, with autonomic signs of abstinence syndrome. The day before the incident, he was placed in three-point restraints. On day 5, he was still judged to be confused but the restraints were removed. A nurse entered his room and he immediately began threatening to throw the urinal at her. The physician on the ward judged the patient to be "actively hallucinating." The security police were called and the patient was again put in restraints.

Staff Response

There has been no rigorous investigation of staff reactions to threatened or actual violence in the medical setting. Ochitill and Krieger's report suggests that before the violent incident some of the patients were felt to be uncooperative, demanding, accusatory, and generally critical of the hospital care. Clearly, there is a rift between these patients and the staff. The staff feels they are dealing with problem patients; patients assert that the staff is insensitive to their needs. By inference, in typifying patients as uncooperative, the staff feels frustrated and stymied in reaching their objectives for patient care. A feeling grows that the patients interfere with their own care. When the patient is regarded as "demanding" the staff is troubled that the patient seems to assume a position of authority, dictating the course of action. Without doubt, for many of the staff this is an unwelcome state of affairs. They refuse or acquiesce with resentment to the patient's demands or vacillate. Staff members working with the patient may respond with hopelessness and avoidance when persistently confronted with impossible expectations. To describe the patient as "accusatory" is to imply a staff struggle to defend itself against the next critique from the patient. contention begins to focus on staff competence. Hostile and hurt feelings are generated which often lead to increasingly perfunctory contact with the patient.

Continuing or escalating pain and requests for analgesics generate many reactions in the staff. By definition, care providers are troubled when patients describe significant discomfort. Elements of diagnostic or therapeutic uncertainty are raised. Staff feelings of exasperation and impotence can contribute to increasing tension and, ultimately, direct or indirect expression of hostility.

The staff working in the emergency department of an inner-city municipal hospital is likely to be at special risk for feelings of irritation and hostility. They are more frequently involved with verbally or physically abusive patients than staff in many other treatment settings. Among the relatively large number of verbally abusive patients, those with a high potential for assault must be identified. Staff members experience conflicting feelings. Simultaneously, the staff want to help the patient, fear personal injury, and feel angry when verbally abused or physically threatened. Even without direct expression of these feelings, such reactions can contribute to an escalation of violence or produce overly harsh treatment of patients and their families. Extended experience in this type of setting can lead to increased insensitivity and cynicism in caring for patients and diminished job satisfaction.

PREVENTION

The foregoing studies suggest certain approaches to the prevention of assaults in the general hospital. Prevention can focus on characteristics of the patient, aspects of the treatment setting, and interaction between the two.

There has been considerable study of those patient characteristics that correlate with increased incidence of street violence,[12] but there has been insufficient study of how valid these factors are in the general hospital setting. Ochitill and Krieger's report supports the notion that the young male substance abuser is at increased risk for violence, although the retrospective, uncontrolled design of the study weakens their argument.[13]

A hospital should document and retrieve information regarding prior hospital violence as well as factors of age, sex, race, socioeconomic and employment status, and drug use history associated with increased risk of violence. Given the nature of these factors, public municipal hospitals are among the most likely to care for violence-prone patients. These institutions have a special need to fashion a more specific approach to these patients. Once an individual becomes assaultive within the hospital, the staff is compelled to pursue specific attempts to prevent further violence. A better approach would be to systematically review relevant information before such a destructive sequence of events develops. The patient at risk could be told of the staff's awareness of past difficulties and their desire to avoid future problems. They might indicate that abuse of the patient or the staff is intolerable and that patient concerns and frustrations will be seriously reviewed if not always completely resolved.

Elements of the treatment setting must also be considered. General frustrations of the working staff can contribute to increased chances of assault. Sources of staff frustration can include short supplies, understaffing, problems in staff communication, and failure to reach consensus about treatment. At the very least, physicians and nurses need to alert each other about manifest patient and staff frustrations. The nursing staff is an often underutilized resource for information about patients and is in a specially vulnerable position to be assaulted. Tending to the specific frustrations of a treatment setting can dramatically improve staff morale and frustration tolerance.

Staff training should explore methods to interdict the escalation of violence between the patient and others. Staff can be assisted to recognize pressures in themselves to respond in a counterprovocative way and, therefore, helped to avoid being participant victims. In-service education can review descriptive models of assaultive behavior, predictive patterns, phase-appropriate interventions, techniques of physical intervention, and documentation procedures.

Conferences can center around responses to the demanding, angry, or threatening patient. Feelings about substance abuse and other health abusing habits can be reviewed. There is no room for moralizing about substance abuse; moral judgements easily lead the staff to chiding or punitive behavior toward patients. Patient complaints should not be reflexly treated as an expression of the patient's character disorder or a pallid recitation of the obvious but inevitable shortcomings of the hospital. While there may be some truth to these statements, the care provider's response to the patient should be characterized by willingness to explore the patient's complaints or to get someone who will; honest appraisal of the validity of patient comments; avoidance of judgement about a co-worker's activity or a conclusion regarding a personally unfamiliar incident or situation; and emphasis on future improvement especially when prior difficulties are poorly defined or elicit mutual blame.

In caring for patients with pain, the staff should avoid challenging the reality of the patient's pain. Such a challenge implies that the patient knows less of what she or he feels than the staff or misreports the truth of the physical experience. Patient discouragement, distrust, and anger are the likely outcome. Particularly for the chronic pain patient, Fordyce has shown that elements other than the pain report can be used in the assessment and treatment of the patient.[6] Since staff members' personal pain experience and clinical experience affect their expectations about patients, there is much potential for divergent approaches to pain management. The staff must come to a consensus; divisiveness means uncertainty and the potential for staff–patient misalliances.

Personnel, such as nurses and staff/attending physicians, with an ongoing involvement in the treatment setting and extensive patient contract are the most likely participants in staff education. Nurses are instrumental in conducting sometimes desired and sometimes uncomfortable treatment of the patient. Collectively, they have the most patient contact and are easily available targets for displaced hostility. Security personnel of the institution require the same careful training in defusing a possibly explosive incident. When the security staff is an effective professional unit, they provide substantial reassurance for the rest of the staff.

Control of patient access to intoxicating substances and weapons is important. Apropos to these concerns, there must be special vigilance in the emergency medical setting in caring for people from the streets, who may be intoxicated and/or in possession of drugs or weapons or both. Obviously, if the clinical situation permits sufficient time for the patient to detoxify, this reduces the possibility of an assaultive episode. Inpatients returning from being AWOL require special scrutiny to rapidly identify intoxicated patients, illicit drugs, or possible weapons.

Other elements of the setting include family and peer relations with the hospitalized patient. Difficulties arising with visitors suggest careful review in order to encourage supportive visits and restrain disruptive visits. A history of violence with family or peers may be predictive of recurrence during hospitalization. On the other hand, families often facilitate harmonious relations between the patient and the staff. They can help the patient to appreciate the intent of the care providers and contribute to the reduction of frustration among all parties.

The differences between the medical and psychiatric settings should be clear to the psychiatric clinician. The medical staff obviously has little training in treating behavioral disorders and typically places little emphasis on preventing them. Often preferring to believe that the problem resides with the patient, the medical staff may have little interest in the interactive aspects of an incident. The staff are not inclined to see themselves as agents for change. With such a formidable set of obstacles, few resources are made available for the problem of assault prevention. While these observations seem stark, they should not be surprising, given even the psychiatric professional's generally unenthused approach to the problem.

Obviously, the psychiatric clinician has little power to change personnel or procedures in medical settings. The setting is not designed for the care of agitated or assaultive patients; the facilities and patients are highly vulnerable to destructive behavior. The conventional psychiatric involvement that occurs is more aptly described as "postvention" than prevention.

There are three means to assist in the prevention of assault: case consultation, programatic instruction, and liaison with mental health resources. The mental health consultant has a preventive role to play in many instances of case consultation: requests to assist with the psychotic, demented, noncompliant or disruptive patient. These are common reasons for obtaining mental health assistance, and each may, through competent consultation, reduce the probability of assault. These examples provide a more likely context for intervention than an explicit request to head off possible violence.

Case Study 8-5

A 26-year-old woman was admitted to the hospital for evaluation and treatment of presumptive bacterial endocarditis. During the first two weeks the patient was treated vigorously and responded well. Her male companion spent considerable amounts of time at her bedside.

As the patient approached her first month in the hospital, the staff noted that she was increasingly irritable and unwilling to allow daily medical and nursing interventions. She became belligerent when reminded of how sick she had been and could become again. The psychiatric consultant was asked to see this "noncompliant" patient. In gathering information, the consultant discovered that the patient's altered behavior coincided with an abrupt reduction in her companion's visits. She was able to recognize several anxieties aroused by his relative absence. Her companion was impressed with the importance of his visits and encouraged to come more frequently. Within a few days, the patient's behavior greatly improved.

The consultation process may contain the seeds of a provocative encounter. The involvement of a mental health professional can be threatening to the patient in several respects. If unexpected, it can increase the patient's confusion and sense of poor communication with the staff. If unexplained, the patient may feel the staff misunderstands him and dismisses his needs as illegitimate. If unwanted, the patient often feels powerless and victimized. To avoid these undesirable responses, the staff and the consultant must inform the patient of the consultation in a proper fashion. That is, the staff review how consultation relates to optimal care and allow the patient expression of his or her feelings before the consultant encounters the patient's room.

Assault prevention can be enhanced through formal staff instruction. Educational conferences and workshops try to reduce the chance that a patient–staff interaction will trigger an assault. Although such exercises are often well received, it is unclear what lasting benefits accrue and what unique role they play in an overall prevention program.

When threats or assaultive behavior continue despite all measures in situ, the staff can insist that prevention of further difficulty requires transfer to a psychiatric facility. The patient's medical condition permitting, the consultant is expected to rapidly facilitate this process. He or she reviews the possibility of a causal relationship between the medical condition and the violence. If none exists, one explores the possibility that a relationship exists between the violence and a mental disorder. If there is no apparent mental disorder, then transfer to a psychiatric facility is more expressive of the medical staff's desire to discharge than to meet the needs of the patient. When a psychiatric transfer is appropriate, considerable thought should be given to the patient's sensitivities and likely reaction. Poorly conducted, the wooden announcement of the patient's imminent transfer for psychiatric hospitalization can provoke further hostility and violence.

FUTURE INVESTIGATION

With virtually no rigorous investigation of assaultive behavior in medical settings available, much soundly designed and implemented research is needed. The need includes a range of outstanding concerns about assault including incidents and description in different health care systems; determinants of documentation; association with demographic, medical, andpsychiatric factors; course and treatment outcome; and its relation to and impact on staff dynamics.

As with so many questions in the mental health field, investigative progress will depend on coherent definitions. Since the assailant and victim are both subject to considerable bias, corroborative data should be sought from others who witness the assault. Descriptive studies could be expanded to routinely include the behavior of various staff members, the patient, and the family before and after the assault. This extended view of the system of relationships promises keener insights into the vulnerabilities of the assailant and victim.

There is a special opportunity in the medical setting to study the psychobiology of assaultive behavior. The influence of illness and its metabolic derangements as well as pharmacologic treatments can be carefully assessed.

Investigation of the comparative incidence of assaults in different health care systems should offer information about the population served and also reveal aspects of the system which minimize or provoke assaults.

Studies of current management of assaultive behavior in the general hospital should begin to address questions of intervention. How effective and feasible are psychological and pharmacologic interventions in the medical setting? Does treatment combining both approaches offer selective advantages? Treatment studies should also investigate appropriate and inappropriate uses of mental health facilities for patients who assault in a medical setting.

Given the interactional nature of much violent behavior, it is vital that we understand more about medical staff dynamics. Through greater comprehension of stressful staff interaction, tension-resolving staff interventions become possible for the liaison psychiatrist. Hopefully, such interventions will reduce provocative and counterprovocative staff behavior.

SUMMARY

There has been very little investigation of the nature and extent of assaultive behavior in the general hospital. Inconsistent definitions and incomplete information impede effective study of the problem.

Although every area of the general hospital is the scene of assaults, the emergency department is likely to be the most dangerous area. Generally, assailants are relatively young male patients whose victims are usually nurses and, less frequently, other patients.

On the inpatient ward, assaultive patients often have relatively benign medical conditions. There is a range of psychiatric disturbance associated with violent patients. For hospitalized patients, substance abuse and acute OBS are the most common diagnoses.

Difficulties in pain management and rule enforcement often provide a backdrop for assaults by hospitalized patients. Some of these patients are seen as uncooperative and demanding well before the violent incident; such patients experience deteriorating relations with the staff before a final series of explosive interactions.

Prevention entails identification of and specific intervention with the individual at risk for hospital violence. Though often overlooked, measures to reduce staff frustration and to bolster tolerance and morale are critical elements. These measures include general improvement in working conditions and specific changes related to the issues that provoke violence. Staff education can focus on sensitivity to their own feelings and avoidance of counterprovocative behavior. The mental health clinician facilitates prevention through case consultation, programatic instruction, and liaison with mental health resources.

Investigators need to explore a range of issues, with special efforts in comprehensive description, psychobiology, intervention, and staff dynamics.

REFERENCES

1. Barnes TR, Bridges PK: Disturbed behavior induced by high-dose antipsychotic drugs. Br Med J 281:274–275 1980
2. Bender D: Seven angry crocks. Psychosomatics 5:225–229 1964
3. Dubin WR: Evaluating and managing the violent patient. Ann Emerg Med 10:481–484 1981
4. Engel G: Psychogenic pain and the pain-prone patient. Am J Med 26:899–918 1959
5. Fitzpatrick JP: Drugs, alcohol and violent crime. Addict Dis 1:353–367 1974
6. Fordyce NE: Operant conditioning in the treatment of chronic pain. Arch Phys Med Rehab 54:399–405 1973
7. Gardos G: Disinhibition of behavior by antianxiety drugs. Psychosomatics 21:1025–1026 1980
8. Gerson LW: Alcohol-related acts of violence: Who was drinking and where the acts occurred. J Stud Alcohol 39:1294–1296 1978
9. Gosnold DK: The violent patient in the accident and emergency department. Roy Soc of Health J 98:189–190 1978
10. Lion JR, Bach-Y-Rita G, Ervin FR: Violent patients in the emergency room. Am J Psychiatry 125:1706–1711 1969
11. Minuchin S, Baker L, Rosman BL, et al: A conceptual model of psychosomatic illness in children. Arch Gen Psychiatry 32:1031–1038 1978
12. Monahan J: The Clinical Prediction of Violent Behavior. Washington, D.C., US Government Printing Office, 1981

13. Ochitill H, Krieger M: Violent behavior among hospitalized medical and surgical patients. South Med J 75:151–155 1982

14. Rada RT: The violent patient: Rapid assessment and management. Psychosomatics 22:101–109 1981

15. Shevitz S: Emergency management of the agitated patient. Primary Care 5:625–634 1978

16. Solomon P, Kleeman ST: Medical aspects of violence. Calif Med 114:19–24 1971

17. Strain JJ, Grossman S: Psychological Care of the Medically Ill: A Primer in Liaison Psychiatry. New York, Appleton-Century-Crofts, 1975

18. Tinkleberg JR: Alcohol and violence, in Bourne PG, Fox R, (eds): Alcoholism—Progress in Research and Treatment. New York, Academic Press, 1973

19. Winterbottom S: Coping with the violent patient in the accident and emergency department. J Med Ethics, 5:124–127 1979

Stephen Armstrong

9

Assaults and Impulsive Behavior in the General Hospital: Frequency and Characteristics

Assaults and impulsive behavior cause trauma, medical problems, and difficulties for large numbers of persons in this country. Assaults also coexist with a number of medical and psychiatric conditions, so the medical care system perforce encounters assaults on a frequent and predictable basis. Since general hospitals form the backbone of the acute care medical system, they are increasingly involved with and concerned about problems of assaultive and impulsive behavior, not only on the physical premises of the general hospital, but also in the community as a whole.

Unfortunately, there are few estimates of the prevalence of assault in general hospital facilities. Reid and his co-workers are now conducting a study of assaults, which includes two general hospitals, and the results will be forthcoming soon. In the meantime there remain about 900 general community hospitals in the country which receive and treat problems associated with assaults and impulsive behavior, including both offenders and victims. This chapter reviews briefly the epidemiology of assaults in the general hospital setting, provides new information about the distribution of assaults in the psychiatric emergency room, and outlines some areas of concern for hospital planners.

THE EPIDEMIOLOGY OF ASSAULTIVE AND DESTRUCTIVE BEHAVIOR

Recent epidemiological studies have documented that violence—suicide, homicide, and accident—is now the leading cause of death in persons under 40 years old.[11] It is commonly understood that the rate of adolescent suicide has doubled since the early 1960s.[24] Moreover, new research indicates that the prevalence of sexual assault, common assault, and child abuse may be far higher than had been previously documented.[9, 27] When we consider only those persons already identified by the health care system as "mental patients," a number of studies after 1965 document higher rates of violence for these persons—and a faster accelerating rate of violence—than for the community as a whole.[7, 10, 14–15, 17, 18, 21, 22] Even when measured by crude indices such as arrest rates, mentally ill persons have relative risk ratios of 1.5–29 times higher than that of the general population for crimes of violence and assault. Arrests tend not to be made merely for minor violations, such as vagrancy, loitering, or inappropriate behavior, but, instead, for seriously deviant behavior.[6]

Two other major data sources contribute to our understanding about the rising importance of assessing and treating violence in the community. The first source is the data on battered wives. Some researchers believe that in most industrialized countries a woman has a 50 percent chance of being beaten at least once severely during her married life.[27] A second data source are studies that examine violence in persons brought to the medical care system for reasons other than assault per se. For instance, general hospital emergency rooms often find that about 2 percent of their female patients have been assaulted, and these women often fail to report to the examining physician that assault is the cause of their medical distress.[1, 16]

There are a variety of speculations about why violence is more common recently, including the theory that there is a higher proportion of persons in the high risk period, and will continue to be until the mid-1990s.[26] A good example of the general hospital's "load" of violence comes from the work at Baystate Medical Center (BMC) of Gelinas and Goodman, who documented that one-third of all women who were hospitalized for psychiatric problems had suffered significant sexual abuse as children or adolescents.[9] In the child psychiatric division, boys with conduct disorders have a high chance of having been abused, as do their mothers; and their adolescent sisters have high risks of being sexually abused.[23] Moreover, the pediatric department may encounter relatively high rates of child abuse that is purposefully masked by the child's parents.

Finally, the high rate of violence in all patients is indicated by the cumulative risk to assault endured by therapists.[13, 25, 28]

There are a host of methodological problems associated with attempts to establish the "true" rate of assault and impulsive behavior in the general hospital setting. The first problem is that many general hospitals operate diverse clinics and facilities, so that any attempt to assess assaultive incidents is very expensive and cumbersome. For example, BMC operates 950 inpatient beds in three geographic units, 10 outpatient clinics, and 3 satellite clinics. Its staff physicians consult at 6 regional hospitals. It employs several hundred staff nurses. Hence, any attempt at accurately sampling to arrive at the prevalence figures for violence would require substantial investment. Another problem is that the incidence of assault in the general hospital may not represent the "true" assault rate in the community, because the hospital often acts as a sink trap for such behavior. As a consequence, any attempts to develop a "screening indicator" of potential assault for use in the general community would tend to overpredict persons likely to assault and thus be inapplicable. (For a discussion of problems in error rates, see Fleiss[8] and Bishop, Fienberg, and Holland.[5])

THE EMERGENCY ROOM ARCHIVE

Patient registers or archives can help establish the existence and distribution of a problem; they also allow for cross-sectional, longitudinal, panel, follow-up, and follow-back studies.[3, 4] Beginning in 1979 I began constructing the BMC Psychiatric Emergency Room Archive, which is a geographically incomplete, duplicated patient count archive of all persons who have used the BMC emergency psychiatric facility. To the extent that the Archive is geographically incomplete, we have no community-wide measure of overall psychiatric emergency room use. However, BMC provides from 60–90 percent of all psychiatric emergency coverage in the Springfield, Massachusetts, statistical area, so the Archive can be regarded as representative of the overall emergency psychiatric "load" in the community. The following report on assaultive persons is based on 3531 psychiatric evaluations of 2732 persons over a 30-month period. From the Archive we can abstract 183 assaultive patients and contrast them to all other patients.

Patients coming to the BMC Emergency Room are first cleared medically and then seen by the Psychiatric Emergency team. The patients and relatives are interviewed for up to three hours; there is a 24-hour "holding unit" available for overnight care, and the patient may be referred to one of the 63 psychiatric facilities in the Springfield area. Beginning in 1979, the following patient information has been coded and stored in a keylocked computer file:

1. Demographic information: age, sex, ethnicity, marital status, and current psychiatric treatment.

2. The "top three" psychiatric problems based on a modified Problem Appraisal Scale.
3. The two most likely probable diagnostic statements, based on the Research Diagnostic Criteria (RDS),[20] modified for use in the Archive.
4. Disposition to a treatment facility or clinic.
5. Psychotropic medications that may have been given in the ER.

The RDC diagnoses are 26 highly refined statements based on formal clinical evaluation and anamnestic records. The realistic limitations of the ER practice, however, forced several modifications. For instance, the diagnoses were coded as "most probable, given the evaluation and historical data at hand." Whenever historical substantiation could not be obtained in the ER, we coded a "downgraded" diagnosis, so that the results would not be contaminated with a number of unsubstantiated cases. (For an example of how this coding was accomplished, see Armstrong.[1])

Assaultive ER patients differ from nonassaultive patients in a number of ways. Fifty-eight percent of assaultive patients are men, which is far more than typically come to the Psychiatric Emergency Service (38 percent). Assaultive patients tend to be unmarried and are slightly younger than nonassaultive persons. Three out of four assaultive persons are white, but ethnic minorities are represented disproportionately in the assaultive group. Assaultive patients are far less likely to complain of depressed mood or feelings of inferiority, but, instead, are overtly angry, belligerent, or negative during the ER evaluation. Assaultive women often report focal problems with spouse or children. A large number of assaultive patients are psychotic at the time of evaluation (about 30 percent, roughly the same as the nonassaultive group). When medications are given in the ER, the assaultive person is likely to get a neuroleptic.

Our analyses indicate that the presence or absence of assaultiveness is the single strongest predictor of treatment disposition. Assaultive patients are far more likely to be committed involuntarily to the state hospital and are far less likely to be offered a voluntary general hospital psychiatric admission. An assaultive patient has a five-fold increased chance of involuntary commitment, over a nonassaultive patient. This relative odds ratio illustrates the interlocking roles of the general community and state psychiatric hospital in containing assaultive behavior.

Problem statements and diagnostic statements can not give us a detailed assessment of assaultive persons and can not contrast assaultive to nonassaultive persons. We therefore inspected in detail the ER evaluations of two subsamples from the Archive, trying to bridge a gap between the data on the ER archive and the specific behaviors and histories of assaultive persons.

Detailed Evaluation of Assaultive and Nonassaultive Subsamples

Fifty patients were selected randomly from the Archive for a detailed analysis of violence or the lack of violence reported in the ER. These 50 patients had a total of 72 ER evaluations, as follows:

- Assaultive evaluation marked in the archive. N = 28.
- Assaultive evaluation, but not marked in the Archive because three other problems superseded assaultiveness. N = 8.
- Nonassaultive evaluation of someone already indexed in the Archive as assaultive. N = 6.
- Assaultive evaluation of a patient indexed in the Archive as nonassaultive because three other problems supervened at the time of the evaluation. N = 2.
- Nonassaultive evaluation of a patient randomly selected from the Archive as nonassaultive. N = 19.
- Nonassaultive other evaluation of a patient indexed as nonassaultive in the Archive. N = 8.

The total number of evaluations in the microanalysis is 72. The total number of nonassaultive evaluations is 27; the assaultive evaluations, 37. The assaultive patients form a 13 percent subsample from the larger assaultive group; the nonassaultive patients, a 0.5 percent subsample from the larger nonassaultive group. Both groups were examined for representativeness to their larger populations on problem statements and RDC diagnoses and found to fit well.

Assaultive Subsample

In the assaultive subsample the assaultive patients are—as they are in the larger Archive—more often male, younger, and currently in treatment elsewhere. They are far more likely to present as angry-belligerent-negative, are given to more frankly homicidal ideation, have an identified target for their aggression and assault, and more often require external controls (such as restraints) while in the ER.

Each patient's evaluation was rated for the presence or absence of 61 risk factors often associated with assault, and these risk factors were grouped into "categories" or scales. Each risk factor and scale was then tested to see whether it discriminated between the assaultive and nonassaultive groups.

Difficulties in the interview process. An assaultive person—or patient expressing anger or belligerence—is difficult to interview, especially when the patient expresses any homicidal ideas and fantasies, or when the patient "teases" the ER clinician with some information and withholds other information. The overall association between "group membership" (assaultive versus nonassaultive) and "the process features of the interview" is .441 (canonical correlation), but this statistical association is not powerful enough to separate the two groups definitively. In a sense, all psychiatric patients are difficult to interview, and assaultive patients slightly more so.

Previous history.   The patient's previous history with respect to violence and assault is by far the strongest correlate of currently assaultive behavior (canonical correlation = .883). In particular, the previous use of violence or the previous endurance of violence (for victims in the sample) is highly associated with current assaults in the ER. Other historical factors contribute significantly to the current situation, and include a history of severe childhood deprivation and brutality, childhood aggression (such as cruelty to animals, fighting, temper tantrums, inability to get along, stubbornness), firesetting, property damage, self-mutilation, suicide attempts, and multiple childhood or adolescent losses.

Psychological factors.   One feature of assaultive persons, as noted by ER clinicians, is that the person on whom they are dependent may be threatening to leave in some way, or the assaultive person has just driven them out. The relationships of assaultive patients have far higher tension levels than do those for nonassaultive patients (t-test = 4.93, d.f. = 62, p < .000). The repetitious pattern of the loss also is evident to the evaluator. Other psychological features of the assaultive person is the use of external standards, such as bravery, defiance, or toughness, and hence the patient may be searching for some external, combative confirmation of self-esteem. Most often this search has begun within the 48 hours immediately preceding the ER evaluation.

Situational factors.   Assaultive persons require a victim, usually a spouse or child, to assault. Having previously abused a victim, or being attracted to a victim, or extreme helplessness in the victim may contribute to an assaultive episode. For the victim, having been victimized previously, having selected a partner with a known history of violence, or having had a brutal father are associated with being the current victim of an assault. It should be noted that few assaultive patients (about 11 percent) report voluntarily whether a victim is currently available.

Disinhibition and means.   The presence of weapons or the use of automobiles, fists, or feet clearly distinguish assaultive persons (canonical correlation = .681). Even given the ER's base rate of assaultive persons (about 5 percent of all ER evaluations are of assaultive persons), knowing whether there are means to hurt someone available to the patient enables the evaluator to correctly classify the patient over 74 percent of the time. Moreover, the use of alcohol or drugs is important. Each factor—the use of drugs or alcohol, and weapons—is extremely important in all assaultive incidents.

Threatened acts. In the ER, patients often state their intentions, or make an overt threat, or respond appropriately to the evaluator's questions about whether they have just threatened someone. When a patient states that he is not comfortable with his aggressive thoughts, the index of suspicion for assault diminishes. It should be noted, however, that nearly half of the imminently assaultive patients in the emergency room see no real alternative for solving their distress than to carry through an assault.

Overall aggression scale. Assaultive patients can be differentiated clearly from nonassaultive patients in the ER (t-test = 5.63, d.f. = 62, p < .000). These differences are very large and can be used to classify correctly about 80 percent of the subsamples. When applied to the larger ER population, use of these indicators increases accuracy by a factor of 10 over chance predictions. In order of importance, the following features should be part of a standard assessment in the presence of anyone suspected of potential for violence:

- Previous use of violence
- Threatened loss of a loved person, or reenactment to drive the loved person away
- Method of violence easily available, or the current or past use of auto, fists, or feet to injure someone
- External evaluation of toughness, bravery, courage, as bolsters to self-esteem
- Homicidal ideation; and, to a slightly lesser extent, suicidal ideation
- Teasing the evaluator with "pieces" of information
- Manifest tension in the relationship between the patient and the one on whom he is dependent; threats, precipitous actions, and so forth
- Childhood deprivation and brutality endured; childhood aggression firesetting, property damage, and self-mutilation
- Emotional crescendo, change in mood or cognition within the 48 hours preceding the ER evaluation; acts or fantasies that increase agitation
- Previous victimization or attraction to a victim; for victims, having previously been victimized, extreme helplessness, absence of alternative housing for self or children
- Violence as ego syntonic; no discomfort with being violent or not seeing any way other than being violent
- Use of alcohol or other drugs

These comments on the ER patients hardly exhaust the domain of violence in the general hospital. In preparing this article, the author met with some staff nurses, who work on the medical units of the hospital. Each nurse could recount episodes of having been pulled, tugged, hit, or spat on by a medical patient. Usually these women had dismissed the incident as regrettable and they each saw no available means of redress. Even senior physicians who have private patients at the hospital can report incidents either in their training or clinical practice in which they were assaulted or pushed around by a patient. The studies of psychiatrists have already been mentioned. Thus, it may be of some benefit to examine events inside the hospital to identify and control such incidents and behavior.

GENERAL HOSPITAL MANAGEMENT OF IMPULSIVE BEHAVIOR

Is the problem of assaultive behavior "recognized" by the institution? At some level, many general hospitals acknowledge that assault is a very real part of their environment. Many urban general hospitals are located in tough parts of town, so incoming patients and visitors are screened very carefully, even to the point of having to pass through metal detectors. Hospital security procedures have been augmented in many hospitals, and the security guards are better trained in crisis management. Additionally, hospital architects are aware of the special needs of certain units, like the ER, for multiple exits, adequate lighting, and segregation of rooms for potentially assaultive persons. For example, in the old Vanderbilt Medical School hospital, psychiatric residents often would have to use the ER orthopedic room to do psychiatric evaluations, so they spent a great effort to clean the room of implements prior to seeing the patient. This design flaw was corrected in the recently constructed Vanderbilt Hospital. Another example comes from BMC, which recently sponsored a training session for nursing unit supervisors on the acute management of assaultive patients on medical or surgical floors.

At another level, however, general hospitals have a very difficult time recognizing the existence of assaultive patients. First, nurses rarely report assaults, or report only the most egregious behavior, for reasons mentioned above. Second, "violence" or "assault" is not a diagnosis, and is not even really thought of as a medical problem, so general hospitals do not have the same investment in establishing a coordinated assessment and treatment protocol that exists, for example, in control of infections. Third, physicians tend to label assaultive behavior as a "psychiatric problem," outside their responsibilities, and hence may not follow through on management plans on nonpsychiatric floors. Fourth, the general hospital tends to "expel" assaultive psychiatric patients to the state hospital system, for a number of reasons, some of which relate to the general hospital's preference to "run a hospital" and not a "loony bin."

There are several generic problems that plague the hospital's efforts to assess and treat patients with assaultive or impulsive programs. The first problem is ideological. Since, as stated above, the general hospital tends to see itself as a medical, not psychiatric, facility, efforts to treat assaultive persons in-house are not favorably received. The ideological stance may be bolstered by a realistic lack of facilities for such patients, and redressing such a lack would require a shift in orientation. Moreover, other physicians in the hospital (who number far more than the psychiatrists) tend to prefer to see medical problems in medical terms—diseases, and treatments—instead of "vague" behavioral phrases such as "assaultiveness," "impulsive disorder," "family troubles," and the like. Indeed, many psychiatrists are not comfortable with these problems, which may be one reason they have chosen general hospital psychiatric practice in the first place. Finally, there is the problem of training psychotherapists to handle problems of violence. Such treatment is difficult and requires careful thinking through and planning (see Armstrong,[1] for a description of some of the skills which a therapist must have in order to conduct treatment with impulsive or destructive persons.)

On the positive side, there certainly are some avenues to approach the institution. For instance, the department of obstetrics and gynecology can be sensitive to adolescents who have been sexually abused and to women who have been subjected to sexual violence. Pediatrics departments can screen large numbers of physically abused children and provide a valuable community service. The emergency or trauma facilities can help identify both victims and potential offenders. I believe that these efforts are all worthwhile but will fail ultimately in a coordinated program, unless the hospital administration accepts a position that assault and violence are public health problems worthy of note and treatment.

Th second problem for the general hospital is departmental, "turf." An example is drawn from BMC, which, as New England's second largest hospital, has a carefully defined administrative structure:

> The Pediatrics Department has managed a screening and assessment program for child abuse for four years. Pediatrics wanted more access to child psychiatrists and child psychologists, but the Psychiatry Department, for a number of important reasons, could not provide the services. So Pediatrics hired outside clinical psychologists to staff its SCAN (Suspected Child Abuse and Neglect) team. At the very same time, a clinical psychologist and a social worker developed the Psychiatry Department's Incest Treatment Program, and another clinical psychologist developed the Impulsive Behavior Program. As a result, BMC has three concurrent programs, all dealing with one or more facets of domestic violence, assaultiveness, and so forth. There are a number of good administrative reasons for the two Departments not to cooperate more fully, but there are also some good reasons why they should.

Since assaultiveness, trauma, and violence are so pervasive in the community, this author feels that it would make good administrative sense to have an overall "destructive trauma" team. The lack of a coordinated voice at the hospital is underscored by the fact that it took the SCAN team over two years to have instituted an official policy that nurses and other line staff workers had to report suspected child abuse and neglect to the team. The hospital still has no official policy on weapons, despite the murder of a boy three years ago in the ER. The hospital has no official policy on nurses' harassment: should they report incidents to the Director of Nursing or to Personnel?

A third problem facing the general hospital is the magnitude of the problem. Members of our Psychiatric Emergency Service can expect to see an assaultive patient every third day on rotation. Residents and staff members in Pediatrics can expect "yet another" abused child every other day or so. The Psychiatry Inpatient unit can expect that one out of three female patients will have some history of abuse. The Psychiatry Outpatient unit anticipates that over half of its patient load will be either destructive persons or victims of abuse. These sorts of numbers lead therapists and staff members to feel burned out, numb, or beleaguered.

Moreover, countertransference to impulsive or destructive persons is difficult to manage.[12] Assaultive persons can be genuinely frightening and distinctly unpleasant to handle, and it often is easier not to see such persons as a general rule than to risk facing the countertransference issues of helplessness, narcissistic injuiry, opprobrium from colleagues, and so forth.

Despite these problems, I am convinced that the general hospital is the community's most important resource—in coordination with other social agencies—in treating impulsive and destructive persons. For one thing, only the general hospital brings together the medical and psychiatric facilities in such a concentrated fashion. Second, the general hospital has immense persuasive leverage in the community to publicize programs for persons who have trouble with their anger of destructive behavior, and to bring other agencies into coordinated programs. Third, only the community general hospital has enough legal clout to support therapists who treat these people and take risks in treatment that would not be taken in a private practice. For instance, BMC is standing behind a therapist threatened with a malpractice suit by a man who abused his son and then did not like having to see his son under supervision. Fourth, the general hospital provides an excellent "laboratory" to assess not only the patients but also the effects of various treatment programs for such persons. Fifth, the general hospital has the resources to provide outside consultation to agencies which may not have the same resources. Such consultation can include work with the local community mental health agencies, social service agencies, police departments, and district attorneys' offices.

REFERENCES

1. Appleton W: The battered woman syndrome. Am J Orthopsychiatry 48:487–494, 1978

2. Armstrong S: Psychotherapy of Impulsive and Destructive Persons. (in press) 1983

3. Babigian HM: The role of psychiatric case registers in the longitudinal study of psychopathology, in Roff M, Robins L, Pollack M (eds): Life History Research in Psychopathology, vol. 2. Minneapolis, University of Minnesota Press, 1972

4. Babigian HM, Jones, DB: The psychiatric case register: a versatile device for the application of multiple methodological approaches, in Strauss JS, Babigian HM, Roff M (eds): The Origins and Course of Psychopathology: Methods of Longitudinal Research. New York, Plenum, 1977

5. Bishop YMM, Fienberg SE, Holland PW: Discrete Multivariate Analysis: Theory and Practice. Cambridge, MA, MIT Press, 1975

6. Bonovitz JC, Bonovitz JS: Diversion of the mentally ill into the criminal justice system: the police intervention perspective. Am J Psychiatry 138:973-976, 1981

7. Durbin JR, Pasewark RA, Albers D: Criminality and mental illness: a study of arrest rates in a rural state. Am J Psychiatry 134:80-83, 1977

8. Fleiss JL: Statistical Methods for Rates and Proportions, 2nd ed. New York, Wiley, 1981

9. Gelinas D, Carr FA, Goodman B, et al: Prevalence of incest in adult women who are psychiatric inpatients. (in press) 1983

10. Herjanic M, Meyer DA: Psychiatric illness in homicide victims. Am J Psychiatry 133:691-693, 1976

11. Holinger PC: Violent deaths among the young: recent trends in suicide, homicide, and accidents. Am J Psychiatry 136:1144-1147, 1979

12. Lion JR, Pasternak SA: Countertransference reactions to violent patients. Am J Psychiatry 130:207-210 1973

13. Madden DJ, Lion JR, Penna MW: Assaults on psychiatrists by patients. Am J Psychiatry 133:422-425, 1976

14. Rappeport JR, Lassen G: Dangerousness—arrest rate comparisons of discharged psychiatric patients and the general population. Am J Psychiatry 121:776-783, 1965

15. Rappeport JR, Lassen G: The dangerousness of female patients: a comparison of the arrest rate of discharged psychiatric patients and the general population. Am J Psychiatry 123:413-419, 1966

16. Rounsaville B, Weissman MM: Battered women: a medical problem requiring detection. Int J Psychiatry Med 8:191-202, 1977-1978

17. Sosowsky L: Crime and violence among mental patients reconsidered in view of the new legal relationship between the state and the mentally ill. Am J Psychiatry 135:33-42, 1978

18. Sosowsky L: Explaining the increased arrest rate among mental patients: a cautionary note. Am J Psychiatry 137:1602-1605, 1980

19. Spitzer RL, Endicott J: Problem Appraisal Scales (PAS). Biometrics Research, New York State Department of Mental Hygiene, 1971. (Available from: Jean Endicott, Ph.D., Director, Research Assessment and Training Unit, 722 West 168th Street, Room 341, New York, 10032)

20. Spitzer RL, Endicott J: Research Diagnostic Criteria (RDC), 1979 Version. (Available from Jean Endicott, Ph.D, as above.)

21. State of California, Department of Mental Health: Violent crime offenders study.

Sacramento, CA, October 12, 1973 (Interdepartmental Memorandum), cited in
Sososky L: Crime and Violence among mental patients reconsidered in view of
the new legal relationship between the state and the mentally ill. Am J Psychiatry
135:33–42, 1978

22. Steadman HJ, Vanderwyst D, Ribner S: Comparing arrest rates of mental
    patients and criminal offenders. Am J Psychiatry 135:1218–1220, 1978
23. Stewart MA, deBlois CS: Wife abuse among families attending a child psychiatry
    clinic. J Am Acad Child Psychiatry 20:845–862, 1981
24. Stuart RB: Violence in perspective, in Stuart RB (ed): Violent Behavior: Social
    Learning Approaches to Prediction, Management, and Treatment. New York,
    Brunner Mazel, 1981
25. Tardiff KJ: A survey of psychiatrists in Boston and their work with violent
    patients. Am J Psychiatry 131:1008–1011, 1974
26. Turner CW, Fenn MR, Cole AM: A social psychological analysis of violent
    behavior, in Stuart RB (ed): Violent Behavior: Social Learning Approaches to
    Prediction, Management and Treatment. New York, Brunner Mazel, 1981
27. Walker LE: A feminist perspective on domestic violence, in Stuart RB (ed):
    Violent Behavior: Social Learning Approaches to Prediction, Management, and
    Treatment. New York, Brunner Mazel, 1981
28. Whitman RM, Armao BB, Dent OB: Assault on the therapist. Am J Psychiatry
    133:426–429, 1976

J. Guy Edwards
William H. Reid

10

Violence in Psychiatric Facilities in Europe and the United States

Aggression has been defined as "any form of behavior directed toward the goal of harming or injuring another living being who is motivated to avoid such treatment."[6] Several contrasting views of the nature of aggression have been expressed; these will be referred to as a theoretical background against which the problem of violence in psychiatric facilities can be understood.

THEORIES OF AGGRESSION

These views regard aggression either as instinctive behavior, an elicited drive, or learned social behavior. Major proponents of the instinctive theory (notably Freud,[26] Lorenz,[37]) see aggression as an innate urge. Lorenz suggested that aggressive energy, derived from the fighting instinct, is spontaneously and continuously produced and thereby accumulates within the organism with the passage of time.[37, 38] Aggressive behavior results from an interaction between

The authors express thanks to Mark James, M.D. for assistance in the preparation of this chapter.

the amount of accumulated energy and aggression-releasing stimuli within the environment. Carrying out noninjurious aggressive acts prevents aggressive energy from accumulating to dangerous levels and therefore decreases the chance of harmful outbursts. Love and friendship from others also helps to prevent such outbursts.

In contrast to this view, the drive theory suggests that aggression originates externally, from frustration or the blocking of goal-directed behavior.[9, 10, 16, 20, 54] Social learning theory sees aggression as a product of previous experience and reward.[2, 5]

There are also social and environmental determinants of aggression. The former include frustration (as already discussed), especially if intense[32] and perceived as being arbitrary or unreasonable;[52] actual or anticipated physical[15, 18, 30, 34] and verbal provocation;[27, 29, 50] and exposure to aggressive models.[3, 4, 8] Environmental determinants include loud and unpleasant noise,[17, 35] unpleasant conditions of overcrowding,[1, 24, 25] and moderate (although not extreme) elevation of environmental temperatures—in the middle to upper 80s°F.

Whichever view is favored, some of the conditions referred to resemble those encountered in at least some psychiatric facilities: frustration, provocation, aggressive models, learned behavior, noise, and heat. Yet, in the literature on violence in psychiatric facilities that has come from Europe and the United States, relatively little attention has been paid to these factors.

SOME METHODOLOGICAL DIFFICULTIES IN ASSESSING VIOLENCE

What has been investigated, however, is the extent to which violent incidents in psychiatric facilities occur, together with some of the characteristics of assailants and their victims. The results of these investigations should be interpreted with caution, because the meaning of such terms as "violent incident" and "violent assault" is not always clear. No one would dispute that an attack with a dangerous weapon leading to serious injury would be universally regarded as a violent assault, but what about the likable, though cantankerous, old man with dementia or an endogenous psychosis who repetitively strikes out at others in a rather gentle, though not gentleman-like, way? To some the incidents would be regarded as inconsequential, perhaps even amusing, although others might not be so tolerant.

There is also no reliable information on the accuracy of reporting. The extent to which incidents are recorded varies considerably, and is influenced by personal, interpersonal cultural, and subcultural factors. It is also influenced by the general level of administrative, medical, and legal concern over violent incidents; the importance attached to their being reported; the motivation, skill, and initiative of staff in recording events, and the extent to which reporting is supervised and monitored.

These influences vary, even within the same facility. If staff are unduly concerned about the reputation of their hospital or any part of it and feel that violence will be seen as a sign of failure of treatment, there is a tendency toward underreporting. There may be pressure on staff to conform, not to "make waves," which prevents the reporting of some incidents, while the paperwork and administrative "hassles" also may be deterrents. The need for individual staff to see themselves as sensitive and competent may conflict with the view of some that being assaulted is a sign of personal failure.

EXTENT OF VIOLENCE IN PSYCHIATRIC FACILITIES

Accepting such methodological difficulties, the limited research that has been carried out in Europe suggests that a considerable number of violent incidents occur, although only a small proportion of the total patient population are involved,[22] and serious incidents are rare.[19,21,23,47] The most recent of this research was carried out in Great Britain at Tooting Bec Hospital, London; Park Prewett Hospital, Basingstoke; and the Psychiatric Unit at Sutton General Hospital, Sutton.[21] These facilities provide a comprehensive psychiatric service for the defined geographical areas they serve and are broadly representative of psychiatric hospitals throughout Britain. The results of this research can therefore be regarded as a reflection of the level of violence that occurs in typical British psychiatric facilities.

Psychiatrists from both sides of the Atlantic have the impression that violence, at least in its most severe form, is encountered much more frequently in psychiatric facilities in the United States than in England. This position is supported by the scanty statistics available. A legislative committee found that there were more than 12,000 violent incidents each year in the 28 psychiatric facilities in New York State.[40] In contrast, the Confederation of Health Service Employees (COHSE), one of the major unions operating within the framework of the British National Health Service, was able to report only 311 violent assaults on staff in Britain over the course of 3.5 years.[12] This seems significant, even if the two countries differ greatly in their definitions and reporting.

In other American research 48 of 115 psychiatrists surveyed by Madden et al.[39] and 15 of 31 psychiatry residents surveyed by Ruben et al.[45] reported being attacked. These and media reports of psychiatrists having been shot or murdered by patients also suggest that there is a higher level of violence in the United States.

Characteristics of Assailants and their Victims

It has been shown in Britain that younger patients are more prone to carry out violent acts than older patients. In the study cited it was also suggested that women behave violently more often than men.[21] This might seem surprising, as one study in the united States revealed that more male, than female, inpatients showed assaultive behavior before admission (although this did not apply to women who had a seventh grade or lower level of education).[48] One possible reason for the apparent difference between the sexes is that violence is regarded as more abnormal in women, and may therefore be reported more often.

Fottrell found that patients with schizophrenia were more often responsible for violent incidents than those with other diagnoses.[21] This is in keeping with the findings of an American study which showed that the majority of patients who assaulted psychiatrists on the staff of the University of Maryland School of Medicine were diagnosed as having schizophrenic illnesses.[39] In the British study, and perhaps also in the American survey, this could have been due to there being more patients with schizophrenia in the hospitals where the research was carried out, and to the tendency for them to remain longer in hospitals than do patients with other diagnoses. In both studies patients with personality disorders and those who were drug or alcohol dependent were responsible for relatively few assaults. This is possibly due to such patients' not being readily admitted and, when they are and they show a propensity for violence, being hastily discharged.

Whatever the relationship between violent incidents and psychiatric disorders, it is difficult to translate findings of the kind described to other countries because of cross-cultural differences in diagnosis, the best-known of which are marked Anglo–American differences in the diagnosis of schizophrenia.[13,14,31,43,46]

The victims of assaults may be patients, relatives or staff—not only those who have close clinical contact with patients but also receptionists and secretaries (see Chapter 7). There has been less research concerning the characteristics of victims than of assailants, although Madden et al. showed in their study that the majority of the 48 psychiatrists who had been assaulted were attacked during the early stages of their careers or while working in high-risk settings such as prisons or emergency departments.[39] These findings were not confirmed by Reid and Haffke in a study of 85 psychiatrists in the Mid-Western U.S.[44]

In another study 31 residents at the Los Angeles County-University of Southern California Medical Center were interviewed concerning physical attacks on them by patients.[45] Fifteen (48 percent) of these had been assaulted at least once during two to three years of residency training. The trainees were assessed on the irritability scale of the Present Status Examination of Wing et al.[51] Significantly higher proportions of those with a score above the mean were attacked compared with those who had a low irritability score. Furthermore, the survey showed that those who said they showed their feelings to others verbally or physically when angry, had higher percentages of having been attacked, compared with those who said they did not show their feelings in this way. The residents who were attacked more than once had higher irritability scores and seemed to be more willing to fight if threatened physically outside the hospital setting.

Time and Place of Assaults

In Fottrell's study conducted in England, violent incidents were most often reported on acute and intensive care wards. Thirty percent of incidents in Tooting Bec Hospital took place between 7 and 9 in the morning, at times when patients were getting up, washing, dressing, and having meals.[21] This was reminiscent of earlier research from Sweden that revealed more incidents occurring during the mornings and evenings, when there was less structured activity, and fewer occurring during the course of more structured occupational and industrial therapy.[19]

Apparent Anglo–American Differences

If the differences between Britain and the United States referred to above are real, and not just apparent, they raise many important questions. For instance, are Americans as individuals basically more aggressive than their European counterparts? Or is their society a more violent one, with violence begetting violence? Do conditions in American hospitals predispose to violence to a greater extent than conditions in European hospitals?

Unfortunately, no comparative studies have been conducted, and the answers to these and other questions must remain speculative. In general, however, there appears to be less peacetime nonpolitical violence in European, than in North American, communities.

The higher rate of violence in America is reflected in its astronomic rates of violent crimes. The Federal Bureau of Investigation's "Crime Clock" for 1980 showed that a case of aggravated assault took place every 48 seconds, a robbery every 58 seconds, a forcible rape (a crime that is grossly underreported) every 6 minutes, and a murder or negligent manslaughter every 23 minutes.[48] Although statistics between the two countries are not directly comparable, recent figures for England and Wales[33] seem to show a much lower incidence of violent crime than those for this United States. This is shown, for example, in the relative figures for homicide. In 1980 there were 23,044 cases of homicide reported in the U.S. (population 222 million). During 1980 there were 620 cases of homicide reported in England and Wales (population 49 million). The annual number of homicide cases (including manslaughter) is 10.2/100,000 total pop. in the U.S.[49] and is 1.3/100,000 total pop. in England and Wales.[33]

Reflecting on violence of this kind in the United States, a former Attorney General, Ramsay Clark (1981) wrote:

> ... America glorifies the power of violence and ignores its pity. Nonviolence is seen as cowardly. For a man to be gentle is for him to be weak. From the school yard fight to "Kojak" on television, we equate might with right. Our folklore is full of criminal heroes like Jesse James and Bonnie and Clyde. We respect force, and it is very human to want respect. Give me death, or life in prison, but don't ignore me, Son of Sam cries out. Few Americans are strong enough to adhere to nonviolence under pressure. "Winning" is everything and force is the way.*

To a certain extent at least, violence in psychiatric facilities is a reflection of violence in the community at large; it is also one of the numerous manifestations of the illnesses treated within these facilities. But studies of the nature of aggression and violence indicate that conditions in psychiatric hospitals and attitudes of staff can also predispose to violence. These conditions and attitudes vary among hospitals and countries and possibly account for some of the Anglo–American differences to which we have referred.

Violent Staff

It is a sad fact, and an ugly blemish on the face of a caring profession, that staff sometimes assault patients. Fortunately, incidents of such brutality are rare. Allegations are not infrequently made, but it is often difficult to learn the truth because of conflicting stories and the difficulties of disentangling fact from fiction, especially when the credibility of the victim—often a psychotic patient—is suspect. Witnesses are often reluctant to help, because of divided loyalties and fears of personal vendettas. Allegations are, however, sometimes referred to the police, and there have been a number of prosecutions and convictions.

A recent example of assault by staff on patients occurred in Britain and received widespread publicity through the mass media. The events took place at Rampton Hospital, which is one of four "special hospitals" in England and Wales that is administered directly by the Department of Health and Social Security for people detained for treatment and conditions of special security on account of dangerousness, violent or criminal propensities. The allegations of physical ill-treatment by male nurses were made in the Yorkshire television film, *The Secret Hospital*. The truthfulness of the allegations has yet to be

---

*Reprinted from Clark R. A few modest proposals to reduce individual violence in America, in Hays JR, Roberts TK, Solnay RS (eds): Violence and the Violent Individual. Proceedings of the Twelfth Annual Symposium, Texas Research Institute of Mental Sciences, Houston, Texas, November 1–3, 1979. SP Medical and Scientific Books, 1981, pp 1–5.

established before the court, but whatever the legal outcome, a review of conditions within the hospital revealed many shortcomings relevant to patient care in general, as well as to the problem of assaults within psychiatric facilities.

Predisposing Conditions and Attitudes

It was found by the review team[39] that Rampton Hospital was not only isolated geographically but, what is worse, isolated professionally.[33] The team was particularly critical of the lack of medical leadership and of the system of nurse management which had not allowed proper leadership to emerge. Nursing practices on the male wards were overstructured, authoritarian, and inflexible, and there was far too much emphasis on security (at the expense of therapy). The hospital had produced an inbred, inward-looking community that perpetuated old-fashioned attitudes. It operated as a closed and secretive institution that was overly defensive and resistant to change. In short, there was too much "institutional inertia."

The same criticisms were not directed toward the female side of the hospital, where assault by staff on patients did not occur. Although the female patients provided more difficult nursing and management problems, there was much less regimentation, more flexibility, and more subtlety in observing patients' behavior.

It was thought that conditions on the male wards predisposed to frustration-induced aggression in patients. Such aggression, whether expressed as violent behavior or shown more passively, could lead to retaliation by staff and hence assaults by staff on patients. Assaults of this kind, made by members of a caring profession, are inexcusable, but so are hospital conditions that predispose to such primitive behavior.

The Review Team's finding is by no means peculiar to Rampton. Earlier authors have commented on the role of authoritarianism and underinvolvement of medical staff as factors contributing to violent behavior in psychiatric hospitals.[11] The part played by nurses in unconsciously provoking episodes of violence has also been addressed.[36] Madden et al. found that 53 percent of the psychiatrists who had been assaulted felt that they had acted in a provocative way, for example by insisting on confronting the patient with upsetting material.[39] Similarly, in the study by Ruben et al. 14 of the 15 residents who had been assaulted thought that they had contributed to the assault by frustrating the patient, for example by refusing admission when requested or admitting the patient against his wishes.[45] It will be recalled also that the more irritable the resident, the greater the chances of being attacked. Of course, in some cases, a psychiatrist might accept blame for an incident as a feature of his or her personality, and not by virtue of any really significant contribution.

Need for Research

Violence is a complex phenomenon involving the assailant, the victim, and the milieu. Some research into assaults in psychiatric facilities has already been conducted, but there are still more questions unanswered than answered. Whenever possible, research should be multidisciplinary. Biologists, sociologists, psychologists, psychiatrists—perhaps even mathematicians with their "catastrophe theory"[53]—all have a part to play. Some of the numerous variables related to violent episodes have already been studied, but there are many others that have not been investigated.

In whatever research is undertaken, it is necessary to define operationally that which constitutes a violent act. In order to differentiate trivial from serious incidents, an attempt should also be made to rate the seriousness of the act. Fottrell referred to three degrees of violence, based on the seriousness of the injury (if any) inflicted. Violence of the first degree occurred when no physical injury was detectable on examination. If there were minor injuries, such as bruises, abrasions and/or small lacerations, second degree violence was said to have occurred. Large lacerations, fractures, loss of consciousness, injuries requiring special investigations (irrespective of the results of the investigations), permanent disability or death called for a rating of violence of the third degree.[21]

PREVENTION OF VIOLENCE IN PSYCHIATRIC FACILITIES

It is clear from what is already known about violence in psychiatric facilities that it should not be examined in isolation, but should be seen within the total social context. Whenever people are grouped together, there will always be a certain amount of violence because man is an aggressive animal. It is logical also to assume that the more violent the society, the greater the potential amount of institutional violence.

In a psychiatric facility violence will sometimes be seen as one of numerous manifestations of the illnesses being treated, although there is disagreement as to whether there is more or less violence among psychiatric patients than among people in general, or no difference.[28, 41, 42]

Acceptance of all violent incidents as being inevitable is fatalistic and nihilistic. Like other problems within psychiatric facilities, attempts should be made to prevent such incidents, as they are symptoms crying out for treatment and because they lead to unpleasant and dangerous working conditions for staff. When staff assault patients they bring shame on a noble profession.

The familiar cry, "more research is needed," should not be an excuse for inactivity. Even in the light of existing knowledge, much can be done to help prevent violence in psychiatric facilities.

It will be recalled that the Rampton Team thought that conditions on the male wards predisposed to frustration-induced aggression. Theoretical knowledge concerning aggression suggests, and common sense demands, that these conditions should be changed. When they are, it is likely that there will be less violence, happier patients, and more contented staff.

Each psychiatric facility should keep an accurate record of violent incidents, which may serve as a barometer of predisposing conditions within the facility. While the routine use of such forms almost certainly underestimates the total number of incidents, the majority of serious attacks will probably be recorded. If there is a significant number of these, or if they are on the increase, there is probably something amiss within the organization, such as outmoded practices, authoritarianism, excessive rigidity, and/or ineffective leadership.

To discuss all the aspects of hospital administration that may predispose to violence is beyond the scope of this chapter; but those social determinants which were highlighted in our discussion of aggression clearly should be assessed relative to violence within any facility. Unpleasant conditions of overcrowding should be corrected, excessive noise diminished, and temperatures adequately regulated. Staffing should be adequate, with attention paid to quality as well as quantity. Staff must be sensitive to potentially violent situations and trained to use techniques of redirecting aggression and gentle containment instead of relying solely on confronting or overpowering the patient, seclusion, or restraint. There should be sufficient structured activity for the release of aggression and for the defusing of potentially explosive situations. Good relationships throughout the organization should be fostered at personal levels and within group meetings. Unless attention is paid to the therapeutic milieu in these ways, the level of violence in a facility is likely to be greater than it should be.

REFERENCES

1. Altman I: The environment and Social Behavior. Monterey,California, Brooks-Cole, 1975
2. Bandura A: Aggression: A Social Learning Analysis. Englewood Cliffs, New Jersey, Prentice-Hall, 1973
3. Bandura A: Social Learning Theory. Englewood Cliffs, New Jersey, Prentice-Hall, 1977
4. Baron RA: Threatened retaliation as an inhibitor of human aggression: Mediating effects on the instrumental value of aggression. Bull Psychonomic Society 3:217-219, 1974
5. Baron RA: Human Aggression. New York, Penham Publishing Corporation, 1977
6. Baron RA: Aggression, in Kaplan HI, Freedman AM, Sadock BJ (eds): Comprehensive Textbook of Psychiatry, III, 3rd ed. Baltimore, Williams and Wilkins, 1980, pp. 409-424

7. Baron RA, Bell PA: Aggression and heat: the influence of ambient temperature, negative affect, and a cooling drink on physical aggression. J Pers Soc Psychol 3:245-255, 1976

8. Baron RA, Ransberger VM: Ambient temperature and the occurrence of collective violence: The "long, hot summer" revisited. J Pers Soc Psychol 36:351-360, 1978

9. Berkowitz L: Some determinants of impulsive aggression: The role of mediated associations with reinforcements for aggression. Psychology Reviews 81:165-176, 1974

10. Berkowitz L: Whatever happened to the frustration-aggression hypothesis? American Behavioral Scientist 21:691-708, 1978

11. Brailsford DS, Stevenson J: Factors related to violent and unpredictable behaviour in psychiatric hospitals. Nursing Times, 69 January 18, Supplement: 9-11, 1973

12. COHSE: The management of violent or potentially violent patients. Banstead, Surey, England, Confederation of Health Service Employees, 1977

13. Cooper JE, Kendall RE, Gurland BJ et al: Cross-national study of diagnosis of the mental disorders: Some results from the first comparative investigation. Am J Psychiatry 125:21-29, (Supplement), 1969

14. Cooper JE, Kendall RE, Gurland BJ et al: Psychiatric Diagnosis in New York and London. Maudsley Monograph Number 10. London, Oxford University Press, 1972

15. Dengerink HA, Schnedler RW, Covey MK: The role of avoidance in aggressive responses to attack and no attack. J Pers Soc Psychol 36:1044-1053, 1978

16. Dollard J, Doob L, Miller N et al: Frustration and Aggression. New Haven, Connecticut, Yale University Press, 1939

17. Donnerstein E, Wilson DW: Effects of noise and perceived control on onging and subsequent aggressive behavior. 1976

18. Dyck RJ, Rule BG: Effect on retaliation of causal attributions concerning attack. J Pers Soc Psychol 36:521-529, 1978

19. Ekblom B: Acts of Violence by Patients in Mental Hospitals. Almquist and Wiksells Boktycheriab Uppsala, Scandinavian University Books, 1970

20. Feshbach S: Aggression in Mussen PH (ed): Carmichael's Manual of Child Psychology. New York, John Wiley and Sons, pp 159-259, 1970

21. Fottrell E: A study of violent behaviour among patients in psychiatric hospitals. Br J Psychiatry 136:216-221, 1980

22. Fottrell E, Bewley T, Squizzoni M: A study of aggressive and violent behaviour among a group of psychiatric in-patients. Medicine, Science and the Law 18:66-69, 1978

23. Folkard MS: A Sociological Contribution to the Understanding of Aggression and its Treatment. Netherene Monographs 1. Coulsdon, Surrey, Netherene Hospital, 1957

24. Freedman JL: Crowding and Behavior. San Francisco, California, W.H. Freeman and Co., 1975

25. Freedman JL, Levy AS, Buchanan RW et al: Crowding and human aggressiveness. Journal of Experimental Social Psychology 8:528-548, 1972

26. Freud S: Introductory lectures on psycho-analysis, Starchey J (ed): in Standard

Edition of the Complete Psychological Works of Sigmund Freud. London, Hogarth Press, 1963

27. Geen RG: Effects of frustration, attack, and prior training in aggressiveness upon aggressive behavior. J Pers Soc Psychol 9:316-321, 1968

28. Giovannoni JM, Gurel L: Socially disruptive behavior of ex-mental patients. Arch Gen Psychiatry 17:146-153, 1967

29. Goldstein JH, Davis RW, Herman D: Escalation of aggression: Experimental studies. Pers Soc Psychol 31:162-170, 1975

30. Greenwell J, Dengerink HA: The role of perceived versus actual attack in human physical aggression. J Pers Soc Psychol 26:66-71, 1973

31. Gurland BJ, Fleiss JL, Cooper, JE et al: Cross-national study of diagnosis of the mental disorders: Some comparisons of diagnostic criteria from the first investigation. Am Psychiatry 125:30-39 (Supplement), 1969

32. Harris MB: Mediators between frustration and aggression in a field experiment. Journal of Experimental Social Psychology 10:561, 1974

33. Home Office: Criminal Statistics, England and Wales, 1980, 1980

34. Kimble CE, Fitz D, Onorad JR: Effectiveness of counteraggression strategies in reducing interactive aggression by males. J Pers Soc Psychol 35:272-278, 1977

35. Konecni VJ: The mediation of aggressive behavior: Arousal level versus anger and cognitive labeling. J Pers Soc Psychol 32:706-712, 1975

36. Levy P, Hartocollis P: Nursing aides and patient violence. Am J Psychiatry 133:429-431, 1976

37. Lorenz K: On Aggression. New York, Harcourt, Brace and World, 1966

38. Lorenz K: Civilized Man's Eight Deadly Sins. New York, Harcourt, Brace, Jovanovich, 1974

39. Madden DJ, Lion JR, Penna MW: Assaults on psychiatrists by patients. Am J Psychiatry 133:422-425, 1976

40. New York State Senate Select Committee on Mental and Physical Handicap. Senator James H. Donovan, Chairman (1975-1976). Violence Revisited . . . A Report on Traditional Indifference in State Mental Institutions Towards Assaultive Activity.

41. Rappeport JR, Lassen G: Dangerousness—Arrest rate comparisons of discharge patients and the general population. Am J Psychiatry 121:776-783, 1965

42. Rappeport JR, Lassen G: The dangerousness of female patients: A comparison of the arrest rate of discharged psychiatric patients and the general population. Am J Psychiatry 123:412-419, 1966

43. Rawnsley K: An international diagnostic exercise. Proceedings of the Fourth World Congress of Psychiatry, Madrid, 1966. Excerpta Medica International Congress Series, Number 150, 2683-2686, 1966

44. Reid WH, Haffke EA: Patient violence against psychiatrists: The Nebraska surveys. Manuscript available from Dr. Reid, Nebraska Psychiatric Institute, Omaha

45. Ruben I, Wolkon G, Yamamoto J: Physical attacks on psychiatric residents by patients. J Nerv Ment Dis 168:243-245, 1980

46. Sandifer MG, Hordern A, Timbury GC: Psychiatric diagnosis: A comparative study in North Carolina, London and Glasgow. Br J Psychiatry 114:1-9, 1968

47. Stierlin H: Der Gualttatige Patient. Bibliotheca Psychiatricia Neurologica (Basel)

97:1-62, 1956

48. Tardiff K, Sweillam A: Assault, suicide, and mental illness. Arch Gen Psychiatry 37(2):164-169, 1980

49. United States Department of Justice: Crime in the United States 1980. FBI Uniform Crime Reports. Washington, D.C., U.S. Government Printing Office, pp 1-39, 1980

50. Wilson L, Rogers RW: The fire this time: Effects of race of target, insult, and potential retaliation on black aggression. J Pers Soc Psychol 32:857-864, 1975

51. Wing JK, Cooper JE, Sartorius N: The Measurement and Classification of Psychiatric Symptoms. An instruction manual for the PSE and Catego Programme. London, Cambridge Univ Press, 1974

52. Worchel S: The effect of three types of arbitrary thwarting on the instigation to aggression. J Pers 42:300-318, 1974

53. Zeeman EC: Catastrophe Theory. Selected Papers 1972-1977. Reading, England, Benjamin, 1977.

54. Zillman D: Hostility and Aggression. Hillsdale, New Jersey, Erlbaum Associates, 1979

PART II

Policy Issues

Gary W. Nyman

11
The Role of Security Personnel in a Psychiatric Facility

Case Study 11-1

A 46-year-old agitated and depressed man was treated for his fractured leg in a small general hospital and needed transportation back to a private psychiatric hospital for continued treatment. Because of his psychological state, nursing service at the general hospital requested their security service to transfer the patient.

Case Study 11-2

A call for immediate assistance from the psychiatric unit of a large general hospital was received by security. On arrival at the unit the two armed security officers were faced with a very large, burly man, seemingly out of control, screaming intimidating aggressive threats from the open doorway of the quiet room. The other patients and three female nursing staff were comforting one of the nurses who seemed to be injured. The focus shifted to the two men from security.

Case Study 11-3

The security unit of a large rural public psychiatric hospital was notified that a 26-year-old male patient with suicidal and homicidal ideation had eloped from one of the closed units and was seen walking toward the road to town. The unit staff urgently requested the patient's apprehension and return to the unit for further treatment.

These three case studies are composites of actual requests that have been made of security personnel in psychiatric units. The actions taken by security will vary and are defined by their role in the hospital. Other factors that determine the function of security personnel are the hospital's location, its governance and funding structure, its size, the types of patients it treats, and any special relationships with community agencies.

MISSION OF SECURITY PERSONNEL

A hospital's security personnel provide protection for patients, visitors, staff, and property. The capacity and scope of protection will vary in the private psychiatric hospital, the general hospital with a psychiatric unit, and the large public psychiatric hospital.

Private Psychiatric Hospital

A private psychiatric hospital often is located in a suburban or rural setting. As such, it is highly dependent on its own security unit to handle incidents and is independent of outside assistance. A sense of tranquility and order usually is associated with these hospitals. Visitors and prospective patients feel as if they are guests within a comfortable, protected environment. The hospital's security unit provides the structure for maintaining the hospital's secure appearance. This secure appearance is accomplished by a comprehensive and detailed security plan. There are an adequate number of security personnel, and they are equipped with radio communication so that their appearance anywhere on the hospital grounds occurs within minutes of request. The concern for staff and patient protection can be consistently depended on. Their competence to handle any incident has a consistent history. Individually, each is known within the hospital and is perceived as an integral number of the hospital's staff. Collectively, they provide a secure, protective environment for the hospital.

Psychiatric Unit in a General Hospital

The psychiatric unit of a general hospital usually has no security unit of its own. It depends on the general hospital's security unit for the provision of a protected environment for its patients, staff, and visitors. An explicit effort between the psychiatric unit and the security unit must be made concerning the additional security needs of the psychiatric unit. The different types of patients, their potentially noncompliant behavior and all legal constraints involved in patient evaluation and treatment must become part of the awareness of every security officer in the hospital. Because of the greater uncertainty about psychiatric patient behavior when compared with other general hospital patients, psychiatric units and their patients are perceived as different by most general hospital security personnel. This difference often contributes to a heightened sense of insecurity of security personnel about interactions with the psychiatric unit and its patients. The insecurity is perceived by both clinical staff on the unit and the security personnel themselves, despite organized communication between both units' personnel and collaboration agreed on by administrative officials. The larger number of staff in general hospitals usually does not permit a personal relationship among unit clinical staff and security personnel. Security often is seen not as an integral part of the psychiatric units, but as an outside policing force. Additional administrative effort and staff time is required to continually work at minimizing potential discordance and increasing familiarity of security personnel with the psychiatric unit's approach to patient treatment.

Public Psychiatric Hospital

The large public psychiatric hospital has a security unit with a mission similar to the two other types of hospitals. However, the scope and capacity of the security unit will more closely approximate the private psychiatric hospital. The public hospital often is in a suburban or rural setting and must count on its own security unit for protection. Budgetary constraints allow for fewer security personnel than the comparable private psychiatric facility would employ. Thus security is far leaner and may even appear incomplete when compared to the private sector. To compensate for the less staff, it is not unusual for nursing, housekeeping, and even maintenance staff to be enlisted to supplement security personnel in the resolution of incidents. This reliance on nonsecurity personnel for security protection often contributes to the difference in the sense of tranquility and order between the private and public psychiatric hospitals. The public hospital cannot as reliably count on the appearance of security personnel within minutes after a request. While the individuals from the security unit usually are well known to clinical hospital personnel and perceived as integral members of the hospital's staff, they often do not collectively provide the same sense of security for the hospital provided by their counterparts in private psychiatric hospitals. In the words of one hospital superintendent, "We just don't have enough of them to go around ..."

Parameters Affecting a Security Unit

Location

A hospital's location can have a significant effect on the function of its security unit. As mentioned, many private and most public psychiatric hospitals are located in suburban or rural settings. The geographic distance between these hospitals and external law enforcement personnel forces a self-sufficiency on the existing security unit. For example, in Case Study 11-3 a patient eloped from a rural psychiatric hospital, and assistance was requested in returning the patient to the unit. In rural settings an arrangement must be made between the hospital's security unit and local law enforcement officers that encourages the hospital's security personnel to help locate and transport eloped patients. Without formal deputization of the hospital security personnel by the local law enforcement agency, hospital personnel can only transport a nonhomicidal, nonsuicidal patient back to the hospital if the patient voluntarily wishes to return. When the patient is an imminent danger to himself and others, this situation is somewhat clearer though local statutes must be consulted regarding hospital personnel's jurisdiction outside hospital grounds.

The general hospital with a private psychiatric unit is more often located in an urban or suburban setting. The boundaries of activity of its security personnel therefore are defined by hospital property more clearly than are the boundaries of psychiatric hospitals. The same eloped patient would infrequently be pursued off hospital grounds by the security personnel of a general hospital. Instead, hospital security would collaborate with local law enforcement officers who would be responsible for any attempt at involuntary apprehension and return of an eloped patient to hospital grounds. Occasionally, when a patient is thought to be very near the hospital, hospital security personnel will assist local law enforcement officers in the latter's efforts to locate and return the patient.

Governance

A hospital's type of governance and funding structure significantly affect the functions of the security unit. Public psychiatric hospitals are governed by federal, state, and local authorities. Private psychiatric hospitals may be privately owned for profit, or may be governed by a board of trustees under nonprofit status. Further, both types of hospitals may have university affiliation, a significant complication for the security unit. The type of governance and funding of the hospital influences the way patients are perceived by the security personnel. For example, it is generally believed that potential patients and their families may not be treated with the same tolerance by hospital staff in the public sector as they are by hospital staff in the private sector. In private hospitals security personnel may be encouraged to deal with disruptive, self-destructive patient behavior with heightened tolerance and perseverance. The security units of public hospitals are often less well staffed, with more strictly defined limitations and greater inflexibility in their behavior. Another example that highlights this difference between the public and private psychiatric hospitals concerns the visits of outside authority to the hospital and the implication of the visits on hospital security personnel behavior. In a private psychiatric hospital, security personnel know the few owners, trustees, or administrators in authority. In a public psychiatric hospital security personnel can never know all the elected executive, legislative, and judicial officials, the appointed budgetary personnel, and administrative officials who impact on the hospital's governance. A security officer in a private psychiatric hospital has clearer lines of authority and consequently is granted a heightened level of staff and administrative as well as trust, flexibility of action, compared with his public psychiatric hospital counterpart. Extremes of behavior may result, as in the situation where security personnel in a public psychiatric hospital did not allow their vehicles to be used by patients and visitors caught in an intense rainstorm because they had been recently chastized for similar kinds of behavior by visiting political officials.

When a university teaching and research affiliation is an integral part of either private or public psychiatric hospitals, significant additional constraints are placed on security personnel. For example, an incident of impending assault was reported to security from one of the psychiatric units of a university general hospital. The two security officers who arrived rapidly on the scene were greeted by a crowd of 20–30 people exiting a conference. As the security officers attempted to intervene, the well-meaning commentary and attempts at assistance from various residents, interns, and assorted medical, nursing, and social work students provoked one security officer to roll his eyes in disgust and walk away from further involvement. The pressures facing security personnel within an environment with an educational or research mission are often intense.

Special relationships sometimes exist between the psychiatric hospital or unit and an external agency or organization. One example may involve the judiciary's referral of its psychiatric evaluations to one hospital or to one unit within one hospital. Security must be aware of the arrival and departure of these patients to insure a minimum of potential incidents. Security's presence in the area at specific times of the day when agents of the court bring in new patients and pick up those ready to be returned to the court may be helpful in fostering a sense of hospital security. Another example may involve a psychiatric hospital or general hospital with a psychiatric unit near a military installation, which finds its emergency services dealing with acute psychiatric illness in youthful military personnel. Security's involvement in restraining disruptive military patients being evaluated or treated will involve their relationship with the military police. The presence of military police nearby or actually within the hospital on Friday or Saturday evenings is often worked out between the hospital and military officials, allowing for collaboration between hospital security and military policy in situations calling for security assistance.

There are places in most hospitals, especially in psychiatric ones, where the presence of security is both useful and reassuring. Major entrance and exit areas, admission suites and emergency service areas are all high patient/visitor flow areas. Security's presence lends a stabilizing influence to these areas, and helps reassure both staff and patients that hospital boundaries and their welfare are being security monitored. Security officers may have designated duties in these areas.

Administration and Staffing of Security Department

As a general rule, it becomes increasingly useful to involve security personnel to clinical decision making, as they spend increasing units of their time with patients. This involvement may be essentially nonexistent for the usual security officer of a large general hospital with a psychiatric unit. In hospitals where infrequent involuntary or court referred patients are transported by security, dialogue about the patient's difficulties, or the clinical staff's perception, is only informal, occurring en route to the patient's destination. In the latter situation, hospital protocol about the handling of these infrequent patients may hope to be reviewed each time by both clinical and security staff, to ensure for the most effective disposition of the patient.

In some private and general hospitals, but in many public hospitals, security officers are consistently involved with clinical staff in the management of large numbers (or high percentages) of involuntary or court referred patients. In these situations, it is important for security personnel to have access to team meetings, clinical staff meetings, and even diagnostic conferences to assist in appropriate patient management. The security chief and other clinical department chiefs (i.e., director of nursing) must meet regularly. For example, on one forensic psychiatric unit, security personnel routinely participate with nursing personnel in team and staff meetings. Responsibility for many unit activities is almost totally shared, and on night shifts, due to personnel and financial constraints, nursing and security personnel share virtually all duties, with a blurring and sometime troublesome overlap of boundaries between the two staff groups.

The hospital's security chief symbolizes the hospital's approach to security. Most large general hospitals with psychiatric units and private psychiatric hospitals have made efforts to employ well-credentialed, experienced security professionals. College and graduate work in both law enforcement and psychology is commonly found as part of the educational background of these professionals. Most have been hired with a background of years of similar work experience, either within other hospitals or from relatively senior positions within external law enforcement agencies. Two common denominators in their backgrounds involve their ability to understand the security needs of the hospital from the vantage point of a trained and experienced security professional and their ability to manage a security unit under their direction.

The approach to hiring a security chief and security staff varies to extremes among general hospitals with psychiatric units and private and public psychiatric hospitals. Some large general hospitals have approached their security needs from a contractual viewpoint. They have designated a number of security functions and duties to be performed, a number of stations to be monitored, and even in some situations designated the specifics of the personnel to be involved (i.e. officer status with firearms, required height, and weight, etc.). They have turned to the marketplace and to bidding procedures to purchase the security "package" that most cost-beneficially meets the hospital's needs. Success with this approach has been mixed. When it works well, it can decrease administrative overhead time with security matters while employing a consistent quality of security professional from an organization whose sole purpose and area of expertise is security. When it works poorly, it can heighten devisiveness between hospital clinical and contractual security staff, foster mistrust and inappropriate utilization of security staff time, and increase the potential for incident occurrence within the hospital. For large general hospitals in urban areas, the number of security incidents and difficulty recruiting adequate numbers of appropriate security personnel has encouraged many administrations to turn to contractual services to meet the hospital's security needs. Other general hospitals and many private psychiatric hospitals approach their security needs differently. They make an effort to hire a security chief whose credentials and background will foster quality security services. The salary and benefit package necessary to attract this type of administration may approach that of the senior hospital administrator. In fact, the hospital may perceive a recently hired security chief as having administrative potential for other hospital administration roles in the future.

The funding available to the security unit for staffing equipment and functional capabilities is also critical.

Security Response to Different Types of Patients

Voluntary and Involuntry Patients

The types of patients being evaluated and treated in the hospital will significantly affect the involvement and constraints facing its security unit. While most psychiatric patients are voluntary in the private sector, this is often not the case in the public sector, where units or the entire hospital may be designated to treat the involuntary patient. Voluntary patients comprise the vast majority of patients treated in the private sector. Security personnel in general hospitals and in private psychiatric hospitals do not seem as concerned about differentiating the types of voluntary patients being treated. They report no difficulties with adult patients whom they believe have voluntarily admitted themselves for treatment. They are far more concerned about the potential dangerousness of the few patients involuntarily admitted for evaluation or treatment; these are the patients about whom most security is most often called.

Public psychiatric hospitals usually have a greater percentage of involuntary patients. Despite the smaller staff-to-patient ratio in the public than in private hospitals, clinical staff in public psychiatric hospitals rarely request security's assistance with involuntary patients. When they do so, it is frequently to help with the return of an eloped patient or the transportation of a patient from one unit to another. When asked why security personnel are infrequently requested to assist public psychiatric clinical staff in the confinement of patients who are "out of control," clinical staff cited the lack of adequate numbers of security personnel available to help with this task. As one psychiatric aide put it, " . . . getting a homicidal patient back into our quiet room when necessary is just part of my job."

Forensic Patients

A special case involves those public psychiatric hospitals that are partially . or completely designated for forensic psychiatric patients. In these units or hospitals, patients are involuntarily committed by the courts for either evaluation or treatment. This patient population contains a higher percentage of individuals who are known to express themselves using nonverbal, physically assaultive behavior. The number of security personnel available to these units or hospitals is much higher, when compared to security personnel available to other psychiatric facilities. However, it usually does not affect the overall staff-to-patient ratio because security personnel are substituted for nursing personnel on the units. As a result, less clinical staff and more security staff are available to the patients. This dovetails with the greater security needs of these patients but unfortunately may allow less clinical staff to be available for active treatment.

Age and Diagnosis

Security personnel may need to adjust their expectations concerning requests for their services according to parameters of age and type of psychiatric illness that the specific hospital unit has been designated to treat. For example, a nursing service request to assist in the handling of an acting-out adolescent on the adolescent unit will require a very different mind set, series of expectations, and stresses when compared with a request from nursing staff on a geriatric unit for help with a disruptive elderly patient. It is unlikely that an adolescent patient, no matter how disruptive, will be incontinent to the point of urinating on the security officer. Likewise it is unlikely that an elderly patient will attempt to or actually bite a security officer in the process of being helped back to her room. A number of psychiatric hospitals have designated specific units for the treatment of different types of patients. In these hospitals, security personnel have become familiar with the heightened uncertainty of patient behavior on an admissions unit. Likewise many find the smells of a chronic men's or women's unit prohibitive or the verbal and nonverbal provocativeness of an adolescent unit continually unsettling.

While specific protocols and training for dealing with the disruptive patient are a necessity, the critical variables for handling these incidents involve the judgment of the security staff. The disruptive, acting-out, yelling, screaming, fist-swinging adolescent can be physically restrained first and placed in seclusion until the outburst spontaneously resolves or is reevaluated by the psychiatrist on call. The frightened, psychotic, paranoid adult backed into a corner must be approached carefully, reassuringly, using effort to verbally encourage the patient voluntarily into a quiet room until psychiatric intervention can resolve the problem. The trust in the competence of security personnel not to over-respond but rather to provide the necessary backup to clinical staffing needs in these situations only comes with time. The psychiatric unit within a general hospital and the larger psychiatric hospitals in the public sector are at a disadvantage here for large numbers of staff and larger staff turnover decreases the development of familiarity and trust potential among hospital staff.

Types of Incidents

Disruptive visitors, assaults, thefts, vandalism, and drug trafficking may all be grouped into two categories. The first concerns the occurrence of any of these episodes in an isolated or small, contained fashion. In this category, the incident is usually dealt with by clinical staff, allowing the patient or family involved the potential for a therapeutic experience. For example, the theft of a toy (doll) from a patient's roommate, by the patient's younger sister during a hospital visit, allowed the family an opportunity to focus on the hospitalization's effects on the sister, during subsequent family therapy sessions.

The second category concerns the occurrence of any of the above episodes in a repeated, widespread or significantly disruptive fashion. Despite the clinical significance of the behavior, its scope will force security and the hospital to approach the incident as a violation of its authority. Discharge or removal from hospital grounds, request for external law enforcement assistance, and legal civil or criminal charges may all individually or sequentially be indicated actions. Again, the judgement of security personnel involved, and the trusting, collaborative history between clinical and security staff, often make the difference between a minor incident and one of major consequences. For example, a series of thefts of small items in one area of a large, rural public psychiatric hospital, and solicitations for soft drug purchases became known to security personnel. With enough information, including two eyewitnesses involving one drug sale attempt, two security officers suspected that one recently hired young male psychiatric aide was responsible. They believed the employee should be confronted, fired, and have legal charges brought against him. The security chief's long hospital work history and trust by hospital clinical personnel provided additional information. The young employee was the son of a prominent and respected licensed practical nurse, with years of service at the hospital. Further, it had been their family tradition to work at the hospital and the young employee was the fourth generation from this family to do so. The security chief sat down informally with the employee, who was of low-average intelligence, and surmised from the discussion that he was trying to make himself known to the hospital, probably to gain more attention from his father. A father-son meeting resulted in the return of the items, a cessation of drug sale attempts, and a shift of the employee's duties, while again on probation, to another part of the hospital. This incident had a fortunate ending for all concerned, and without the intervention of security the results might have been drastically different.

Visual Identification of Security Personnel

The effectiveness of uniformed security personnel in general and psychiatric hospitals is worthy of consideration. Uniforms help rapidly identify the employee as part of the security unit. The visibility of security is a crucial ingredient to the accomplishment of its mission, functions, and duties, and the appearance of a uniform may help maintain appropriate hospital decorum. However, many clinical staff working in psychiatric facilities believe uniforms are detrimental to their clinical, therapeutic work. The staff in many public and private psychiatric hospitals, as well as in psychiatric units in general hospitals, oftern do not wear traditional white uniforms so prevalently worn in nonpsychiatric hospitals or units. They question the uniforms for security staff at their hospital and often encourage its abandonment. The question of whether clinical staff should or should not wear uniforms continues to be debated among clinicians. Do keys at one's side or in one's hand, or a tie or jacket represent a uniform? The issue as related to security staff should depend on whether the uniform assists security personnel in the performance of their mission, functions, and duties; it often does. Uniforms can be tasteful and nonmilitaristic, conforming to the needs and decorum of the hospital. For example, the small private psychiatric hospital may choose a blazer and slacks outfit for security uniforms. In contrast, the large, urban general hospital may choose uniforms similar to those of the local law enforcement agency. This latter choice may help maintain the hospital's decorum and the functioning of its security unit by association with the protective role of the external policing agency.

The designation of security personnel as officers, with the wearing of firearms, has both support and opposition. In general, the private psychiatric hospitals, especially when they are located in rural settings, do not employ security officers with firearms. In contrast, there are some public psychiatric hospitals that utilize security officers with firearms, and other public psychiatric hospitals that do not. The importance of removing and securing their weapons, under lock and key, when entering specified patient areas in the hospital or when assisting in the acute management and transportation of some psychiatric patients cannot be overemphasized.

William Snyder, III

12

Administrative Monitoring of Assaultive Patients and Staff

This chapter describes the activities of a committee concerned with incidents of violence and assaultiveness within a large mental hospital. The committee was concerned with a broad range of violence, from the common-place—the daily slaps, scratches, and bites suffered by staff in the process of restraining a combative, acutely disturbed patient—to the relatively infrequent, illegal, and reprehensible form of violence known as patient abuse.

The author would like to express special recognition and appreciation of the current Patient-Staff Abuse Committee members for their assistance and support: Robert Lippy, L.P.N., Nursing Services Supervisor; Ellis McClelland, M.D., Staff Psychiatrist; Catherine Poff, L.P.N., Nursing Staff Supervisor; Robert Walker, M.A., Staff Psychologist; and Shirley Zarfos, R.N., Associate Director of Nursing In-Service Education.

ORIGIN OF THE PATIENT ABUSE COMMITTEE

In 1979 the Springfield Hospital Center, Maryland's largest mental hygiene facility (inpatient census approximately 1300), sought to improve its policies and procedures regarding patient abuse. The hospital's response to allegations of patient abuse had evolved in a piece-meal fashion over a number of years and needed to be consolidated into a cohesive policy. The Patient Abuse Committee (PAC) was formed in an attempt to standardize the hospital's definitions, teaching guidelines, and administrative procedures regarding allegations of patient abuse.

This author was one of the members of the original committee, which consisted of a psychologist, a psychiatrist, and four representatives from the nursing department. Through hospital experience, each member was acquainted with the complexities presented by allegations of patient abuse. One member, for example, taught student nurses who had many questions regarding the propriety of some of the behavior they observed while on their field placement on various hospital wards. Another member supervised nursing staff in a busy admission area known for its active, aggressive milieu, while a third screened new employees and had experience with the administrative response to allegations of abuse.

As the committee was being formed, we learned that the Maryland legislature was debating proposed legislation that would make patient abuse in mental health and retardation facilities a felony. The eventual passage of this law (see Appendix 12-1) in July 1979 provided some much needed follow-up to the hospital's response to patient abuse allegations.

Defining Abuse

Physical Abuse

The meaning of the word "abuse" may appear obvious and self-evident, but as the committee discussed past allegations and incidents, we realized that the concept is seldom simple and straightforward. We wought to make the definitions of abuse useful in two ways. First, we wanted practical definitions that could be translated into "do's" and "don't's" for teaching purposes. Second, we wanted the definitions to be as clear and unambiguous as possible. The clearer the rule, we reasoned, the easier to interpret and enforce it, keeping in mind that the hospital must protect staff from erroneous accusations as well as prevent and correct instances of abuse.

Physical patient abuse was defined as follows: a patient is physically abused by staff when he or she is the object of assault, sexual abuse, or corporal punishment, and/or when so harmed by another person at the instigation of an employee. The next and more difficult step was to broaden that statement to include an appreciation of the interpersonal and situational contexts unique to the mental hospital milieu which further obfuscate the boundaries in this area of patient–staff interaction.

For example, very violent and combative wrestling and restraining may be unavoidable in the process of physically controlling an agitated patient. On some of our wards, primarily admission wards, physical restraint is almost a daily occurrence, and it is viewed by the staff as a necessary treatment procedure for a patient during a disruptive and unstabilized point in his or her hospitalization. Patients, however, do not always view being restrained in like manner; in fact, restraint may seem to them to be an instance of abuse and mistreatment. One need not be delusional to feel that way—the average person would probably agree that restraint is abusive. The public seems to have little realization of the extent of aggressive interaction within some mental hospital wards and of the consequent need for or frequency of physical restraint. Thus, in developing an understanding of physical abuse in a mental hospital, it is essential to distinguish treatment procedures involving physical restraint or seclusion from punishment, retaliation, and excessive physical control.

The committee described the limits of acceptable action committed by staff in self-defense; physical response by staff would not be considered abusive if the act met the patient's offensive or aggressive force with a counter-defensive force intended to control the patient and protect people from harm. The desired tone of the staff's behavior during the physical restraint of a patient should be defensive rather than aggressive, controlling rather than punitive, and with no more forcefulness than the situation requires. Overreaction in the name of self-defense or the use of improper defenses or holds to subdue a patient are considered to be forms of physical patient abuse. In summary, the staff in hospital areas in which frequent aggressive or restraint procedures occur need the most protection from wrongful accusations of abuse and the greatest sensitivity to the physical contact aspect of their work. Not only are they more likely than staff working in less aggressive wards to be mistakenly accused of patient abuse, but they are exposed to more frequent violent encounters in which their own skill and self control is severely tested.

Psychological Abuse

Psychological abuse was defined as mistreatment or harm that can occur in the course of interpersonal relationships or in response to detrimental socioenvironmental surroundings. Psychological abuse may occur through acts of commission or omission, thus, to clarify the nebulous quality of psychological abuse one must appreciate as much of the total situation as possible. The effects of psychological abuse are rarely as visible as the bodily harm of physical abuse; nevertheless, it may be equally painful and have a lasting damaging impact. (For the sake of this discussion physical and psychological abuses are artificially separated, but in reality physical abuses leave psychological as well as bodily scars.) Psychological abuse may take the form of humiliation through the loss of human dignity, a psychological assault damaging to one's self concept and sense of worth, or the creation of a sense of despair and hopelessness regarding one's plight and well being. The complex subtleties of a term as broad as psychological abuse are impossible to enumerate; therefore, the committee tried to define major subtypes.

Exploitation. A patient is exploited when he or she is used by a staff person for reasons of selfish gain. Exploitation occurs when food, gifts, or personal belongings of a patient are unnecessarily restricted, stolen, or given away. It is also exploitation to employ a patient without fair pay for his or her services or to bribe a patient to engage in activities that are unrelated to his or her treatment.

Verbal abuse. Verbal abuse is probably the most common form of psychological abuse that is alleged in a mental hospital. A patient is verbally abused by staff when he or she is subjected to harsh, profane, derogating, or harassing remarks that are void of any redeeming therapeutic value. Verbal abuse as one might suspect, is fraught with individual subjectivity and interpretation, particularly since it is possible to be verbally abusive without using conventionally vulgar or insulting words. A person's tone of voice, inference, and manner can be psychologically abusive even though the choice of his words is not. As a further precaution staff are advised to exercise discretion in the use of pet names or nicknames since some may be objectionable or have offensive connotations to a patient. One benefit of stressful verbal abuse was to sensitize staff to the potential psychological help or harm they could bring to their social interaction with patients, since it is not true in our setting that only "sticks and stones can hurt you."

Demeaning treatment. Demeaning treatment was defined as acts of commission or omission which disregard a patient's rights, exert a dehumanizing influence, or diminish his or her dignity through coercion, ridicule, or insensitivity. The basic safeguards protecting a patient from demeaning treatment were found in our hospital's declaration of patient's rights and responsibilities. To summarize our hospital's philosophy: any violation or deprivation of a patient's rights could be considered to be demeaning treatment; however, clearly documented limitations and controls placed on those rights could be authorized by the patient's treatment team. For example, it may be necessary to deny a patient the use of writing utensils, one of the designated "rights," when it is clinically determined that pens or pencils would pose an imminent danger to that patient or others in his or her environment.

Demeaning treatment can occur when a patient is the object of ridicule or teasing. Examples of this type of abuse would be the creation of situations where patients are made to appear foolish at the request or persuasion of a staff person, e.g., asked to run nonsensical errands, dress inappropriately, or behave improperly.

Misuse of treatments. The misapplication of bonafide treatments and services in ways that would undermine or defeat their therapeutic purpose were defined as misuse of treatment. Examples of treatment misuse can be reflected in the purely arbitrary denial of treatment requests made by a patient, or through failure to honor a treatment contract. Another area sensitive to misuse involves the stablishment of rules, limit setting, and use of disciplinary measures within behavioral contracts. These are important ingredients that make the group living situation a therapeutic experience in many hospital wards. However, these procedures may, at times, appear to be punitive and in violation of a patient's rights. Staff therefore need to be sensitive to the ways in which these elements of a therapeutic milieu can be misused abusively.

It is not considered an abuse to employ rule making, limit setting, and discipline if the methods and purposes are consistent with acceptable treatment procedures and are a part of the treatment team's efforts to assist the patient toward healthier functioning. Treatment teams usually develop rules and guidelines for their patients and need to correct misbehavior, although care must be taken not to use grossly unfair restrictions nor overly coercive treatment contracts. A corrective step regarding this type of abuse is to sensitize the staff to the overall context that they share with their patients.

Insensitivity to psychological abuse of patients through misuse of treatment usually has two sources: staff's failure to appreciate (1) that inpatients may be likened to a "captive audience" who are dependent on the staff for meeting their basic needs, and (2) that some therapeutic techniques are very powerful tools that can be misused or harmful if applied in a clumsy, unthinking, or heavy handed way. The difference between an abusive misuse of a treatment and a well-intentioned but improper application of a treatment is a crucial distinction regarding allegations of this type.

Social and environmental inadequacies. The committee was concerned with the hospital milieu and its effect on the psychological well-being of patients and staff alike. A patient is psychologically abused when his or her hospital environment is substandard or antitherapeutic, since humane surroundings constitute a minimum requirement for effective care and treatment. A hospital environment that is overcrowded, understaffed, inadequately furnished, or lacking in privacy is psychologically abusive. Such environmental inadequacies contribute to patient abuse both directly, in the form of a dehumanizing psychological impact on the patient, and indirectly by lowering morale and providing insufficient resources to accomplish this task. The committee felt that understaffing or other chronic environmental inadequacies can create a breeding ground for many types of patient abuse.

Dissemination of Definitions

After the state's Resident Abuse Law was enacted, a summary of the law along with the recommended hospital procedures was attached to each staff member's pay check (see Appendix 12-2). In reaction there were numerous inquiries concerning the suggested chain of responsibility and communication since an allegation of patient abuse can be initiated at any point in the hospital or police hierarchy. Sometimes the superintendent's office, the state police, or even the central office of the Department of Mental Hygiene are the first to be informed of an allegation of abuse, through a patient's relative for instance. At other times, a health aide or part-time student may be the first to learn of an allegation. Thus, the communications of the initial allegations seldom conform to a particular structure or policy, and the less rigid the expectations regarding a specific sequence of communications, the better.

Data on Abuse

The committee has compiled follow-up information about allegations of patient abuse for two years, 1980 and 1981. In that time 44 allegations (25 in 1980 and 19 in 1981) have been formally documented; 31 cases, or about 70 percent, have alleged physical abuse, and 13 cases, 30 percent, have alleged psychological abuse. Most of the allegations of physical patient abuse were unsubstantiated after investigation. However, a total of 7 out of the 31 (approximately 23 percent) of the physical patient abuse allegations resulted in further legal and/or administrative action. In contrast, almost half (6 out of 13) of the psychological abuse allegations were substantiated. Unfortunately we have no comparable data regarding allegations of patient abuse before Maryland's resident abuse law. We also have no way of tabulating the many "false alarm" or informal and undocumented allegations that are reported to the hospital. For instance, the hospital superintendent may receive a phone call from someone who alleges he saw a patient physically abused, but when questioned the informant refuses to give his name, or any constructive data to follow up. It is estimated by the superintendent's office that twice as many informal allegations, those that are without sufficient data to begin an inquiry, occur as formal or documented allegations.

POLICY ISSUES IN PROBLEM AREAS

The procedures we advised were intended to highlight the most relevant features of the law, such as the need for promptness, the inclusion of a formal law enforcement agency, and the hospital's need to notify and involve certain supervisory and administrative staff. The following example illustrates the unpredictable and unexpected course of events which some allegations can take:

A 40-year-old black female, diagnosed bipolar disorder, mixed, unspecified with psychotic features resided in a locked admission area. During the early weeks of her hospitalization she made numerous allegations about being assaulted by other patients. Some of her allegations had some credence while others were the products of her psychosis. At one point she was allowed to be escorted by three staff to the State's Attorney's office in a nearby town for the purpose of placing formal charges against certain patients. However, instead of filing charges against the patients as initially planned, when she met the State's Attorney she alleged an assault by one of three employees who had just escorted her to his office. The employee was falsely charged with assault before anyone at the hospital had any knowledge of the incident.

Weeks of corrective communications and investigation were finally successful in exonerating the accused staff without the stress and expense of a trial. Nevertheless the case illustrates the extent to which an allegation can defy the best laid plans of hospital policy and procedure.

As seen in the example cited above, false reports that are the product of a psychotic thought disorder are among the most problematic aspects concerning allegations of abuse in a mental hospital. When such allegations occur the erroneously accused employee may understandably be in a very awkward and vulnerable position. To make matters worse, nonhospital persons can also be involved, as sometimes happens when a relative or the police are the first to be informed of a bizarre and erroneous allegation. It is also true, on the other hand, that a psychotic person may be quite capable of making an accurate report of patient abuse. Thus, the presence of a severe thought disorder by an alleged victim or witness does not automatically discount any allegation. Each allegation, regardless of its content, we felt, should be reported to the hospital superintendent accompanied by all the preliminary information that can be collected by the supervisory staff in charge of the accused employee and patient. The superintendent then is required to notify the appropriate law enforcement agency. Such a course of action has helped to lessen the unnecessary involvement of the police in response to an allegation that is totally frivolous and/or the product of a psychotic thought disorder. The hospital administration does not want to prejudge an allegation before the involvement of the police, but it perceives a responsibility to screen out those allegations that are totally without merit. For example a male patient claimed an employee used a laser beam and killed the unborn fetus he was carrying; a female patient alleged that an employee (not on duty) struck her while she was asleep; and a female patient alleged that she was raped by male staff when in reality she was locked in seclusion and supervised by all-female staff.

Between the extremes of bizarre allegations and those that are uncontaminated by any thought disorder, are the majority of reported allegations.

Many allegations are initially vague and lack the type of evidence needed in order to file criminal charges; they are, nevertheless, reported to the police and then followed up within the hospital by the employee's supervisors and the personnel department who undertake administrative actions, if necessary. To repeat, since the hospital can not prejudge a patient abuse allegation, it notifies the law enforcement agency of all allegations (except those that are clearly frivolous or the product of a thought disorder). The result is the reporting of some allegations for which data is scant. Consequently, there are instances when the police investigation of a vague and ultimately erroneous allegation proves to be a disturbing experience for the accused employee. In response to such situations, the hospital now undertakes the responsibility for achieving closure and notifying the employee when he or she is exonerated of culpability.

A second issue our committee confronted concerned the proper law enforcement agency to be notified in response to patient abuse allegations. The Patient Abuse Law specified that "the appropriate law enforcement agency" should be notified of allegations of abuse. Large hospitals such as Springfield have their own special police department. Some committee members felt that our hospital police would be the logical choice while others opted for the State Police. There were several reasons why we finally recommended the Maryland State Police as the appropriate law enforcement law agency to be called. First, it was felt that the involvement of the State Police would increase the deterrent effect of the patient abuse law. Second, the use of an outside, neutral investigative agency would reduce the likelihood of one possible criticism: that an in-house investigation may not have been fully impartial and objective. Third, the utilization of the Maryland State Police would permit an investigation to be conducted on or off hospital grounds, since our hospital police are not empowered to conduct an investigation beyond the hospital's property. Finally, a most difficult problem involved potential cases where security personnel within the hospital itself might be accused of patient abuse. Considering the above rationale, we recommended that the State Police be the law enforcement agency routinely notified of allegations of physical patient abuse, reserving the assistance of our own police department for those allegations where the immediate attention of the law enforcement agency was required.

The last major area of discussion regarded the committee's potential role as an investigative resource to the hospital, in effect, responding to each allegation of abuse and assessing information and evidence. While it was tempting to consider the prospects of providing a direct and immediate investigative response to an allegation of abuse, there were some drawbacks, including the likelihood of interfering with the formal investigation by the police as the most obvious. Furthermore, limitations concerning deterence, perceived objectivity, and breadth of investigative powers that were cited in regard to the hospital police department could also be applied to the abuse committee. Finally, since all information regarding an allegation of abuse proceeds to the accused employee's department head and subsequently to the personnel department where further administrative action may or may not be warranted, the inclusion of another investigative step did not appear necessary.

The committee's discussion of patient abuse was frequently coupled with the topic of staff abuse (more accurately called assaults on staff) since allegations of both seem to cluster in those hospital areas in which the more disturbed patients reside. Some admission wards, for example, were known for their active and aggressive patient–staff interaction. In addition, some members of the committee had taken part in an earlier study of the incidence of assaults on staff at Springfield hospital (Lion, et al, 1981) and as a result were aware of the correlated risk of patient abuse allegations and assaults on staff. Thus, the committee recommended that its task and focus be broadened to include attention to the issues concerning violence directed toward staff as well as patient abuse. By incorporating a focus that included both types of violence, we gained in knowledge and sensitivity. The direct care staff was already well aware of the extent of violence in their work and a study that focused only on patient abuse and ignored assaults on staff would not have accurately reflected their working environment. Finally, promotion of concern for the safety of patients without like concern for staff suggests a lack of appreciation of the problems and stresses common to both. Thus, approximately six months after the committee's inception, it was renamed the Patient–Staff Abuse Committee (PSAC).

Assaults on Staff

It is significant that there had been no previous efforts to officially report or discuss assaults on staff. This is probably due in part to bureaucracy; there have been genuine efforts at catching individuals who abuse staff or exploit the hospital, but the emphasis has not been sustained positively oriented toward the staff. Related to this, perhaps, is the issue of accountability; if one addresses that problem, then one has the responsibility to do something about it. Another consideration comes from an actuarial point of view; although the assaults on staff that create the greatest concern are those involving severe physical injury, these assaults are of statistically low frequency so that momentum is not generated between incidents to mount the sustained effort that might produce more lasting corrective changes. There is a tendency to view those seemingly isolated assaults (excluding the hundreds of less severe assaults that also occur) as extraordinary and unique, hardly the sort of problem from which benefit and change might be derived. Finally, there is the prejudicial attitude of the "deserving victim" that connotes blame for an assault; It is assumed that the assault was to some degree self-induced by the victim. Such a point of view severely inhibits open discussion or investigation and all but excuses others from accountability.

In one of our more severe assaults, a nonpsychotic, court committed, male adolescent attacked a female member of the nursing staff without warning and caused multiple facial fractures. Every effort ensued to transfer the patient to a maximum security institution, and once that was accomplished the matter was laid to rest. While that response may have had considerable merit, there may also have been additional constructive outcomes from that incident, and others like it, that were unexplored. In follow-up to an attack it is sometimes necessary to review the incident for the purpose of exploring constructive changes that possibly would prevent further violence by other patients. Such an intervention should be conducted with sensitivity to the staff involved, and the focus should not be on blaming particular staff members for the incident. A hypervigilant, overreactive attitude will alienate staff. Utilizing trained staff who are already assigned to various subsections of the hospital may be a more effective method of providing follow-up to assaults than to send one member of a central committee into each area of operation.

PREVENTION OF ASSAULTS

Review of Data on Assaults

At the inception of our committee, members met biweekly to discuss patient abuse. As the discussion phase was completed and policies became augmented, the committee's functions changed, and the committee met less frequently with a more varied agenda. At the beginning of each year we review the results of the incidence of patient abuse and assaults on staff from the previous year and submit a summary of findings to the hospital administration. In follow-up to that data, which is admittedly in its infancy, we pursue some particular facet for more detailed study. Some of our supplementary tasks have dealt with the patterns of assaults on staff within various sections of the hospital, a demographic study of patients who commit assaults on staff, and the interaction of staffing patterns and assaults.

Our best source for the annual sampling of data concerning assaults on staff is the 24-hour daily ward report, which is a log of the activities and noteworthy occurrences on each ward. As a data source it is admittedly vulnerable to many types of error, e.g., omissions, understatement, and overstatement; we therefore use strict guidelines in qualifying an incident as an assault on staff. The ward report must at least indicate that a physical act of aggression occurred between a patient and a staff person, i.e., "patient hit and kicked nurses" or "patient was combative to staff".

In our first two years of data collection, we have obtained almost identical estimates of assaults on staff: 1276 for 1980 and 1284 for 1981. Many factors impinge upon the issue of assaults on staff, and as these are explored the information becomes available to the training workshops. In some cases the data is sufficiently compelling to influence clinical and administrative programs within the hospital. Data concerning injuries that staff receive from assaults by patients is another form of information that helps complete the picture of the extent of staff risk.

Data are also maintained for patient abuse allegations, mentioned earlier, and instances in which staff members place criminal charges against patients following an assault by the patient. With regard to patient abuse allegations, the desire to collect information was partly to learn about the legal process brought about by the new Patient Abuse Law as well as to develop a data base regarding this sensitive and relatively uncharted domain.

For similar reasons data has been compiled concerning the process and outcome of cases in which hospital staff seek legal retribution from a patient following an assault by that patient. This is a relatively new phenomenon for hospital staff and its acceptance and value is still in doubt. Too few cases have occurred to warrant an educated guess as to the future of this type of legal recourse; its early appeal, however, suggests that it may have been employed as a counterreaction to the newly enacted Patient Abuse Law with the sense that "staff's rights" needed to be balanced with "patients' rights." Since we have not experienced a deluge of patient abuse allegations, the frequency of efforts to formally charge patients with assault has declined.

Staff Safety Programs

Members of our committee train staff in safety, and conduct workshops, which are open to all staff, concerning the prevention, management, and control of violent behavior. The workshops are given on a monthly rotating basis in various sections of the hospital, although the admission areas receive the most concentrated attention, for obvious reasons. Taught by male and female nursing supervisors, participants are given practical do's and don'ts with an emphasis on preventing physical confrontation, if at all possible. About half of each three-hour session is devoted to practicing holds and demonstrating approved restraint procedures. All new nursing staff undertake this training, and experienced staff from all disciplines are also encouraged to attend for periodic review and practice.

As an outgrowth of these training sessions, staff members from various departments have been prepared to train other staff in violence-management techniques. These trainers, who may be psychologists or social workers as well as nurses, serve, in addition to their regular duties, as on-site instructors or coaches to their co-workers, conduct mini-workshops for teams of employees, or serve as resource persons in behalf of patients and staff. These types of educational programs are vital to promote an awareness of safety, the therapeutic management of violent behavior, and instructions regarding patient abuse issues.

Developing Institutional Policies to Prevent Assault

At this time the committee is viewed primarily as an advisory and consultative group with a research and evaluation orientation, and it has no specific authority in administrative decisions. The absence of a more influential administrative role stems from several sources: (1) the hospital is divided into semiautonomous units that operate with a minimum of centralized authority, (2) members of the committee are not unit directors or department heads, and have no identifiable status in the organizational hierarchy, and (3) "staff safety" as a determinant of hospital policy remains a variable with a generally low order of priority among all the pressing concerns of a large mental health facility.

The patient–staff abuse committee advises the hospital and undertakes special problems. The forerunner of this committee, the research group that originally assessed the extent of underreporting of assaults on staff, provides the clearest example of the extent to which advisement can contribute to hospital programs for patients. One unanticipated finding from that particular study was that an inordinate proportion of assaults on staff were committed by a group of patients who were persistent offenders. Furthermore, these chronically aggressive patients resided in several unitized admission areas. These patients needed the security afforded by the locked ward living area but did not benefit from the rapid turnover of incoming new admissions nor could they receive as much of the attention and specific treatment they needed while in such a busy and demanding setting. The data was sufficiently compelling to suggest the formation of a separate residential area, the Center for Behavior Management, for those intractably aggressive patients. There they could receive the concentrated attention and therapeutic efforts necessary to modify their dangerous behavior. The Center for Behavior Management originated as a highly staffed behavior modification program with specialized treatment and continues to accept new referrals of aggressive and violent patients from the various admission areas of the hospital.

Another example of the committee's involvement occurred in response to two reports in which nurses working in fairly remote cottages called for assistance via the hospital telephone system but were unable to get the needed connection in prompt fashion. One can imagine the helpless feeling generated by an unresponsive telephone at such a critical time. The committee attempted to act as an advocate in that situation, and the hospital was able to devise a more reliable and responsive telephone emergency system.

Conclusion

For those who might develop a patient–staff abuse committee, a few closing comments, precautions, and suggestions are offered.

First, and perhaps most obvious, is the valued contribution of in-service education. The ambiguities of patient abuse and patient–staff violence are difficult to communicate, particularly by memo or administrative lines of authority. Classes and workshops for direct care staff as well as any other employee who might need to know the procedures for safely restraining patients and minimizing the risk to others are a priority. Participation by ancillary ward staff (e.g., housekeepers or ward clerks) and professional staff (e.g., physicians, social workers, occupational therapists, psychologists, and so on) is just as important as participation by direct care and nursing staff since the safety of patients and staff involves the entire treatment team.

Second, while the collection of patient abuse and hospital violence data can be a helpful learning tool, it also has potentially complicating elements. The initial exploration and research of patient–staff violence can create the impression (or suspicion) among staff, whose encounters with violence are being studied, that they are doing something wrong or are mistreating patients. Violence in a hospital setting can be an emotionally sensitive area for staff, and can be an area difficult to open for inspection. Such research consequently has the potential to arouse displeasure and defensiveness. Investigators collecting such data should be aware of the feelings of the staff being studied, who may sometimes feel "damned if you do and damned if you don't." Basic safeguards, such as confidentiality and anonymity, may lessen staff uncertainty about the future use of the information collected as well as help to minimize intrahospital rivalry and competition.

The membership of our patient–staff abuse committee has been varied, tailored somewhat to the talents of the staff as well as the type of problems we were addressing. Our initial tasks, definition, policy recommendations, and follow-up were undertaken by a diverse group from several disciplines, such as nursing education, psychiatry, psychology, and nursing supervision. It is important to engage a diverse membership since there may be a mistaken tendency toward the narrow view that assaults on staff and patient abuse are "nursing's problem." All members of the hospital staff who have a working relationship with patients share in the responsibility to provide a safe and therapeutic environment including physicians who prescribe medication and order restraints and direct care aides who implement the physician's orders. Special contributions from the personnel department, security staff, and hospital administration are added to the committee when needed since violence in a hospital touches numerous facets of a patient's and an employee's life. One type of contribution that we have lacked is a member who could address the numerous legal issues that interface with abuse and violence.

The patient–staff abuse committee has been in existence about two years, not long enough to accumulate sufficient feedback to demonstrate the kind of impact it can make in a large mental hospital setting. Although we would like to be able to demonstrate reduction in the frequency of patient abuse and assaults or injury to staff, in all probability that kind of data may not be available for a considerable time. Despite the absence of supportive hard data there can be contributions that justify the time and efforts of this type of committee, not the least of which is the moral support it offers to the many employees who share a strong concern for the safe and humane treatment of mental patients.

REFERENCE

Lion JR, Snyder W, Merrill GL: Underreporting of Assaults on Staff in a State Hospital, Hospital and Community Psychiatry, 32:497–498, 1981

APPENDIX 12-1

Maryland State Resident Abuse Law

FOR the purpose of providing for a method of reporting suspected incidents of abuse of the residents of mental health facilities, mental retardation facilities, and certain other residential facilities; providing for a written report by the law enforcement agency to be prepared within a certain period of time and to be sent to certain officials; and providing immunity from civil liability for certain persons making a good faith report.

BY adding to

>Article 59—Mental Hygiene
>Section 52A, to be under the new subtitle "Resident Abuse"
>Annotated Code of Maryland

SECTION 1. Be it enacted by the General Assembly of Maryland, That section (s) of the Annotated Code of Maryland be repealed, amended, or enacted to read as follows:

>Article 59—Mental Hygiene

>RESIDENT ABUSE

52A.

(A)   As used in this subtitle, the following words have the meanings indicated:

(1)   "Abuse" means any physical injury or sexual abuse sustained by a patient of a mental health facility as a result of cruel or inhumane treatment. It does not include the performance of accepted medical procedures ordered by a licensed physician.

(2)   "Sexual Abuse" means sexual acts, sexual contacts, and vaginal intercourse as those terms are defined in Article 27, Section 461 of the code.

(3)   "Mental Health Facility" means any clinic, hospital or other institution, public or private, other than a veterans' administration hospital, which provides treatment, residential care, or other services for mentally disordered or mentally retarded persons. This definition includes group homes, halfway houses and other community residences for the mentally ill or mentally retarded.

(B)   Any person who has reason to believe a person in a mental health facility has been abused shall report the abuse to the appropriate law enforcement agency, or to the superintendent of the facility who shall promptly forward it to the appropriate law enforcement agency. The report may be oral or in writing and shall contain as much information as the reporter is able to provide.

(C)

(1) The law enforcement agency shall make a thorough investigation of the reported abuse and shall attempt to insure the protection of the victim.

(2) The investigation shall include a determination of the nature, extent, and cause of the abuse, if any, the identity of the person who may have caused the abuse, and all other facts or matters found to be pertinent.

(3) The law enforcement agency shall render a written report of its findings to the states attorney and the superintendent of the facility as soon as possible, but not later than 10 working days after the completion of the investigation.

(D) Any person except an abuser, who makes a report pursuant to this subtitle in good faith, or participates in an investigation or in a judicial proceeding arising from a report is immune from any civil liability for this action.

Section 2. AND BE IT FURTHER ENACTED, That this ACT shall take effect July 1, 1979.

APPENDIX 12-2

Information Distributed to Hospital Staff Concerning
Resident Abuse Law

RESIDENT ABUSE

Article 59, Section 52 A

A new law (S.B. 186) concerning patient abuse went into effect on July 1, 1979. The purpose of this law is to provide a method of reporting suspected incidents of patient abuse in mental health facilities and to provide for investigation by a law enforcement agency.

The law states: "abuse" means any physical injury or sexual abuse sustained by a patient as a result of cruel or inhumane treatment. It does not include the performance of accepted medical procedures ordered by a licensed physician.

Anyone who has reason to believe a person in a mental health facility has been abused shall report the abuse to the appropriate law enforcement agency (State Police), or to the superintendent of the facility who shall promptly forward it to the State Police. The report may be oral or in writing and shall contain as much information as possible.

The State police shall make a thorough investigation of the reported abuse and attempt to insure the protection of the victim.

Any person, except an abuser, who makes a patient abuse report in good faith or participates in an investigation of patient abuse arising from a report is immune from any civil liability for this action.

Recommended Procedure

In compliance with this patient abuse law, hospital staff should report patient abuse promptly to the patient's unit director *and* the abuser's supervisor. It is the duty of the unit director and/or supervisor to present the reported information to the hospital superintendent and the director of personnel as soon as possible. The superintendent shall contact the State Police.

It is expected that all employees will cooperate with the State Police during any subsequent investigation.

Paul S. Appelbaum

13

Legal Considerations
in the Prevention and Treatment of Assault

Assaults in mental hospitals pose a classic dilemma for the law: to resolve a confrontation between conflicting and seemingly irreconcilable rights. Patients have the right to be treated appropriately and with the least possible loss of liberty, yet both patients and staff members have the right to be protected in their persons. This chapter will examine the legal principles that govern the reconciliation of these competing interests and—since in practice this reconciliation is usually the responsibility of clinicians and not judges—will attempt to construct a clinically oriented framework in which such decisions can be made.

THE LEGAL SETTING

Legal involvement in mental health care is not a new phenomenon. The law has been intimately concerned with the regulation of psychiatric practice since the second quarter of the nineteenth century with the development of state hospital systems led to the construction of a regulatory framework that still exists today.[4]

A clear qualitative change has occurred in the nature of legal regulation of mental health care. Until approximately the late 1960s, legislatures and courts were primarily concerned with standards and procedures for confinement and release of patients. Laws intruded into the everyday practice of hospital-based psychiatry generally in order to ensure that patients were not illegally detained. For example, in the middle of the nineteenth century, a number of states altered their involuntary commitment statutes to guarantee patients the right to communicate freely with their attorneys, even if mail directed elsewhere continued to be censored.[37]

During roughly the last 15 years, however, the law has widened the scope of its attentions. Impelled by general societal concerns with the civil rights of the less fortunate and stimulated by the abysmal conditions in many state hospitals, the activist mental health bar has helped to expand substantially the acknowledged rights of the mentally ill. Litigation over a right to treatment has resulted in courts laying down detailed guidelines for staffing, physical plant, management, and methods of treatment in entire state systems.[56] Patients have been granted a right to refuse unwanted medications[42,45] and to be treated in the least restrictive way.[56]

Perhaps of even greater importance than the court decisions—many of which are limited in their impact to relatively narrow jurisdictions and few of which have been affirmed by the U.S. Supreme Court—have been the proliferating state statutes and regulations concerning patients' rights. Often called "Patients' Bills of Rights," these acts and regulations grant rights including rights to refuse treatment, to participate in planning treatment, and to the preservation of confidentiality.[38] Such bills of rights often go far beyond rights granted in court decisions. They are an indication that much of society now accepts the principle that psychiatric treatment requires close regulation to prevent abuses of patients' rights.

The more rights granted to psychiatric patients, however, the greater the chance of conflict between these rights. Nowhere is that conflict more apparent than in the issue of assault. A number of federal courts, including the U.S. Supreme Court, have found that patients, whether voluntary or involuntary, have a constitutional right to be protected from harm.[35,46,51] This right is, in part, a *quid pro quo* granted the patient in exchange for the deprivation of his liberty. In addition, all patients may have a common-law right to be protected from assault, especially that caused by the negligence of the professional staff.[1] On the other hand, since steps taken to prevent violence, such as secluding or restraining patients, often result in an infringement on patients' liberty, clinicians may be forced to walk a fine line between treading on the rights of the potentially assaultive and ignoring the rights of potential victims.

Epitomizing the particularly acute nature of this dilemma is the legal maxim, "No right without a remedy." The law concretizes rights by exacting penalties for their violation, confronting clinicians with the prospect of liability for invading or neglecting either set of rights.

GENERAL RIGHTS AND LIABILITIES

The Patient as Victim

The patient's right to be free of negligent treatment is vindicated in an action for *malpractice*, the most common category of potential liability for clinicians.[19] Malpractice is a civil action classified as a negligent tort and ordinarily requires that four elements be proven: 1) that the professional had a duty to care for the patient; 2) that he was negligent in the performance of that duty; 3) that the patient suffered some harm; and 4) that the harm was directly (or "proximately," in legal terminology) caused by the negligent act or omission. Ordinarily, in the case of prevention of assault in mental hospitals, a duty of care has already been established and some obvious harm to the patient has motivated the suit. Causation, in some cases, may be in dispute, but most allegations of malpractice in this area must stand or fall on the question of whether the clinician's behavior was negligent.

In malpractice cases negligence is usually described as a deviation from the ordinary behavior of one's professional peers. Using doses of barbiturates, for example, that exceed the levels usually recognized by the psychiatric profession to be appropriate for the control of violence may, if a poor result ensues, leave the psychiatrist open to a finding of negligence. Failure to conform to existing hospital policies may constitute powerful evidence of a deviation from the accepted standard of care. Hospital policies themselves should be carefully formulated and compared with guidelines in the professional literature[27,47] to ensure that they correspond to generally accepted standards. On the other hand, in cases in which common sense is more appropriate to the situation than any professional standard, a clinician may be found to have been acting negligently on the basis that *no* reasonable person would have acted similarly in the same situation.

Malpractice suits, in an application of Sutton's Law (the incorrigible bank robber Willie Sutton said "I rob banks because that's where the money is"), are most likely to be directed against those professionals with the most malpractice insurance. Psychiatrists are most likely to be named as defendants with psychologists, social workers, nurses, and other professionals less frequently the targets. In addition the clinicians responsible for a given patient or ward may be sued for the actions of their subordinates under the doctrine of *respondeat superior*.

One need not perform an act to commit malpractice; the failure to act, particularly in situations in which violence is threatened, may also constitute negligence. In such cases the clinician may face a suit filed by the victim of the assault charging that stronger measures should have been taken to prevent the outburst. Again, the usual standard of care comes into play, although keeping all patients locked in their rooms around the clock might diminish the level of violence in a psychiatric hospital, that is not generally accepted as a proper method of treating the mentally ill. The courts have recognized that risks may have to be taken, such as allowing potentially assaultive patients to walk freely through the wards, in order to maintain an optimal hospital milieu and to effect treatment of the potentially dangerous patient himself.[46] There are accepted limits to such risk-taking. Allowing a repetitively assaultive patient to mix freely with other patients may constitute negligence if most clinicians would have restrained, secluded, medicated, or transferred such an individual.

A hospital staff member might also find himself accused of an *intentional tort*. For example an attendant involved in restraining a threatening patient might be sued for the intentional tort of battery, i.e., having committed an unconsented touching. The likelihood of this happening, however, is extremely low, because the courts have generally felt that psychiatric hospitalization of necessity involves a good deal of unconsented touching and that staff members should be held liable for such acts only if they fail to conform to professional norms. Such actions are usually measured by a negligence standard (as actions for malpractice) rather than being considered as intentional torts. (Some states also have immunity statutes that may protect state employees from civil suit.[23]) For the same reason, it is highly unlikely that criminal charges of battery would ever be brought against a staff member who participated in the restraint of a patient, as long as that person was acting in good faith.[45]

Civil rights suits for *constitutional torts* reflect the recent expansion of patients' rights and now constitute a potentially significant form of liability for the clinician.[2] Federal statutes allow suits to be filed against individuals who, acting "under color" of state law, deprive patients of their rights.[7] A recent Supreme Court decision expanded the scope of these statutes to include rights granted by federal laws, not only those embodied in the constitution.[29] (An effort to use this latter rationale to support a statutory right to treatment has been turned back by the U.S. Supreme Court.[20]) Victims of assault or patients who feel they were unfairly restrained or medicated in an effort to prevent assault would therefore seem to have a potential remedy in civil rights litigation, based on either statutory or constitutional principles.[14,15]

A recent, major decision by the U.S. Supreme Court, however, has substantially limited the potential for successful suits in this area. In *Youngberg v. Romeo* the Court recognized constitutional rights to freedom from harm and from unnecessary restraint, but held that professionals exercising clinical judgment could abridge those rights legitimately in the interests of care and treatment.[51] Patients thus are entitled to have professional decisions made about limitations on freedom from harm and restraint, but have no recourse to the courts unless those decisions fall sufficiently short of the standard of care to constitute malpractice.

Despite the decision in *Youngberg*, civil rights suits remain potent means of enforcing a variety of patients' rights. In general, actions or failures to act must transcend mere negligence in order to reach the level of constitutional review; maliciousness or wanton disregard of an individual's rights is usually required.[13,23] Ordinarily, some substantial harm must have resulted from the negligence for a civil rights action to be tenable.[26] Clinicians may take some additional solace from the so-called "good faith" exception to liability in civil rights suits: individuals who acted in performance of their duties and had no reason to know that they were violating a patient's rights will not be held liable for monetary damages. That does not mean, of course, that they will not be subjected to the rigors of a trial to determine whether they were, in fact, acting in good faith.

Staff as Victim

Staff members are of course also the frequent targets of patients' outbursts.[28] Although staff members have no constitutional rights at stake (after all, they are free to leave their job if they do not like it), they, too, may have the common-law right to be free of assaults caused by clinicians' negligence, especially if the assault is predictable.[9] Negligence in this case may mean failing to predict and to take measures to prevent patient violence. The author knows of no reported appellate cases in which staff members of mental hospitals have successfully sued therapists or the hospital as a result of assault, but the possibility of such an occurrence can certainly be envisioned.

RIGHTS AND LIABILITIES ASSOCIATED WITH SPECIFIC TREATMENTS

Medications

Antipsychotic medications, most notably the phenothiazines and the butytrophenones, have become invaluable additions to the psychiatric pharmacopeia. In considering the actions of these drugs in the prevention of assault, two properties need to be distinguished. First, these medications have a true antipsychotic effect; second, because of their sedative properties, many of these drugs are useful for the nonspecific control of disruptive behavior. Although this distinction is frequently difficult to make in practice, the legal consequences of administering antipsychotic medications to a violent or potentially violent patient may depend heavily on which of these two properties is sought.

The simplest case involves the use of medications for their antipsychotic effects alone. An assaultive patient's medication dose may be increased after the assault if the staff views the patient's act as an indication of inadequate treatment of his or her psychosis. In such cases the medication is being used for its long-term antipsychotic effect rather than for its short-term sedative effect. Additional measures may be used at the same time to prevent an immediate recurrence of violence; e.g., the patient may be restrained or secluded until the imminent threat has passed. When medication is being used in this way, the clinician's potential liability and the legal controls over his or her actions are no different than when treatment is being prescribed for a nonviolent patient.

When antipsychotic medications are being used for their immediate, sedative effect, a different legal environment is operative. Mere sedation is not ordinarily considered treatment, and therefore the limits of the clinician's actions are demarcated by legal controls on the "restraint" of patients. These controls may take the form of statutes or regulations establishing guidelines for the use of "chemical restraints."[32] Use of medications in this way is often limited to narrowly defined emergencies. Violation of the statutes or regulations may carry penalties in themselves, or may serve as *prima facie* evidence of a deviation from the standard of care in a suit for malpractice.

It is, of course, an oversimplification to dichotomize medication effects into pure categories of antipsychotic or sedative. Frequently, perhaps even most often, medications are used both for their sedative and for their antipsychotic effects. Some regimens, such as those involving "rapid neuroleptization," explicitly involve the titration of dosage until sedation is achieved, in the service of determining optimal dosages for the treatment of the underlying psychosis.[31] Many clinicians feel strongly that such treatment should be considered essentially therapeutic and not restrictive. The courts, however, are sensitive to the possibility of sedation being substituted for treatment and the taint of restriction associated with sedation may determine the court's decision. Medications given in response to a violent act at least in part for their immediate sedative effect, even if also intended to have long-term effects may be considered as coming under the particular regulations of the jurisdiction in which the clinician works that govern the use of "chemical restraints."

In the absence of state regulations, clinicians should be guided by professional standards of reasonable treatment. It is clear that many authorities advocate the use of antipsychotic and other drugs in moderate doses for the sedation of acutely agitated patients.[54] On the other hand, there is evidence to suggest that massive doses of phenothiazines are not, in themselves, effective for the prophylaxis of assault.[5] Although little data are available on how psychiatrists actually respond to violent acts, there is some evidence that dramatic changes in drug regimen or the use of large doses of medication are eschewed.[3] In actions for malpractice it is probable that clinicians will be expected to have conformed to this level of moderate use of medication.

The use of antipsychotics solely for the purpose of sedation may also raise constitutional issues. If patients are being deprived of their right to liberty, guaranteed by the Fourteenth Amendment, the state must have a strong justification for its action; for example, an imminent threat to the safety of the patient or others must be demonstrated.[45] The state may also be require that the deprivations be the least possible to accomplish the intended goal. In jurisdictions in which the courts have declared a right to treatment, nonemergency sedation, if "unnecessary or excessive," also may be seen as infringing on that right.[56] These issues are still being actively litigated, especially in the right-to-refuse-treatment suits discussed below. Definitive guidelines for when the clinician oversteps the bounds of constitutionally permitted actions are, therefore, impossible to formulate. Nonetheless, the spectre of civil rights suits attends the nonemergency use of medications solely for sedation.

Inherent in the use of antipsychotic medications for this purpose is another risk. Clinicians have been held liable for malpractice when extensive use of antipsychotics for the purpose of behavior control alone (as in nonpsychotic, mentally retarded patients) has led to the development of tardive dyskinesia.[8] Antipsychotics should probably never be used strictly for sedation. Other sedatives (for example, benzodiazepines and barbiturates) with a much lower incidence of serious long-term side effects are available for that purpose, as are mechanical means of restraint. On the other hand, when both properties of the antipsychotic medications, sedation and true antipsychotic effect, are desired, antipsychotics should be preferred over less-specific sedative drugs.

Voluntarily and Involuntarily Medicated Patients

It is not unlikely that a fair number of patients who have been assaultive will refuse medication and will be involuntarily medicated. The law governing patients' right to refuse antipsychotic medication is in a state of flux, but it is undisputed that in emergencies medication may be administered against the patient's will. (The definition of emergency is the subject of considerable dispute. Psychiatrists often argue for a broad standard, i.e., any situation in which the risk of deterioration of the patient's condition is present, while the courts have generally favored limiting the definition to situations in which the patient or others face imminent harm.[45])

Unfortunately, there is little else that can be said about this subject with nearly that degree of clarity. A variety of lower federal courts have found, in nonemergent situations, an absolute right for both voluntary and involuntary patients to refuse any treatment with psychotropic medications.[11,25,45] This right is generally grounded in Fourteenth Amendment rights to liberty and privacy. Other courts have interpreted state constitutional provisions or statutes as granting similar rights.[14,16,43] Many states provide a statutory right to refuse medication that varies according to the patient's legal status, the clinical situation, or the treatment proposed.[40] The Supreme Court has twice declined to make a definitive statement on the issue.[42,45]

In the meantime some guidelines can be proposed. Every clinician should be aware of whatever court decisions, statutes, or regulations are controlling in his jurisdiction. The failure of other staff members or the facility as a whole to abide by these rules, as frequently occurs, should not be understood as imparting immunity to the clinician to similarly disregard them. In the absence of clear-cut rules in a given state, clinicians ought to proceed carefully. Use of involuntary medication for the prevention of assault should occur only when there is a reasonably high likelihood that assault will in fact occur without it. The prevention of assault should not be used as an excuse to accomplish long-term involuntary treatment, unless a legal opinion can be obtained from the facility's counsel that current state law permits such treatment with antipsychotic drugs. Even then, review of patients' objections by independent psychiatrists is advisable. Without such an opinion, medications should be administered only when assault is believed imminent. The current mood of the courts appears to place the clinician at risk of civil rights suits for indiscriminate treatment of unwilling patients.

Seclusion and Restraint

The legal issues involving the use of seclusion and restraint are similar to those for medication. Although clinicians recognize that seclusion and restraint can be used as therapeutic modalities that decrease the amount of sensory input to which an acutely agitated patient is subject, the law has been resistant to seeing these measures as anything other than means of controlling behavior.[17,18] Consequently, the legal restrictions that attend their use resemble the restrictions on the use of medication for the same purpose.

Many states have statutes limiting the use of seclusion and restraint to certain indications, usually emergencies. There may be restrictions on the amount of time a patient is allowed to be secluded or restrained and requirements for routine checks on his conditions. Documentation and centralized reporting of the use of these modalities is also frequently required. As with the use of medications for restraint, a clinician violates these standards only at the risk of penalties contained in the laws themselves or of a charge of malpractice. In states without regulations, a general standard of negligence will apply.

Use of seclusion and restraint may also rise to the level of constitutional violations if they are employed in nonemergencies solely for the purpose of behavior control.[46] Violation of state standards may constitute an infringement of patients' constitutional rights to due process.[45] Even when used to prevent imminent harm, constitutional principles may require that seclusion or restraint be the least restrictive means of achieving that goal.[11,46,56] Several courts have found constitutional reasons to require a number of specific procedures attending seclusion or restraint, among them: patients must be personally examined by a qualified mental health professional prior to restraint and by a psychiatrist within two hours of restraint;[11] patients must be checked every 15 minutes[12] and reevaluation must occur within 12 hours;[11] careful records must be kept on the use of seclusion and the grounds therefore;[34] patients must be allowed to use a bathroom once an hour and be bathed every 12 hours.[56] Although these particular criteria apply only to limited jurisdictions, many of them are merely elaborations of good clinical practices that should be followed everywhere.

Electroconvulsive Therapy

Electroconvulsive therapy (ECT) may be the only effective means of preventing violence in a small number of circumstances. Catatonic and manic excitement, for example, even when refractory to drug therapy, may be quite responsive to ECT. Unfortunately, ECT has acquired a generally bad reputation with the public, and legislators have responded by hedging its use with a large number of restrictions. These vary among the states, but patients are sometimes given statutory procedural rights and rights to refuse ECT even when similar rights are not granted for other forms of treatment.[32]

The use of ECT in emergencies is controlled by the same principles outlined above for medication (barring statutory exceptions). Given that a patient must be restrained and medicated before ECT can be used, some might argue that its involuntary use is never justified by the presence of an emergency, since the emergency must be under control before its administration. Nonetheless, it seems reasonable to view some situations—for example, prolonged states of catatonic excitement that can be controlled only temporarily with sedatives—as instances in which ECT might be used as an emergency measure to prevent further violence. Some states' statutes recognize this explicitly.[36]

Except when otherwise provided for by statute, the right of a patient to refuse ECT in a nonemergency generally conforms to the outline of the right to refuse medication in that jurisdiction. At least one court, however, has found a constitutional right to refuse ECT, based on the Fourteenth Amendment principles, in the absence of a similar finding for antipsychotic medications.[16] Other courts have required judicial review of ECT treatment of patients who refuse ECT or who are incompetent[41] or review of all ECT use by a committee especially established for that purpose.[55]

Discharge

Although rarely discussed openly, discharge of a potentially or actually violent patient is probably a relatively frequently employed means of preventing in-hospital violence. A variety of justifications are offered for it: a staff that is frightened of a patient cannot treat him (or other patients) successfully; in some cases the hospital milieu fosters regression and violence, and discharge will be therapeutic; and dangerous people ought to be dealt with by the legal system, not by psychiatric facilities. Whichever of these rationales is used, discharge poses some complicated legal issues.

From the point of view of the discharged patient, the hospital assumed a duty to care for him when it accepted him for hospitalization. A precipitous discharge following or in anticipation of an assault may represent an abandonment of the patient and open the possibility of a malpractice suit. Charges of abandonment are enhanced if the patient is still in need of psychiatric care, especially if psychotic. When such patients can no longer be handled by a mental hospital, they should be transferred to more secure settings and not released to the street. For patients whose need for continued inpatient care is less pressing—and especially for those of whom it is said that hospitalization is contributing to their regression—discharge can be considered, but only when arrangements are made for aftercare or referral. Such arrangements should preclude charges of abandonment.

This latter group of patients, however, presents another risk of liability. By virtue of the therapeutic relationship, a clinician and a mental hospital may assume responsibility for preventing the patient from injuring third parties.[19] If the discharged patient actually commits a violent act on the outside, the clinician might find himself sued by the victim for failure to detain the patient. The author knows of no cases in which this issue has been raised in context of the deliberate discharge of a patient thought to be assaultive, but there is a large body of case law in closely related areas. When patients have been released as nondangerous and subsequently committed violent crimes, or when patients negligently have been permitted to escape from a facility and then been assaultive, courts have usually held the clinicians and the facility liable for the damages suffered by the victim if the act could be said to have been foreseeable.[24, 48, 49] Clinicians who deliberately discharge assaultive patients would seem to be at even higher risk of liability because the reason for discharge confirms the danger posed by the patient. Obviously, the greater the length of time between discharge and the violent act, the less foreseeable the violence can be said to have been. When the potential victim is identifiable, the obligation to protect him or her, such as by warning the potential victim of the danger, may be even stronger.[30, 53]

Patients who are potentially assaultive, but do not have major mental illnesses can be categorized as a subgroup of patients that poses a still more difficult problem concerning the hospital's obligations to the patient. Many of these patients may be classified as sociopaths or as having other character disorders. Violence may have been a precipitant to their admission, or may have occurred during their hospitalization, but a careful evaluation has ruled out any other diagnosable disorders. Psychiatrists argue whether such patients are really "mentally ill," and the utility of inpatient treatment is equally in dispute. Clinicians frequently claim that assaultive, character disordered patients should be discharged to the street, since their lack of benefit from hospitalization and the disruption they cause make them more fitting subjects for the criminal justice system than for psychiatric facilities.

Again there is a dearth of case law on this subject. Although the argument for discharge may seem clinically persuasive, it is unclear if the legal system would agree. Judges or juries often find it hard to understand why hospitalization is not of benefit to all "troubled" people. Similarly, it may be difficult to explain in court why someone said to have an "antisocial personality disorder"—a diagnosis listed in DSM III—is not "really" mentally ill. In 1971 at least one court upheld discharge in these circumstances,[6] but currently the many precedents holding clinicians liable for foreseeable acts may be more influential.

All that can be said at this point is that discharge of nonpsychotic but dangerous patients, though often clinically indicted, may place the facility at some risk. Given the sensitive nature of the question, such a patient should not be released without careful discussions with the hospital administration and its legal counsel.

The question of whether a patient in seclusion should ever be discharged directly to the street is much argued. Some legal-psychiatric experts shun such action entirely, believing that it is almost negligence *per se* for a patient who cannot even be controlled on a hospital ward to be released into society. There are, however, occasions when discharge from seclusion directly to the street may be appropriate. When it is believed that the regressive pull of the hospital milieu has provoked the patient's violence, and especially when the patient had not been violent prior to admission, discharge from seclusion to the street might represent the safest way of separating the patient from a potentially harmful setting. Needless to say, this procedure should be employed only after careful consideration and consultation with other clinicians.

AN APPROACH TO THE PREVENTION AND TREATMENT OF VIOLENCE

Predicting Assault

The conflict of rights between potentially assaultive patients and their potential victims places clinicians in a difficult position. If clinicians could accurately predict who will be violent and take only those measures necessary to prevent the assault, they would have little difficulty meeting this challenge. Complicating the picture, however, is the difficulty clinicians have in accurately predicting violent behavior.[33] Although the most relevant type of studies have not been done, currently extant data suggest that psychiatrists are not good predictors of future violence.[33] One study that examined the frequency of violent acts in the hospital by patients who were committed because of a likelihood of assault found they had a significantly higher rate of violence than did a control population.[44] Even here, however, substantially less than half of the sample became sufficiently threatening to require restraint at any point during an average 45-day hospital stay.

The attitude of the courts toward clinical prediction of future violence is rife with ambivalence and ambiguity. Recognizing the difficulty of the task, one court has rejected efforts at prediction in a context—namely, death penalty hearings—where there is little tolerance for error.[39] On the other hand, in cases in which liability for the acts of their patients is at issue, and the courts are primarily concerned with compensating the victim, psychiatrists have been presumed to be capable of some measure of prediction.[30, 53] Thus the clinician is faced with the prospect of being held liable for over- or underpredicting something that most clinicians are not very good at predicting at all.

Some approach to prevention nonetheless must be charted among these legal shoals. The first step for the clinician is to determine as accurately as possible which patients are likely to be at high risk of violence. Monahan has recently reviewed those factors associated with violent behavior in an effort to systematize clinical evaluations.[33] Gutheil and Appelbaum have outlined a clinically oriented approach.[19] In the absence of good data that any approach has solid predictive validity, the most important thing for the clinician is to choose one model that can be defended on theoretical grounds and to use it consistently. Many courts still accord a great deal of deference to clinical judgment, as long as it stands on some reasonable foundation.

Second, having made the prediction, the clinician must carefully document the basis for it. A record developed at the time of the decision is many times more valuable for courtroom purposes than retrospective recollections.

Third, once violence is predicted, the clinician must take all appropriate steps to prevent it. Nothing leaves a caregiver more open to charges of negligence than failing to take measures in the face of his own prediction that violence would occur. This was exactly the situation in the famous *Tarasoff* case and it probably played an important role in the outcome of the case.[53] Half-way measures are of little use to anyone: they simultaneously deny the assaultive patient his liberty, and leave his victim defenseless.

Fourth, if at all possible, consultation should be requested. It is much harder to accuse a clinician of poor judgment when the record shows that another clinician, preferably one not directly involved in the patient's care, concurred with the original decision.

Fifth, the patient's status must be carefully reviewed over time. Measures taken to prevent violence by a newly admitted manic patient may be much less appropriate after a week of neuroleptic treatment has rendered him practically nonpsychotic.

Preventing Assault

It may be useful to emphasize at this point the cases under discussion are cases in which it has already been determined that steps to prevent assault are necessary. When assault seems unlikely, of course, even a minimal infringement of patients' rights is unwarranted.

As difficult as it is to determine when preventive measures should be taken, the worst outcome is for the clinician to lapse into a state of fearful paralysis. The decision is difficult, but not making a decision and thus failing to act is also a decision of sorts. In general, there is much to be said for leaning, when in doubt, toward taking measures to prevent assaults. Although room restriction or locked seclusion represent some encroachment on a patient's liberty, the diminishment is not as great as it would be for someone who was not already being held in a psychiatric facility. Compared to the harm that might result from an assault, temporary seclusion, restraint, or increased medications are a relatively small price to pay.

It should be stressed, of course, that not only the victim benefits from the assault being prevented. The potentially or actually assaultive patient also gains in the long run. Containing this violent patient's feeling of being out of control may decrease his or her anxiety level and aid resolution of the acute episode. The remorse that many patients feel about violent acts committed during acute psychoses is also precluded. Prevention of violence, whether it involves space restriction or medication, is often impossible to dissociate from effective treatment of the patient's underlying condition.

Even if one were to examine the issue from a narrower point of view, concerned only with the potential liability for the clinician from restraining or not restraining a potentially violent patient, the analysis favors restraining when in doubt. Suits for inappropriate restraint are much less likely to occur than suits for injuries suffered by the patient's victim. Should a suit be filed, a judgment for infringement of rights, particularly if motivated by legitimate clinical concerns, is likely to be much less than the damages for serious injury or death of a patient who was left negligently unprotected. In fact, since patients have sued clinicians for not restraining them when psychotic, restraint may represent good defensive medicine from that point of view as well.[9]

Instituting measures to prevent further violence leaves the clinician in the position of having to determine when those measures should be removed. Such judgments, though difficult, are rarely challenged. However, in a recent Massachusetts case dealing with the use of seclusion, the court was unusually willing to second guess psychiatric decision making in this area. The decision noted that although the first few days of seclusion following a patient's violent outburst had been warranted for the purposes of secondary prevention, the slow weaning of the patient from the seclusion room over a period of several weeks constituted a violation of his rights.[45] Such Monday-morning quarterbacking is unusual in court decisions, but this case points out that it can occur. Clinicians should therefore be able to justify not just the reason that restrictions have been imposed, but also why they continue to be needed. There is, of course, always a gray zone in which it is unclear if preventive measures continue to be warranted. At such times, the rule suggested above of usually erring on the side of caution would seem to be applicable.

The primary pitfall of which the clinician must beware is responding to the patient's act in a punitive way. Many varieties of theoretical formulations can be offered to defend actions that in reality derive from nothing more than a desire to strike back at the offensive patient. A careful self-examination by the clinician is probably the surest means of preventing such a response, but outside consultation may be of use, as well. Punitive, nontherapeutic responses, their detrimental effect on a patient's clinical state aside, leave therapists open to suit for such intentional torts as assault and battery and to charges of infringing the Eighth Amendment's prohibition against cruel and unusual punishment.

Using the Legal system to Prevent and Treat Violence

A few ingenious efforts have been made to use legal mechanisms for the prevention and treatment of violence. These have generally involved forcing patients to take responsibility for the consequences of their acts, for example, billing patients for property damage incurred as a result of aggressive acts they commit.[20] The theoretical basis for this maneuver is the belief that holding patients responsible for their actions limits the regressive pull of the hospital environment, but the hospital's response when patient's refuse to pay—since third party payers will not accept bills for broken windows or unhinged doors—is problematic. One suspects that such efforts work best in hospitals whose milieus are most able to exploit the issue of responsibility for psychotherapeutic purposes, without necessarily expecting that the bill will be paid. Legal means of collecting payment for these bills, particularly if the amounts involved are small, would not usually be worth the time and money expended.

More frequently discussed is the possibility of filing criminal charges against patients who commit assaults. The enthusiasm with which hospital staff members respond to such suggestions is probably a function of both the sense of impotence they feel to control repetitively assaultive patients and the opportunity prosecution offers to respond in a punitive but socially accepted fashion. Despite one Canadian report of a successful prosecution,[50] the technique faces a number of legal obstacles that reflect society's feelings about the culpablity of the mentally ill and render prosecution unlikely to succeed.

First, prosecutors must be persuaded to file charges against the patient. In most cases, they will be reluctant to do so, because simple assaults by mentally disturbed individuals represent the type of case overworked prosecutors are most eager to be rid of. Outside the hospital setting, such cases would usually be handled by dropping charges in return for an agreement to seek psychiatric care. Even in the face of evidence to the contrary, many lawyers and judges continue to believe that sending a mentally ill, minor offender to a psychiatric facility is always preferable to processing him through the legal system.

If the assault is relatively serious, or an unusually cooperative prosecutor is involved, the case may move to the pretrial stage. Here, there may be renewed pressure from a clogged court system to drop charges or to accept a plea bargain. Failing that, the aggressive defense attorney will inevitably raise the issue of the defendant's competency to stand trial, examination for which may need to be performed at a neutral facility, with further attendant delay. Throughout this period, the staff member who is pressing charges may feel the trauma occasioned by the assault recede into the distance. He may begin wondering whether whatever can be gained from these prolonged legal maneuvers is worth the time and strain on him, or whether he is acting inappropriately in seeking to "punish a sick person." Disapproval from other staff members and patients may compound these feelings.

Assuming the case makes it to court, the patient has a variety of legal arguments at his or her disposal. Psychotic patients, and even many patients with character disorders, may claim that they meet the criteria for being found criminally nonresponsible by reason of mental illness. If the patient was involuntarily committed, the court may believe, as did one judge, that "to convict the involuntary committee of a quasi-criminal offense for displaying the symptoms of his illness while in a place intended to treat that illness and upon the complaint of one whose duty it is to have the care and custody of such patient imposes punishment where none can either constitutionally or morally be justified."[52] Judges may feel that just as clinicians are granted a certain leeway in preventing violent acts by means, such as seclusion, that would not be tolerated in open society, so patients should be permitted to be assaultive on occasion without facing punishment for it. This notion is an extension of the idea of "asylum," and is related to a feeling that mental health professionals should expect to withstand an infrequent assault as part of the anticipated hazards of their job.

Given all this, the so-called "therapeutic prosecution" is unlikely to come to much. Even if found guilty, the defendant-patient is likely to be returned to the mental health system. How much the process actually forces him to internalize responsibility for his acts is in doubt. At best, prosecution of assaultive patients should be reserved for more serious acts of violence, in which the chances of success are likely to be greater.

CONCLUSION

Legal efforts to accommodate conflicting rights when psychiatric patients become assaultive have yet to yield many definitive guidelines for clinicians. Since many clinicians are terrified by the spectre of potential liability regardless of the course they choose, it may be useful to emphasize that actions taken in conformance with existing law and professional standards, with the patient's best interests at heart, and with sensitivity to the rights of all parties involved are most likely to lead to liability. Clinicians have been delegated an unusual amount of power to act in emergencies. In situations that are not emergent, i.e., when the threat of assault or self-injury is more remote, clinicians' powers are more circumscribed but still substantial. As the law in these areas continues to evolve, particularly concerning involuntary treatment in nonemergencies, the clinician's best protection is to remain conversant with the changes that affect his or her jurisdiction and, when in doubt, to seek competent clinical and legal consultation.

REFERENCES

1. Annotation: Liability of one releasing institutionalized mental patient for harm he causes. 38 ALR 3d 699
2. Appelbaum PS: Civil rights litigation and mental health: section 1983. Hosp Community Psychiatry 32:305–306, 1981
3. Appelbaum PS, Jackson AH, Shader RI: Psychiatrists' responses to violence: pharmacologic management of psychiatric inpatients. Am J Psychiatry 140: 301–304, 1983
4. Appelbaum PS, Kemp KN: The evolution of commitment law in the nineteenth century: a reinterpretation. Law and Human Behavior 6:343–354, 1982
5. Appleton W: Massive doses of chlorpromazine: effectiveness in controlling psychotic behavior. Arch Gen Psychiatry 9:586–592, 1963
6. Cameron v. State, 37 A.D.2d 46, 322 N.Y.S.2d 562 (1971)
7. Civil Rights Act, 42 U.S.C., section 1983.
8. Clites v. Iowa, 322 N.W.2d 917 (Iowa Ct. App. 1982)
9. Cole v. Taylor, 301 N.W.2d 766 (Iowa 1981)
10. Coleman v. Mercy Hospital, 373 So.2d 91 (Fla. App. 1979)
11. Davis v. Hubbard, 506 F. Supp. 915 (W.O. Ohio 1980)
12. Eckerhart v. Hensley, 475 F. Supp. 908 (W.D. Mo. 1979)
13. Estelle v. Gamble, 429 U.S. 97 (1976)
14. Goedecke v. Colorado, 603 P.2d 123 (Colo. 1979)
15. Goodman v. Parwatikar, 570 F.2d 801 (8th Cir. 1978)
16. Gundy v. Pauley, 519 S.W.2d 735 (Ky. Appl. 1981)
17. Gutheil TG: Observations on the theoretical basis for seclusion of the psychiatric inpatient. Am J Psychiatry 135:325–328, 1978
18. Gutheil TG: Restraint vs. treatment: seclusion as discussed in the Boston State Hospital case. Am J Psychiatry 137:718–719, 1980

19. Gutheil TG, Applebaum PS: Clinical Handbook of Psychiatry and the Law New York, McGraw-Hill, 1982
20. Gutheil TF, Rivinus TM: The cost of window breaking. Psychiatr Ann 7(2): 47–51, 1982
21. Halderman v. Pennhurst State School & Hosp., 466 F. Suppl. 1295 (E.D.Pa. 1978), 612 F.2d 84 (3d Cir. 1979), 451 U.S. 1 (1981)
22. Harver v. Cserr, 544 F.2d 1121 (2st Cir. 1976).
23. Jacobs v. Dept. of Mental Health, 276 N.W.3d 627 (Mich. App. 1979)
24. Januszko v. New York, 404 N.Y.S.2d 486 (Ct.Cl.1977), 391 N.E.2d 297 (N.Y. 1979)
25. In re K.K.B., 609 P.2d 747 (Okla. 1980)
26. Knight v. Colorado, 496 F. Supp. 779 (D.Colo. 1980)
27. Lion JR: Evaluation and Management of the Violent Patient: Guidelines in the Hospital and Institution. Springfield, Illinois, Charles C Thomas, 1972
28. Lion, JR, Snyder W, Merrill G: Under-reporting of assaults on staff in a state hospital. Hosp Community Psychiatry 32:497–498, 1981
29. Main v. Thiboutot, 488 U.S. 1 (1980)
30. McIntosh v. Milano, 403 A.2d 500 (N.J. Super. Ct., 1979)
31. Mason AS, Granacher RP. Basic principles of rapid neuroleptization. Dis Nerv Sys 37:547–551, 1976
32. Massachusetts General Laws, Chapter 123
33. Monahan J: The Clinical Prediction of Violent Behavior. NIMH, Rockville, MD, 1981
34. Negron v. Preiser, 382 F. Supp. 535 (S.D.N.Y.1974)
35. New York State Association for Retarded Children, Inc. v.Rockefeller, 357 F. Supp. 752 (E.D.N.Y. 1973)
36. Ohio regulation requires informed consent prior to administration of ECT. Mental Disability Law Reporter 3:39–40, 1979
37. 1869 PA. Laws, Act of April 8, 1869, Pub. L. No. 78
38. 55 PA Code, section 7100.113.4
39. People v. Murtishaw. 175 Cal. Rptr. 738, 631 P.2d 446 (1981)
40. Plotkin R: Limiting the therapeutic orgy: mental patients' right to refuse tretment. Northwestern University Law Review, 72:461–525, 1977.
41. Price v. Sheppard, 239 N.W.2d 905 (Minn. 1976)
42. Rennie v. Klein, 462 F. Supp. 1131 (D.N.J. 1978), 476 F. Supp. 1294 (D.N.J. 1979) aff'd in part, 653 F.2d 836 (3rd Cir. 1981), vacated and remanded, 102 S. Ct. 3506 (1982)
43. In the Matter of the Guardianship of Richard Roe III, 421 N.E.2d 40 (Mass. 1981)
44. Rofman ES, Askinazi C, Fant E: The prediction of dangerous behavior in emergency civil commitment. Am J Psychiatry 137:1061–1064, 1980
45. Rogers v. Okin, 478 F. Supp. 1342 (D. Mass. 1979), aff'd in part, 634 F.2d 250 (2st Cir. 1980), vacated and remanded sub nom Mills v. Rogers, 102 S. Ct. 2442 (1982)
46. Romeo v. Youngberg, No. 76-3429 (E.D. Pa. 1978), 644 F.2d 147 (3d Cir. 1980), vacated and remanded, 102 S. Ct. 2452 (1982)
47. Rosen H. DiGiacomo JN: The role of physical restraint in the treatment of

psychiatric illness. J Clin Psychiatry 39:228–232, 1978

48. Ross v. Central Louisiana State Hospital, 392 So.2d 698 (La. App. 1980)
49. Rum River Lumber Co. v. Minnesota, 282 N.W.2d 882 (Minn. 1979)
50. Schwarz CJ, Greenfield GP: Charging a patient with assault of a nurse on a psychiatric unit. Can Psychiatr Assoc J 23:197–200, 1978
51. Spence v. Staras, 507 F.2d 554 (7th Cir. 1974)
52. State v. Cummins, 403 A.2d 67 (N.J. Super. 1979)
53. Tarasoff v. Regents of the University of California, 131 Cal. Rptr. 14, 551 P.2d 334 (1977)
54. Tupin JP: Management of violent patients, in Shader RI (ed): Manual of Psychiatric Therapeutics: Practical Psychopharmacology and Psychiatry. Boston, Little, Brown and Co., 1975, pp 125–136
55. Wyatt v. Hardin, No. 3195-N (M.D.Ala.Feb. 28, 175, modified July 1, 1975)
56. Wyatt v. Stickney, 325 F. Supp. 781, 344 F. Supp. 373 (M.D. Ala. 1972)

Bruce Dennis Sales
Thomas D. Overcast
Karen J. Merrikin

14

Worker's Compensation Protection for Assaults and Batteries on Mental Health Professionals

In the social science literature, the word "assault" is commonly used to describe a physical attack on a mental health professional, with resulting physical injuries.[33,35] In legal terminology, however, "assault" has a precise meaning that must be distinguished from that of "battery;" an *assault* is a *threat* made by one person against another with an apparent intent to inflict bodily injury by force. Legally, an assault includes only the threat (not the fact) of physical injury. It must, however, appear that the threat will be carried out, putting the victim in reasonable fear of bodily harm. A *battery*, is an unjustified application of physical force to the person or body of the victim. Thus, a battery may be a complicated assault (resulting in the common phrase, "assault and battery").[30] To avoid confusion, the words "assault" and "battery" will be used in their legal sense throughout this chapter.

Assaults and batteries by patients on mental health professionals are neither new nor trivial phenomena. Bernstein reports that in Germany, the first known case of a fatal battery by a patient occurred in 1849.[2] A number of investigators have attempted to gather current data on the incidence of patient assaults and batteries.[4, 13, 22, 34, 36] The reported frequency varied from 24 percent of 101 therapists[36] to 42 percent of 115 therapists surveyed.[22] More recently, Bernstein reported that, out of 422 therapists surveyed, a total of 60 (14.2 percent) indicated that they had been battered; a total of 150 (35.6 percent) reported being personally assaulted; and finally, a total of 257 (60.9 percent) reported generally being physically afraid of certain of their patients.[2] According to Lion and co-workers, however, the incidence of batteries against staff in mental hospitals may be far higher than previously reported. Over a three-month period, their data showed only 40 reported batteries. An examination of the daily ward reports for the same period of time, however, showed the occurrence of 237 incidents of potential battery.[19]

Lion et al. also reported that, although the finding of a high incidence of battery had potentially serious implications for hospital care,[1,5] there was no clear agreement among mental health professionals about how to handle such incidents.[19] For instance, Lion[17] and Lion and Pasternak[18] have suggested that clinicians often resort to denial when confronting a violent patient, whereas Schwarz and Greenfield describe the criminal prosecution of a violent patient who battered a hospital staff member.[32]

In addition to a lack of information about management of violent behavior directed against hospital staff, little has been written about compensation for injuries sustained by the victims of such behavior. Lion and co-workers[19] note parenthetically that, in order to protect hospital staff, the concept of victim compensation[24] may be appropriate for hospital staff who are the victims of patient assaults and/or batteries. There are, however, at least two important limitations to applying victim compensation concepts to the situation of the mental health professional who is the victim of a violent patient. First, some victim compensation plans provide assistance only for those cases in which a perpetrator is officially charged with a criminal offense, and as Schwarz and Greenfield imply criminal prosecution of psychiatric patients is often not the therapy of choice for violent behavior.[32] Second, many victim compensation plans award compensation based only on a legislatively imposed schedule of damages, with no regard for the actual injuiries suffered, the actual expenses incurred in treating the injuries and rehabilitating the victim, or the actual wages lost during this time.

There is, however, another legal approach—worker's compensation law— that more directly addresses the issue of recompense for employees who are injured on the job. Under these state plans, compensation is generally awarded without regard to fault, i.e., there is no need to determine whether the employer or the worker was the cause of, or contributed to the injury. As long as the injury is "work-related" (a concept that is explored in greater detail below), the worker is entitled to compensation. Thus, depending on the nature and extent of his or her injuries, the injured worker can expect to receive full medical and mental health care, physical and vocational rehabilitation, or, if necessary, retraining and job placement services. In addition, as opposed to victim compensation plans, which may award only a lump sum cash payment and may be subject to a maximum benefit ceiling, worker's compensation benefits are virtually unlimited and are bounded only by the limits of being able to return an injured worker to his or her highest level of productivity in gainful employment.

THE DEVELOPMENT OF WORKER'S COMPENSATION LAWS

Before the first worker's compensation laws were enacted in the late nineteenth and early twentieth centuries, employers were considered legally responsible only for injuries to their employees that resulted from the employer's negligence. In addition to placing the legal burden of proof on the worker, the law also allowed the employer to interpose a number of affirmative defenses. For the injured or disabled worker, compensation or recovery through the legal system was a slow, costly, and uncertain process.

As the pace of industrialization accelerated and the number of work-related injury suits concomitantly increased, it became apparent that the prevailing legal structure imposed too harsh a burden on the injured worker. After several attempts to remedy this situation, the first modern worker's compensation laws were enacted in 1911.

Today each jurisdiction has a worker's compensation law through which injured workers receive compensation for injuries that arise "out of and in the course of employment."* These laws are based on the theory that employers should, without regard to the fault involved, assume the costs of industrial injuries to workers, and pass the increased costs on to consumers as a cost of doing business.

Because mental health personnel are employed in such a wide variety of settings and conditions, it is important to understand how coverage under worker's compensation is determined. For example, most regularly employed professionals on the staff of a school, hospital, or other institution most likely will be covered by worker's compensation. On the other hand, self-employed mental health professionals or partners in a small mental health business may not automatically be covered.

---

*This is a test of legal causation. It usually requires the employment situation to create a risk of injury for the worker. The interpretation of the phrase has become less rigorous since the inception of worker's compensation statutes.[6] Clearly, however, diseases or illnesses that are characteristic of life in general are not within the included range of coverage as they involve no risk arising out of employment. In addition, in order to be compensable, a disability must result in a workers' being unable to perform a job in keeping with his or her qualifications. The concept thus involves more than just a medical injury; that injury must have an adverse effect upon the worker's earning power.[15]

The statutes and case law of the fifty states, the District of Columbia, and the federal system were reviewed to determine whether and under what conditions mental health personnel are eligible for compensation for both physical and mental injuries under the state worker's compensation systems. This material is divided into two sections: 1) the types of employment situations covered by worker's compensation, and 2) the nature of injuries covered under worker's compensation.

Mental injury is a term that is likely to be unfamiliar to mental health practitioners and researchers. As a concept in law, it encompasses the full range of more familiar psychological and psychiatric diagnoses from simple personality disorders and neuroses to the more serious psychoses. Synonyms that sometimes arise in worker's compensation cases include such terms as *psychological trauma* and/or *disorder*, and *mental disability*. To avoid confusion the term "mental injury" is used throughout this chapter.

REVIEW OF CURRENT LAW*

Employment Situations Covered by Worker's Compensation

State workers compensation statutes can be divided into two major categories: 1) those states that *require* employers to carry coverage on their employees and in which a large portion of the working population is automatically covered; and 2) those states in which coverage is largely *elective*—employers may carry worker's compensation insurance on themselves and their employees at their option. The majority of states require that many employers provide worker's compensation for themselves and their employees. Even in those states with "compulsory coverage," however, certain types of workers are exempted. For example, no state requires coverage of domestic and agricultural workers. Many small businesses, independent contractors, charitable and nonprofit institutions, and many forms of public employment also are exempt from compulsory coverage. In addition, jurisdictions have different coverage requirements for employment in the private and public sectors.

Private Sector

In 41 jurisdictions the statutes provide that privately employed persons (except for certain types of exempted employment, discussed below) must be covered by worker's compensation (Table 14-1). In six jurisdictions, coverage for private employers and employees is elective (for firms larger than a specified

---

*This review encompasses statutes and cases current as of September 1, 1981. Readers should consult the specific laws of their own states for the latest statutes and judicial interpretations.

size), and the decision to be covered lies with the employer. In three jurisdictions, coverage is required only for workers in certain listed "hazardous" or "ultrahazardous" occupations, none of which specifically include the mental health field or other settings in which mental health professionals might be expected to work, and in one state coverage is elective for all types of private employment, regardless of firm size. Table 14-1 provides a detailed analysis of the coverage and exemptions in each jurisdiction. (The reader should refer to Table 14-1 for the data cited throughout the following discussion.)

Breakdown of Coverage Requirements by Employment Category

Small business—few employees. Even in the 41 jurisdictions requiring coverage for most types of private employment, small businesses are exempted if the employer has fewer than a specified number of regularly employed workers. These numbers range from one or more employees (in nine jurisdictions) to five or more employees (in three jurisdictions).

Sole proprietors. Arkansas, Delaware, Florida, and Washington require coverage for sole proprietors and their employees. Of those four states, three (Arkansas, Florida, and Washington) require coverage only for those sole proprietors who devote a certain percentage of their time to the business. Five jurisdictions allow sole proprietors to elect coverage *only if* they devote a certain percentage of their time to the business. The rest of the jurisdictions fall into one of two categories: 1) coverage for sole proprietors is entirely elective, with no restrictions, or 2) no mention is made in the statutes of special coverage requirements for sole proprietors.

Partners. Six jurisdictions require that partnerships be covered by worker's compensation. Of those, coverage is compulsory in four states *only if* (as with sole proprietors) the partners devote a certain amount of time to the business of the partnership.

In four jurisdictions coverage is elective for partnerships in which the partners devote a certain amount of their time to the business of the partnership. In 22 jurisdictions coverage for partnerships is entirely elective, with no such restrictions. In the remaining states there is no mention whatsoever of coverage of partnerships.

Independent contractors. This category includes those mental health professionals who serve as consultants for others in a wide variety of settings, including public and private institutions. In many cases it may not be clear who is acting as the employer. If the professional is not a regularly employed worker of the person or the institution for whom he or she is providing a service, coverage under worker's compensation may be denied.

Table 14-1
Worker's Compensation Coverage and Exemption Requirements

		PRIVATE EMPLOYMENT			PUBLIC EMPLOYMENT		
State	Type of Coverage/ No. of Employees	Sole Proprietors/ Partners	Charitable and/or Nonprofit Institutions	Independent Contractors	Compulsory for All Public Employees	Elective— Based on Size of Town or County	Effective for All Governments
Alabama	E/3 or more	E/E				E—Not Birmingham	E
Alaska	C/3 or more				C		
Arizona	C/3 or more				C		
Arkansas	C/3 or more	C*/C*			C		
California	C/all, with exceptions	E*/C*			C		
Colorado	C/all, with exceptions		E		C		
Connecticut	C/all, with exceptions	E/E			C		
Delaware	C/1 or more	C/C			C		
Florida	C/3 or more	C*/C*	C*	E	C		
Georgia	E/5 or more	E/E	E	E	C		
Hawaii	C/all, with exceptions			C	C		
Idaho	C/all, with exceptions	/E	E	C	C—Including Ind. K		
Illinois	C/extrahazardous employment	E/E—hazardous	E	E	E	Not elected officials	E

196

State						
Indiana	C/all, with exceptions	E/E	E	C	C	
Iowa	C/all, with exceptions	E*/E*		E	C	
Kansas	C/all, with exceptions	E/E			C	
Kentucky	C/1 or more	E/E			C	
Louisiana	C/all, with exceptions	E/E	E	E	C	Not elected officials
Maine	C/all, with exceptions		E*		C	
Maryland	C/1 or more	E/E			C	
Massachusetts	C/all, with exceptions				C—Including Ind. K	E
Michigan	C/3 or more			C	C	
Minnesota	C/all, with exceptions	E/C			C	
Mississippi	C/5 or more		E		C	E
Missouri	C/5 or more			C	C	
Montana	C/all, with exceptions	E/E			C	
Nebraska	E/all	E/E	E	E	C	
Nevada	C/all, with exceptions			X	C—Including Ind. K	
New Hampshire	C/1 or more			C	C—Including Ind. K	
New Jersey	E/all				C	
New Mexico	C/3 or more	E/E	C		C	
New York	C/1 or more				C	

(continued)

Table 14-1 (continued)

State	Type of Coverage/ No. of Employees	PRIVATE EMPLOYMENT			PUBLIC EMPLOYMENT		
		Sole Proprietors/ Partners	Charitable and/or Nonprofit Institutions	Independent Contractors	Compulsory for All Public Employees	Elective— Based on Size of Town or County	Effective for All Governments
North Carolina	C/4 or more	E/E			C		
North Dakota	C/hazardous work	E*/E*—haz-ous	E	E	C	C	
Ohio	C/1 or more	E/E			C	C	
Oklahoma	C/all, with exceptions	E/E			C	C	
Oregon	C/all, with exceptions	E/E		C	C	E—Except Portland	
Pennsylvania	C/all, with exceptions	E/		E	C		
Rhode Island	C/all, with exceptions				C—Only state and city of Providence	E—all others	
South Carolina	C/4 or more	E*/E*			C		
South Dakota	C/all, with exceptions		E		C		
Tennessee	E/all	E/E	E				E
Texas	E/all	E/E	E	E			
Utah	C/1 or more	E/E		E	C		

Vermont	C/all, with exceptions	E/E	C	C	C
Virginia	E/4 or more	E*/E*			C
Washington	C/all, with exceptions	C*/C*			C
West Virginia	C/all, with exceptions				C
Wisconsin	C/3 or more	/E		C*	C
Wyoming	C/extrahazardous employment				C—extrahazardous only

C   = Compulsory
E   = Elective
C*   = Compulsory—if devotes certain time to business
E*   = Elective—if devotes certain time to business
Ind. K = Independent Contractor

In nine jurisdictions employers are required to include independent contractors as their employees for purposes of worker's compensation coverage. In forty-one jurisdictions, there is either no mention of worker's compensation, it is elective, or the provisions would not be applicable to mental health practitioners.

The issue of coverage for independent contractors is confusing; however, this confusion is typically resolved in favor of coverage for the injured worker. All of the jurisdictions have language in the statutes describing the worker's compensation acts as "remedial," meaning that the laws were designed to aid injured workers. Further, the statutes of all of the jurisdictions indicate that the definitions of "employer" and "employee" should be liberally defined in a way that will benefit all workers, for whom the acts were intended. Thus, any confusion about whether a person or institution was acting as the employer of a consulting professional is most often resolved in favor of the worker.

Private charitable or nonprofit institutions. A minority of jurisdictions provide that coverage shall be elective for employees or officers of such institutions. This would include most social service agencies, some private hospitals, halfway houses, and the like. Florida and Vermont require that officers and/or employees of such institutions be covered by worker's compensation.

Public sector. Mandatory coverage for public employees is much broader than that in the private sector. The majority of jurisdictions require that public employees be covered by worker's compensation. Three specifically require that those who contract with public bodies must be covered and must cover their employees as well. Wyoming requires worker's compensation coverage only for those public employees engaged in hazardous employment. Missouri, however, requires that employees of its Mental Health and Welfare Departments be covered.

In Illinois, Massachusetts, Mississippi, and Tennessee, coverage for public workers is entirely elective. In Illinois and Louisiana, elected public officials are not covered.

Coverage of Personal Injuries Under Worker's Compensation

Once it is determined that a person is covered by worker's compensation, the next question is whether he or she is eligible for benefits for the injury. As previously noted, worker's compensation laws were designed to compensate an employee who sustains a work-related injury without consideration of who was at fault for the injury. The legal test or formula used by all of the jurisdictions to determine whether a worker may receive compensation is that the injury must "arise out of and in the course of employment." All jurisdictions have adopted either identical or similar language.

Type of Injury and Causation

In many early cases under the worker's compensation statutes, courts tended to adhere to the common law principle which conditioned compensability on a physical impact on the body of the injured worker, even though the contact may not have been directly related to the injury which the worker received. For example, two workers could both be deafened by the explosion of a boiler, but only one touched slightly by a piece of flying metal; under the older interpretations of the law, only the worker touched by the metal could be compensated for his or her deafness. Later decisions, however, indicated judicial awareness of inequities arising from a strict adherence to the "physical contact" rule, and courts instead began to condition compensability on convincing evidence of a causal relationship between the injury and the workplace.

Because the statutory language itself is vague and therefore subject to wide judicial latitude in interpretation, the compensability of injuries under state worker's compensation law is best examined in relation to the specific categories of injuries which have developed out of the case law. The extent to which such injuries are recognized as compensable is best understood when the injuries are categorized by their *cause* and *effect*. Compensation was first awarded to claimants with injuries in which the cause and the effect were both physical, i.e., when a physical cause resulted in a physical injury.

More recently, courts have been willing to allow compensation when work-related *mental* causes have resulted in either physical or mental injuries. Thus, for the purposes of discussion, the four major categories of compensable injuries are: 1) *physical-physical injury* (a physical cause resulting in a physical injury); 2) *physical-mental injury* (a physical cause resulting in a mental injury); 3) *mental-physical injury* (a mental cause resulting in a physical injury); and 4) *mental-mental injury* (a mental cause resulting in a mental injury). The reader is cautioned that these categories are purely a result of legal distinctions; they are not intended to represent classifications made outside the legal arena.

Physical-physical injuries. Injuries in the physical-physical category, so long as they meet the other requirements of the statutes, are compensable in all jurisdictions.

According to Larson the trend among the jurisdictions in awarding compensation for physical-physical injuries is toward the adoption of the most liberal view.[15] That is, if a worker was in what later was determined to be a dangerous situation by virtue of his or her employment and was harmed as a result, the injury will be considered work related. The courts in four jurisdictions (Illinois, Missouri, New Mexico, and Utah) have, however, expressly stated that they cannot adopt the view that claimants should receive compensation for any remotely connected injury or attack. In those states there must be a very close connection between the injury and the employment. In a recent New Mexico case a worker finished his shift and was leaving the building in which he worked when he was attacked.[27] It was determined that he was not entitled to benefits because the attack was not technically during work time.

A smaller number of jurisdictions have not rejected the liberal view, but still require a stronger connection between the injury and employment than do those adopting the most liberal view. In these jurisdictions compensation has been awarded for workers attacked by co-workers or other persons. Such compensation has been awarded in Alaska, Arkansas, California, Arizona, Delaware, Florida, Indiana, Kansas, Maine, Maryland, Massachusetts, Minnesota, Nebraska, Nevada, New Hampshire, North Carolina, North Dakota, Ohio, Oregon, Pennsylvania, South Carolina, Tennessee, Vermont, and Virginia.

Physical–mental injuries.   All jurisdictions currently allow compensation for a mental injury resulting from a physical cause. Where a work-related physical cause results in a mental injury based on diagnoses such as traumatic neurosis, hysterial paralysis, or conversion hysteria, the jurisdictions uniformly treat the full disability, including the effects of the mental injury, as compensable. For example, compensation has been awarded for a depressive reaction sustained by an iron worker after a fall from the roof of a building,[11] psychoneurosis following a severe physical reaction to a tetanus shot administered after a dog bite,[3] and a conversion reaction in a claimant whose back was injured in the collapse of a roof.[12]

A preexisting weakness, such as a neurotic tendency, does not bar or lessen the compensation awarded to a worker who suffers a disabling mental injury as a result of a physical cause.[23] The courts generally hold that the employer takes the worker as he or she is, including weaknesses and predispositions. A preexisting condition does, however, make it more difficult for a claimant to establish the requisite degree of causation, since the claimant must prove that the employment aggravated or combined with the preexisting infirmity to produce the disability for which compensation is sought.[15] Moreover, the theory that a traumatic neurosis or similar mental injury is not an "injury" covered by worker's compensation legislation is not a valid ground for denial of compensation.

Mental–physical injuries.   This category of injuries is characterized by those in which a mental or psychological stimulus results in a physical injury. For example, during a consultation and in the presence of the psychiatrist, a patient shot and killed himself. The psychiatrist, although physically untouched, suffered an extremely serious heart attack as a result of the incident and was unable to work for nine months. Like physical–mental injuries, mental–physical injuries are compensable in every jurisdiction (with the single exception of Ohio, discussed below).

Cases within this category can be further subdivided into three groups on the basis of the nature of mental stimulus. The resulting injury in all three groups is of a physical nature, such as a heart attack:

1. *Intense stimulus of short duration.* Cases in this group generally have the most readily apparent causal nexus between the mental stimulus and the physical result.

2. *Intense stimulus of prolonged duration.* These types of cases also have a readily ascertainable "cause" and are typified by *The Matter of Gray Truit*,[8] in which an embassy worker was compensated for a heart attack he suffered as a result of the fear of mob violence directed against the U.S. Embassy in Formosa.

3. *Less intense (i.e., less stressful) stimulus of prolonged duration.* Typical compensable injuries in this category include the stroke and resulting paralysis suffered by a labor arbitrator after 65 days of intense contract negotiations,[9] and the heart attack of an employee who suffered prolonged emotional stress over clerical errors that occurred in his office.[20]

Ohio courts disallow compensation for injuries in the third category, basing their decision upon a peculiar interpretation of the word "injury."[29] Other jurisdictions may also limit recovery to claims in which the moderate mental stimulus is of an "unusual" nature. Under such statutes, compensation is denied when injuries are precipitated by mental stimuli common to the ordinary or everyday stresses of a job.

Mental-mental injuries.   By far the greatest amount of legal confusion surrounds the category of cases in which a mental stimulus results in a mental injury, particularly in those cases where no *specific* blameworthy incident or event can be pin-pointed as the "cause" of the mental injury.

A number of reasons are offered to account for the lack of uniform acceptance of mental–mental injuries as compensable injuries under worker's compensation laws. For example, Render notes that:[21]

in most states there is little or no legislative history to guide courts and most statutes were written before the advent of the psychiatrist or psychologist. Add to these the difficult questions of proof in this kind of case, and the fear of an avalanche of this kind of litigation once the door is opened, and one can readily understand the sharp division of opinion.*

Variations in the language of the worker's compensation statutes also influence the courts' willingness to forego the requirement of some degree of physical contact or impact in cases of mental–mental injuries. A key phrase is the particular statutory definition of "compensable injury." The definitions range from "any work-related change in the human organism,"[14] or an

---

*Reprinted with permission from Render ER: Mental illness as an industrial accident. Tennessee Law Review, 31:299, 1964.

Table 14-2
Compensability of Mental–Mental Injuries[1]

No Case Law on Mental–Mental Injuries	Denying All Mental–Mental Injuries	Compensating at Least Sudden Onset Injuries	Compensating at Least Some Forms of Gradual Onset Mental–Mental Injuries	Compensating Sudden Onset Mental–Mental Injuries, No Case Law on Gradual Onset Mental–Mental Injuries
Alabama	Florida	Arizona	Arizona	Connecticut
Alaska	Georgia	California	California	Illinois
Arkansas	Kansas	Connecticut	District of Columbia	Missouri
Colorado	Louisiana	District of Columbia	Federal System	Virginia
Delaware	Nebraska	Federal System	Hawaii	West Virginia
Idaho	Oklahoma[2]	Hawaii	Kentucky	
Indiana		Illinois	Maine	
Iowa		Kentucky	Massachusetts[6]	
Maryland	Maine	Michigan		
Nevada		Massachusetts	New Jersey	
New Hampshire		Michigan	New York	
New Mexico		Minnesota[3]	Oregon	
Maine	Michigan			
Nevada		Massachusetts	New Jersey	
North Carolina		Mississippi[3]	Pennsylvania	
North Dakota		Missouri	Tennessee	

204

Rhode Island	Montana[3]	Wisconsin
South Carolina	New Jersey	
South Dakota	New York	
Utah	Ohio[3]	
Vermont	Oregon	
Washington	Pennsylvania	
Wyoming	Tennessee	
	Texas[4]	
	Virginia	
	West Virginia[5]	
	Wisconsin	

---

[1] This categorization by state may be overbroad because the actual case relied on for the categorization may be an appellate decision and hence appealable in a higher court and/or binding in only some jurisdictions within the state. However, unless otherwise indicated, the appellate decisions are uniformly for or against compensability in any one category.

[2] In Georgia, such injuries may, however, be compensable "occupational diseases." See, Sawyer v. Pacific Indemnity Co., 141 Ga. App. 298, 233 S.E.2d 229 (1977).

[3] The case law in these states denied compensation in some types of gradual onset mental–mental injury cases, and did not rule on sudden onset claims. However, the grounds for refusal would seem to allow sudden onset claims.

[4] The Texas Courts, however, may be willing to entertain what would normally be classed as a gradual onset claim if the worker can point to one specific incident which functioned as the "straw that broke the camel's back." See, Gloor v. U.S. Fire Insurance Co., 457 S.W.3d 925 (Tex. Crim. 1970).

[5] West Virginia case law is not directly on point. However, in Montgomery v. State Compensation Commissioner, 116 W. Va. 44, 178 S.E. 425 (1935), there are indications that sudden onset injuries would be compensable. The case involved a coal miner who suffered either a physical or mental injury as a result of being lost in a coal mine for seven days. The opinion did not clearly indicate whether the injury was a purely mental one, but stated that the injury was covered if it was attributable to a specific event arising out of employment.

[6] Because of other legal doctrines, compensation in gradual onset cases is limited to circumstances where the claimant can show a series of specific incidents occurring over a relatively short period of time. See, Albanese's Case, 389 N.E.2d 83 (1979).

"accidental injury arising out of or in the course of employment."[10] to an "injury by violence to the physical structure of the body."[21] The last definition is the most restrictive; yet even this type of language has not prevented some courts from compensating mental–mental injuries.

Although 21 jurisdictions have no case law on the compensability of mental–mental injuries, the states which do can generally be divided into three major groups, including those which: 1) deny compensation for all mental–mental claims; 2) compensate for sudden onset claims; and 3) compensate for gradual onset claims. Table 14-2 shows the distribution of states into these categories.

1. *Denying all mental–mental claims.*   Of the 31 jurisdictions with case law on the subject, only six specifically rule out compensation for *both* gradual and sudden onset mental injuries. The courts in these cases generally argue that the statutory definition of "accident" or "injury" does not encompass injuries with no physical component.

2. *Allowing claims for sudden onset.*   The remaining 25 jurisdictions allow compensation for mental–mental injuries of sudden onset. Courts recognizing the right to compensation when the employee suffers a mental injury as a result of a sudden, work-related stimulus generally reason that compensability should result from the disabling effect on the worker, not from the nature of the injury itself or its cause. In these jurisdictions, courts will award compensation in sudden onset mental injury cases when they find that: 1) the claimant is disabled by an injury; and 2) the injury was caused by the employment.

3. *Allowing for gradual onset.*   The 15 jurisdictions awarding compensation of gradual onset mental injuries are a subset of those 25 allowing sudden onset claims (see Table 14-2). While six of these jurisdictions currently treat gradual and sudden onset mental injuries the same (California, the District of Columbia, Hawaii, Kentucky, Michigan, and the federal system), the others have placed additional conditions on recovery in cases of gradual onset. In these, the work-related stress may have to be proven to be: 1) a material contributing factor, 2) a substantial contributing cause, 3) the predominating cause of the injury, or 4) in Oregon, the sole explanation of the injury (Oregon courts require that no other substantially similar causes exist in the claimant's nonwork environment). Several jurisdictions use a combination of all or some of these limitations.

CONCLUSION

There is little doubt that, given fulfillment of the applicable requirements, a mental health worker would be compensated for the *physical* injuries sustained as a result of an assault and/or battery by a patient. It is not clear, however, that all jurisdictions would compensate the mental health worker for *mental* injuries arising out of the same events; nor is it clear that a mental health worker could receive compensation for mental injuries sustained as a result of an assault or otherwise stressful employment conditions in a mental health facility. The right to compensation in these latter cases would depend solely on the statutory language and case law interpretation of each jurisdiction. For example, as discussed above, some courts have been unwilling to deny such claimants compensation, even in the face of restrictively worded statutes. However, since these courts generally are bound by the language of the statutues, they must often devote considerable attention to "otherwise unnecessary statutory construction" in order to compensate the mentally injured claimant.[27]

While the statutory insistence on the "physical" presents problems for both the claimant and the worker's compensation system, many legislatures and courts have neither advocated nor implemented change. Several factors can be identified which have contributed to this legal lag. First, both courts and legislatures are well aware that mental injury claims involve establishing what appears to the layperson to be an intangible injury. When faced with a compensation scheme which is pregnant with possibilities for malingering, they may hesitate to deem an entire class of injuries compensible.

Second, clinical research indicates that, at present, very few individual factors can be isolated as the sole precipitators of mental disabilities. At best such research has identified some factors which may increase the *likelihood* (or the probability) that a mental disability will result.[27] Thus, the disabled worker who must prove a causal connection between a mental disability and the workplace simply may not have the means to do so. Consider, for example, the mental health professional who suffers a "nervous breakdown" under objectively stressful work conditions. The worker has almost certainly also experienced nonemployment related stress, but how does the court determine which source of stress was the "real" or "major" cause of the mental injury? The problem of proof in this example is compounded when the claimant is especially sensitive to stress and suffers a mental injury under working conditions which the average person would not find stressful. Even if the court is philosophically willing to compensate the "eggshell" claimant, and accepts the injury as bona fide, the claimant in most jurisdictions must still prove the work connection; no mean feat considering the absence of evidence of an objectively stressful work environment.

Until research develops accurate techniques for identifying malingering in compensation cases and delineates the relationship between job pressures and mental injuries, and until the legal community modifies the worker's compensation system to take account of the multiple causation of mental injuries more adequately, courts and legislatures will continue to make compensation decisions that are based not on the actual presence or absence of a work connection, but rather on artificial causation criteria, outright bans on compensation for gradual onset mental injuries, or legal allocations of the burden of proving work connection. For example, at least one court[7] solved the issue of work connection by awarding compensation to a worker whose mental injury was established but whose work connection was established by nothing more than the claimant's subjective belief that the work situation caused his injury. The Michigan legislature, presumably reacting to this solution, narrowed the class of compensible injury by requiring that the injury "arise out of actual events of employment rather than unfounded perceptions thereof."[25]

In effect, the courts must steer an uncharted course between the hazard of assuming the work connection unless the employer can prove otherwise (and thus possibly burdening the system with payments for malingering and nonwork-related injuries) and the equally hazardous use of arbitrary exclusion criteria (and instead subjecting the genuinely disabled worker to potentially destructive financial hardship). Depending on the mechanics of the compensation system, either the employer or the employee is shortchanged.

Equity to the employer, the taxpayer and the worker, as well as administrative considerations demand greatly increased accuracy for the criteria and the standards of proof used to establish the injury and the work connection.[16] These legal standards and criteria will be impossible to set, however, until the nature of the relationships between work-related stress and the myriad types of mental injuries are better understood by mental health professionals, and until that understanding is disseminated to the decision makers within the legal system. Once this goal is achieved it should result in a law that sensibly recognizes the sole issues of injury and work-related causation, without recourse to the artificial and unnecessarily cumbersome classifications of physical and mental injuries.

But even if the mental health professional could qualify for workers compensation for all work-related injuries, would the compensation be sufficient? Unfortunately, the answer is no. Although workers compensation does cover the cost of rehabilitation for the immediate physical and/or mental affects of an injury it does not cover the income lost as a result of an injured mental health professional's inability to work. Thus, further research must identify other alternatives that mental health professionals can use to cover more of the true costs of an injury.

An alternative that should be explored is that of a civil suit in cases of assault and/or battery. Civil prosecution has the distinct advantage of allowing the recovery of all expenses including lost income resulting from the injury. As with all other civil claims, however, in the case of an assault and/or battery by a mental patient, there are numerous elements to the offenses which may be difficult to prove. In addition, even if the mental health professional prevails in the court, it is unlikely that a patient in a state institution would have the resources necessary to pay the damage judgment. Finally, there is one alternative—professional disability insurance—which is outside the realm of legal remedies, that may provide the mental health professional with more appropriate coverage both for injuries and the indirect costs associated with them. Disability insurance coverage may be purchased independently by the professional, or a provision for such coverage may be negotiated for inclusion in the professional's employment contract. The applicability and appropriateness of these and other alternative to worker's compensation protection need to be explored in greater depth.

REFERENCES

1. Armstrong B: Conference report: Handling the violent patient in the hospital. Hosp Community Psychiatry 29:463–467, 1978
2. Bernstein HA: Survey of threats and assaults directed toward psychotherapists. Am J Psychother 35:542–549, 1981
3. City of Austin v. Crook, 162 Tex. 189, 346 S.W.2d 115 (1961)
4. Climent C, Ervin F: Historical data in the evaluation of violent subjects. Arch Gen Psychiatry 27:621–624, 1972
5. Cornfield R, Fielding S: Impact of the threatening patient on ward communications. Am J Psychiatry 137:616–619, 1980
6. Duckworth ME: Injuries arising out of and in the course of the employment. Drake Law Review 30:861–871, 1981
7. Deziel v. Difco Laboratories Inc., 403 Mich. 1, 268 N.W.3d 1 (1978)
8. Employee Compensation Appeals Board, Doc. No. 61-131, May 11, 1961.
9. Fireman's Fund v. Industrial Accident Commission, 39 Cal. 2d 831, 250 P.2d 148 (1952)
10. Florida Statutes Annotated, § 440.02
11. Gunnerson v. Kansas City Structural Steel, 535 S.W.2d 585 (1976)
12. International Yarn Corporation v. Carson, 541 S.W.2d 150 (1976)
13. Kalogerakis MG: The assaultive psychiatric patient. Psychiatric Q 45:372–381, 1971
14. Kansas Revised Statutes, § 342.004 *et seq*
15. Larson A: The Law of Workmen's Compensation. New York: Matthew Bender, 1978
16. Ledue J, Mulyar LE, McCarthy K: Cumulative injury or disease claims: An attempt to define employers' liability for worker's compensation. Am J Law Med 6:1–28, 1980
17. Lion JR: Evaluation and Management of the Violent Patient. Springfield, Illinois, Charles C. Thomas, 1972
18. Lion JR, Pasternak SA: Countertransference reactions to violent patients. Am J Psychiatry 130:207–210, 1973
19. Lion JR, Snyder W, Merrill GL: Underreporting of assaults on staff in a state hospital. Hosp Community Psychiatry 33:497–498, 1981
20. Little v. Korber & Co., 71 N.M. 294, 378 P.2d 119 (1963)
21. Louisiana Revised Statutes Annotated, § 23:1021

22. Madden DJ, Lion JR, Penna MW: Assaults on psychiatrists by patients. Am J Psychiatry 133:422–425, 1976
23. Meador v. Industrial Commission, 2 Ariz. App. 382, 409 P.2d 302 (1966)
24. Meiners R: Victim Compensation. Lexington, Massachusetts, Lexington Books, 1978
25. Michigan Code of Law, § 418-301 (Amended 1980)
26. Morse SJ: Crazy behavior, morals and science: An analysis of mental health law. South Cal Law Rev 51:527–654, 1978
27. Mussoff J: Determining the compensability of mental disabilities under worker's compensation. South Cal Law Rev 55:193–253, 1981
28. (New Mexico) 91 N.M. 788, 581 P.2d 128 (1978)
29. (Ohio) 160 Ohio 1, 113 N.E. 2d 81 (1953)
30. Prosser W: Law of Torts: Handbook of the Law of Torts. St. Paul, Minnesota, West, 1971
31. Render ER: Mental illness as an industrial accident. Tenn Law Rev 31:288Ç299, 1964
32. Schwarz MB, Greenfield GP: Charging a patient with assault on a nurse on a psychiatric unit. Can Psychiatr Assoc J 23:197–200, 1978
33. Skodal A, Karasu T: Emergency psychiatry and the assaultive patient. Am J Psychiatry 135:202–204, 1978
34. Tardiff KJ: A survey of psychiatrists in Boston and their work with violent patients. Am J Psychiatry, 131:1008–1011, 1974
35. Tardiff KJ, Sweillam A: Factors related to increased risk of assaultive behavior in suicidal patients. Acta Psychiatr Scand 62:63–68, 1980
36. Whitman RM, Armao BB, Dent OB: Assault on the therapist. Am J Psychiatry 133:426–429, 1976

PART III

Management

Denis J. Madden

15

Recognition and Prevention of Violence in Psychiatric Facilities

All facilities that treat psychiatric patients have "quiet rooms" and "seclusion rooms." The justification for such rooms is that if a patient begins to act out and presents a problem for ward personnel and other patients the patient will more easily regain control by being made to be quiet and secluded from adverse stimuli. There are also some facilities that have special "security areas" for more assaultive and dangerous patients. These patients are recognized to need closer scrutiny with regard to safety factors. While one can not object to such procedures, they do raise the interesting question of who is being protected. It is also questionable whether or not seclusion or segregation are good treatment. Such procedures place much of the treatment burden directly on the patient. It is a known fact that patients placed in seclusion also present suicide risks.[1]

The segregation of violent patients may well reflect our hesitancy to address all of the issues that are associated with violent behavior. Violence has not been understood because it is most often responded to by avoidance, ambivalence, denial, and attempts to snuff it out.[5] A lack of understanding of violent individuals make us more fearful and makes them appear to be more threatening.

This chapter attempts to offer some understanding of the issue of violence in facilities by examining the patients who present risk factors, personnel who might be at risk of being assaulted, and facilities themselves that might be at greater risk for such behavior. Statistical results of controlled studies will not be presented. Such studies are rare and often present data on a specific aspect of violence that presupposes a more general understanding of this phenomenon. This chapter presents material intended to aid mental health professionals in making an appropriate personal response to the kinds of assaultive behavior already described in the previous chapters.

CHARACTERISTICS OF THE VIOLENT PATIENT

Violence does not occur in a vacuum, and it is multivariate.[7] There are many reasons for assaultive acts: the sight of a policeman might be reassuring for most persons but for some it can be threatening; a crowd might not be threatening for most persons but for some it is. While we are not able at this time to describe well all of the factors that lead to violent behavior, we do have some understanding of the dynamics involved and the themes repeated in the lives of such persons.[8]

Those who most frequently respond in an assaultive manner are usually young. They are often aged between approximately 18–33 years. They are individuals who have been victimized themselves, either physically or psychologically. They are persons who have not been able to made adequate adjustments in forming relationships, holding jobs, or persevering in education.[10] They have histories of violent responses.[6] Some have organic brain disorders that make it difficult for them to understand and to delay action.[12] Some are given to substance abuse and some have had frequent contact with social agencies including courts. They are individuals not given to insight and do not as a rule display the ability to empathize or to be altruistic.

Violent individuals often have deprived backgrounds. While some attention has been paid to the effects of material deprivation, less has been given to the internal deprivation of persons who have not learned life skills. Such deprivation is like living in a foreign country where the individual does not know the language or customs and is looked on with suspicion. This leads to a defensive posture often manifested by hypervigilance.

Trust is one of the basic life-skills that violent individuals have not mastered.[2] This aspect of the personality is developed early in life. If it is not, only with great difficulty can any knowledge be hoped for in this area. Violent persons do not trust others because they do not trust themselves. Violent individuals have been unsuccessful and thus have not been encouraged to go a little further in this area. They need to defend themselves from getting too close and being hurt. Violent persons are very vulnerable and their best defense is to be assaultive and take no chances.

It is often difficult for persons working with violent persons to see them as weak because they present such a powerful facade. Observation of their behavior, however, reveals the pathetic quality of their stance. Such individuals have an inner sense of weakness but lack understanding of true weakness. Violent patients have come to believe that if they appear strong they might be strong and not have to face what is most threatening to them. They intend to impress others with their own importance and that they are to be taken seriously; they most often do this through violent behavior.

The Violent Patient in Treatment

Modifying the behavior of a violent individual is an arduous task. It depends on the patient's motivation to change what may have become a life-long response pattern.[15] Most violent individuals are coerced into treatment. This coercion is a neutral event that can help or even worsen the situation.[9] However, even the patient coerced into treatment is provided a time to relearn.

Violent patients must learn to establish more consistency in their lives and this learning can only occur when their treatment is reasonably consistent. Consistency depends on the honest willingness of those most concerned with the violent individual to work toward some resolution of this problem.

Persons with histories of violent behavior are not honest or trustworthy. Any treatment that is not honest therefore is doomed to failure from the start. Honesty is not always easy and there are times when confusion exists about whether one can be completely honest with an assaultive patient.[13]

Therapists generally think that it may not be beneficial to the process to let a patient know how the behavior of the patient effects the therapist. Therefore, when the patient's behavior is threatening the therapist attempts to hide his or her reaction. However, patients should be told when they are threatening, frightening or make the therapist angry. This can be communicated to the patient without arguing or threatening; such patients should be informed of the reaction he or she illicits in order to increase self-awareness of his or her own behavior.

Patients who are labile and unable to control themselves are frightening. Experienced clinicians respect this feeling and take the necessary means to protect themselves and the patient. It may be necessary to have support personnel in the area when working with such individuals. Patients usually are aware of the presence of these persons and should be told why they are there. Most clinicians are not skilled in managing physical confrontation, and their strength lies in their ability to communicate verbally. Most violent patients are more skilled at physical confrontation than verbal exchange, and it is not helpful to deny this. If the therapist feels safe he or she is better able to help the patient learn new means of relating to others.[5]

Some clinicians believe that informing the patient that he or she will need hospitalization creates danger of further exciting the patient. When a patient must be moved to another more secure hospital or a more secure area within a given facility, the patient also is at risk for excitability. However, providing the patient the opportunity to be more controlled is helpful even when a more secure environment is required. Patients seek to be controlled by others, and they manifest this by attempting to control others with their behavior. Providing a secure environment for these patients is directly related to the therapeutic limit setting.

There is greater risk of assault when there is inconsistent limit setting. A rigid demand for conformity and a lax attitude toward this assaultive group of patients signals them that they are going to have difficulty learning balance in that particular setting. Therapists must keep in mind that they are dealing with an impulsive group of individuals who are in treatment because they have not been able to effectively control their impulses. This is demanding work because the therapist and the setting will be tested and tried repeatedly. Consistency and time are the crucial elements in this process. Historically, teachers have made demands on their students that demand a certain discipline. This external pressure is used to aid in establishing of internal principles that otherwise would not emerge.

Therapists occasionally will also influence the degree of freedom that the patient will have when he or she is not in the direct care of the therapist. In some settings, such as prisons or security hospitals, the therapist plays an important role in making decisions about release or type of release, and then this information—including whether case records will be reviewed—must be made known to the patient.[13] Patients who have not been dealt with honestly on all levels will not respond honestly to therapists. This means that they will attempt to "con" the therapist and the setting. An example of this follows.

Case Study 15-1

A 27-year-old white male was hospitalized for violent behavior. His history of assaultiveness included breaking furniture within his home and assaulting his wife on many occasions. He also had attempted suicide on several occasions. Staff members knew his history and observed him with a certain degree of fear. After a relatively short period of time this man became a model patient on the ward. He participated actively in group sessions, appeared to demonstrate insight into the nature of his problem and seemed to have good judgement with regard to plans for the future. This rather tough individual sat in the day room watching television and doing needle point. In addition to or as a part of his problem with violence, he also had problems with substance abuse. This patient presented no management problems and was soon considered for release. A consultant from a specialized clinic that deals with violent individuals alerted the staff that the patient might not be as calm as he appeared. Staff regarded this observation was as perhaps being true in principle, that is, violent individuals do not change overnight, but was not recognized as having much validity with regard to this particular individual. The patient was released from the hospital and after a short period had to return again for inability to control violent impulses.

Although the prediction of future violent behavior is not always easy, the patient with a history of violent behavior who apparently and abruptly changes this mode of interaction should be held suspect. Clinicians must pay close attention to their own feelings when working with violent patients; at times clinical intuition may be the most important consideration and may even outweigh observed behavior.[4] The impact of denial is explored in the following discussions.

Violent patients are most prone to use the defense mechanism of denial. They will deny they have a problem with assaultiveness or that it is as serious as others perceive it. This denial is also manifest when they state that they do not care what happens to them. This reaction may be expressed after being told that they must be secluded or moved to a more secure setting. Here the denial serves, among other things, as a defense for a fragile ego that is sensitive to any form of rejection. Persons who do not care what others say about them or do to them display a disregard for relatedness and intimacy. While this defense should not be dismantled too quickly, an offering should be made to the patient to begin to entertain alternate views especially regarding intimacy.

Violent patients usually have not been able to maintain relations with others. In treatment they will have difficulty engaging in the intimate process of psychotherapy. Therapists and staff moving too quickly in this area can easily threaten a patient and such behavior can be as provocative as any other form of confrontation. Therapy is indeed a confrontation at a level at which the patient is ill equipped to respond. Violent patients do not view themselves as being good or as being worthy of or even capable of being liked by others. This attitude needs to be respected because such respect acknowledges the patient's feelings and offers the opportunity for growth.

Violent patients need to learn to be more tolerant, flexible, able to live with a certain amount of ambiguity, and, more immediately, able to delay. If the violent person is viewed as a highly charged individual one is better equipped to deal effectively with him. The violent individual often quickly responds to insults—real or imagined—with that most primitive of responses, attack. This quick response set must be undone. One method employed is group psycho-therapy where the patient learns that "just talking" does help.[6] Within the group an individual can learn through social constraint to delay physical attack and later even verbal assault. An example of this process follows.

Case Study 15-2

One group member had a history of assaultive behavior, including street fights, bar-room brawls, and fights with employers. As a result this individual had great difficulty holding a job. He was viewed by the group leaders as being easily insulted, quite sensitive, and having a brittle self-image. He responded to any insult by engaging in fights.

The patient had just recently lost a job as a warehouseman. His main task had been to keep the loading area clean. In one group session, role playing focussed on the patient's former job. Some of the group members served as fellow employees and one of the group leaders acted as the platform manager. The "platform manager" told the patient to be very careful of the way he swept the platform because there seemed to be a lot of debris. This was said in a neutral manner and a conscious attempt was made not to be overly critical. The patient nevertheless ceased participating in this role playing and began a verbal attack on the therapist. He accused the therapist of being overly critical of him as an individual and of not liking him. He continued to express distress at not being helped more in the group and attributed this to the lack of concern on the part of the therapist. The patient's harangue centered on group material and not on the role playing.

This case demonstrates how difficult it is to change ingrained response patterns. Patients who have a lifelong history of a specific pattern perception do not easily learn to listen and to try to understand what another individual is really saying to them. This role playing also demonstrated however that the patient was able to delay physical attack, something that he had not demonstrated in the past, and was now able to express his feelings of anger verbally.

It is important for violent patients to have a safe forum for expressing anger.[14] This often is not possible outside the hospital or therapy because too often verbal attacks have led to physical assaults and those closest to the patient become fearful that the patient's expressions of anger once again will result in violence. The absence of expressions of anger in a session or a hospital may be a sign that therapy is not progressing.

When patients express anger they may categorize staff and therapists as being "good" or "bad." These patients seem unable to accept the fact that there is a certain amount of good and bad in most individuals. They feel that certain "bad" staff members refuse to meet any of their demands while other "good" staff are more sympathetic. Violent patients also have difficulty perceiving and accepting both good and bad within themselves, and they want to free themselves from this internal dilemma. Demanding instant gratification is one mode of escape. Again, on a rather primitive level, they want to be worthwhile and demand to be told that they are and treated as though they are worthwhile. This leads them to demand instant gratification. They demand medicine to help them sleep, remain calm, control their feelings, and, essentially, remove their pain. They demand privileges and trust before having demonstrated that they can effectively regulate their own behavior. They exhibit an unreasonable demand to be cured immediately and to be compensated by the therapist for all of the deprivations of the past. This plea for resolution of internal strife can be seen as an expression of the healthier part of the person.

The healthier part pushes to recognition but the individual does not yet know how to be recognized. Many violent patients feel that through violent behavior they will be recognized as being important.

Violent patients can be helped to modulate their behavior in more appropriate ways by therapists and in hospitals. Therapists may, however, through lack of experience or concern add to the problems and at times even provoke violent behavior on the part of their patients.

THE THERAPIST TREATING VIOLENT PATIENTS

While violent patients are recognized as having certain propensities for violent behavior, the question of whether or not therapists have similar propensities has not been researched. Since violence does not occur in a vacuum and since therapists often have close relationships with their patients, we should be concerned over whether or not therapists overtly or covertly provoke violent behavior in their patients.

A small study of this question surveyed 115 full and part-time psychiatrists at a University hospital.[11] This group represented a variety of clinical and administrative positions including private practice, mental health clinics, medical school appointments, forensic and prison settings, and state hospital positions. Psychiatrists were asked whether or not they had, in the course of their career, ever been assaulted by patients and then further questions were asked regarding the nature and quality of the assaults. Of the 115 psychiatrists sampled, 48 responded that they had been assaulted and the total number of assaults was 68. Most psychiatrists who were assaulted by patients were attacked when they were in the early stages of training. The majority of the patients who assaulted were in active treatment with the particular therapist assaulted.

In reviews of incident reports on the assaults, and in retrospectively examining these assaults with the therapists, most of the therapists stated that they could have anticipated the assault, and 53 percent felt that they had acted in a provocative manner. Some therapists felt that they had made comments or interpretations in the course of therapy that were unfavorably received by the patients and perhaps were untimely. Among the reasons given for the assaults were refusing to meet a patient's request, forcing patients to take medication, setting too many limits, not setting enough limits, transference reactions, homosexual panic, and the material being dealt with in therapy. Many therapists felt, at least in retrospect, that they had been at times too insistent that a patient confront upsetting material. Such therapists felt that the incident might not have occurred if they had backed off. Several therapists reported quite candidly that they did not particularly like the patient who assaulted them and might have projected this feeling to the patient. Therapists also felt that inexperience and fear of patients, which at times was translated into an omnipotent facade, might trigger an assault. One senior psychiatrist said that it had been his experience that residents who allowed patients to act out in therapy sessions were most frequently assaulted. Some of the clinicians felt that therapists sometimes act in a seductive manner that projects an unconscious expectation that an assault will occur or sometimes attempt to veil an underlying hostility with kindness, all of which can lead the patient to assault the therapist.

Some clinicians work in what might be deemed high-risk settings, such as prisons, forensic units of state hospitals, or emergency rooms. A number of clinicians who work in such settings see the danger of being assaulted as part of working in such settings. Although the risk may be higher in such settings, clinicians must be aware that their expectancy also plays a role in whether or not they will be assaulted. There is indeed a greater need for staff vigilance in recognizing that they work with assaultive individuals. This does not mean that assaultive behavior should be regarded as commonplace or should be expected; such an attitude can easily be translated by patients to mean that violence is not serious.

Patients can be told directly what sort of behavior will or will not be tolerated. For example, one maximum security state hospital, where the author has consulted, has patients who are considered too dangerous to be treated in the other state hospitals. Individuals often are brought there from the correctional system because they were considered too disruptive to be housed even in a maximum security prison. When individuals are admitted to this facility, they are evaluated and informed of the hospital's rules and regulations. The security personnel are unarmed and there are no gun turrets. The number of assaults and "escapes" from this setting is very small. The patient is told on arrival that such behavior is not tolerated, and the effectiveness of such a stance is borne out by the low incidence of assaults.

Denial plays a heavy role in both the ways clinicians deal with patients who might be assaultive and in their recollection of assaults. An example of the use of denial follows.

Case Study 15-3

A clinician in private practice had been treating a patient who had severe problems in controlling his temper. This patient began to leave threatening statements on the clinician's answering service. These threats were directed not only against the clinician but against his family as well. The patient informed the therapist that he was aware of where the therapist's family shopped, went to school, and so on. Despite these direct threats the therapist did not bring up this matter while meeting with the patient.

Denial veils fear and anger. This anger may be directed toward the patient or at times toward other staff. In hospital settings staff may be angry with each other, and when this anger is not dealt with it may be allowed to be played out through the patients. There have been instances when a particular staff member was not well liked by other staff. Staff may then "allow" the patients of this therapist to fail, to act out, as a means of getting back at the clinician. This places the staff, as well as the patients, at greater risk.

As mentioned previously, unexpressed anger in the assaultive patient increases the risk that the patient will assault. Similarly, unexpressed anger in the clinician increases the risk that the clinician will be assaulted. Unexpressed anger leads to denial, anxiety, and projection. These responses increase the likelihood that a therapist will be assaulted. An ambiance of anger needs some resolution. If the resolution is not provided through the use of appropriate psychotherapy, it will most likely occur through less appropriate means.

THE TREATMENT SETTING

Changes must be made in some of our treatment settings so that the assaultive patient will learn to better negotiate with life's demands. External and internal approaches need to be used so that the patient may begin to exercise internal control and better modulate his own external environment.

It is not always easy to discern which institutions are at greatest risk for violence. The name or stated function of the facility more correctly describes the intended function than it describes daily activities within the setting. Denial impedes institutional effectiveness in meeting stated goals and reasons for existence. Institutions practice denial in two major ways: first, they deny that the patients are as assaultive as careful study would show them to be, and second, they deny dysfunction careful scrutiny would reveal within the system. In the first form of denial, assaultive incidents are underreported and poorly documented. Occasionally, a particular therapist or a particular ward may have more assaults and there is hesitancy to examine this important piece of data.

In the second form of denial, the assaultive behavior of patients is recognized, but no reflective examination is made of the possible causes of such behavior. Two examples of this second form of denial follow:

Case Study 15-4

A state hospital sought consultation from clinicians who had experience in working with violent patients because, according to the hospital, "there had been an outbreak of violence in the facility." The staff and administration felt that they needed to learn how to deal more effectively with this problem. On the first day the consultants arrived at the hospital, they read in the local newspaper that several staff members were under investigation for charges of physical and sexual assault against some of the patients. This information had not been given to the consultants by the administration in the initial request for the consultation. A walking tour of the hospital reveals obvious areas of concern, such as a ward where all of the patients beds were pushed into one small area while repairs were being made in another area. One ward administrator questioned a request to review some of the charts, asking why such a review was necessary; "what are you looking for anyway." In meetings with staff the consultants became aware of disharmony among staff. This disharmony appeared to exist on all levels within the hospital, and there was also a noted disharmony between the hospital administrators and the state officials and legislators.

Obvious factors of poor treatment practice and staff problems were not viewed by this institution as being in anyway related to the disruptive behavior of the patients.

The state of the art in psychiatry is such that violent incidents often are unexplainable. There are times, however, that such acts are closely related to other factors over which clinicians and staff could exercise more control. There are times when patients appear to "go sour" when the clinician's personal life is in upheaval. For example, one clinician known to the author was in the process of separating from his wife. In the course of this separation three of that clinician's patients attempted suicide. Although an experienced clinician, he failed to recognize any connection between what was going on in his own life and the acts of his patients. He viewed their acts as "just one more thing that had gone wrong" in his life.

Human beings indeed affect one another. There may or may not be a direct connection between the assaultive acts of patients and the personal problems of clinicians or institutional problems, but there is a need to honestly examine the possibility that there might be a link between the two.

University or training facilities must be aware of the level of experience of its staff. Problematic patients admitted at the beginning of a psychiatry rotation need to be watched by the more experienced staff members. Clinicians in private practice are aware of this issue when deciding where to admit a patient, and training facilities must be equally sensitive.

It is recognized that individuals who are overcontrolled or undercontrolled can present a greater risk of being assaultive. This is also true for clinicians and for institutions. Fear, anger, and anxiety can lead to assaultive behavior on all levels. It can happen that our patients are responding more to overcontrol or lack of control in the institution than to these same qualities within themselves.

It has been known since the early 1900s that the economy of a nation also affects the crimerate and homicide rate. Economic factors within institutions also play a role in assaultive behavior. Poor physical facilities, understaffing or poorly trained staff play a role in assaultive behavior. A poorly trained staff does not feel safe, they do not know what to do, and do not have confidence in themselves and other staff members for their own safety. In some facilities each incident seems to be treated as a new event and no set of established procedures are followed. Hospital settings that do not have adequate space for patients and places for staff to meet and unwind make for difficult working conditions and can be seen as playing a role in the assaultive behavior of patients. Assaultive patients who have not yet learned through experience that "just talking" does help and are more accustomed to physical activity need to have space and time to engage in physical activity that will help to displace inner tensions. Unless these opportunities are provided, the patient is forced to ruminate over his life and there will be little hope of making therapeutic interventions in this thought process.

REFERENCES

1. Benesohn HS, Resnik HL: "Suicide proofing" a psychiatric unit. Am J Psychother 27:204–212, 1973
2. Carney FL: Treatment of the aggressive patient, in Madden DJ, Lion JR (eds): Rate, Hate, Assault, and Other Forms of Violence. New York, Spectrum, 1976
3. Kozol HO, Boucher RJ, Garofalo RF: The diagnosis and treatment of dangerousness. Crime Delinquency 18:371–392, 1972
4. Kozol H: The diagnosis of dangerousness, in Pasternack SA (ed): Violence and Victims. New York, Spectrum, 1975
5. Lion JR: Evaluation and Management of the Violent Patient. Springfield, Ill, Charles C. Thomas, 1972
6. Lion JR, Christopher RL, Madden DJ: A group approach with violent patients. Int J Group Psychother 27:67–74, 1977
7. Lion JR, Madden DJ: Management of the violent patient, in Balis GU, Wurmser L, McDaniel E, et al. (eds): Psychiatric Problems in Medical Practice, vol. 6. Boston, Butterworth, 1978
8. Madden DJ: Psychological approaches to violence, in Madden DJ, Lion JR (eds): Rage, Hate, Assault, and Other Forms of Violence. New York, Spectrum, 1976
9. Madden DJ: Voluntary and involuntary treatment of aggressive patients. Am J Psychiatry 134:553–555, 1977
10. Madden DJ, Lion JR: Clinical management of aggression, in Brain PF, Benton D (eds): Multidisciplinary Approaches to Aggression Research. Elsevier, Holland, Biomedical Press, 1981
11. Madden DJ, Lion JR, Penna M: Assaults on psychiatrists by patients. Am J Psychiatry 133:422–425, 1976
12. Monroe R: Episodic Behavioral Disorders. Cambridge, Harvard University Press, 1970
13. Roth LH: Correctional psychiatry, in Curran WJ, McGarry AL, Petty CS (eds): Modern Legal Medicine, Psychiatry, and Forensic Sciences. Philadelphia, F. A. Davis 1980
14. Rothenberg A: On anger, in Pasternack SA (ed): Violence and Victims. New York, Spectrum, 1975
15. Schmideberg J: Re-evaluating the concept of "rehabilitation" and "punishment". Int J Offender Therapy 12:25–27, 1968

Mary Ellen Kronberg

16

Nursing Interventions in the Management of the Assaultive Patient

Nursing staff are with patients throughout hospitalization and therefore can observe a patient's routine behavior and assess any deviations from it. This contact also exposes nurses to the possibility of assault, since assaultive behavior often is displayed by patients on an inpatient psychiatric unit.

When nurses enter employment they should be informed that the management of assaultive behavior is included in their job description. In virtually every hospital the hospital's policies and procedures for dealing with assaultive behavior are taught during the orientation program. All nursing staff are expected to know relevant policy and to be able to intervene in assaultive situations when emergencies arise. Staff training programs are discussed by Penningroth as one aspect of an organizational policy to control violence. That organizational policy also includes an accurate method of reporting and an impartial system for reviewing violent incidents.[4] He states it is the organization's responsibility to formulate and communicate this policy and gives several basic assumptions necessary to effect it:

- All staff who accept employment in a mental health facility also accept an obligation to control violence.
- When the violence inflicts injury to the self or others, it must be controlled immediately, regardless of personal risk. If only property is being destroyed, one can wait until assistance arrives to control the violence.
- The organization will support the staff when the control of violence is carried out according to policy. The policy should be reviewed, updated, and revised as necessary to provide for quality patient care.[4]

Nurses need to be specially trained to work with assaultive behavior, but they are not specially salaried, since dealing with assaultive behavior is one of their accepted duties. If, however, a nurse is hired to deal only with violent patients, as on a specialty team, then salary compensation should be made.

Health care professionals must work as a team when dealing with assaultive behavior. Nurses, for example, have the skill and front-line experience necessary to determine the need for emergency seclusion and/or restraint. Psychiatric aides and technicians also are involved and must react quickly. There may be time to contact a physician for seclusion room and/or restraint orders, yet often the patient's assaultive behavior needs to be dealt with immediately. A decision usually can not be postponed until a physician is called and arrives on the unit to deal with the situation. In these cases the nurse makes the decision to seclude or restrain the patient, takes the action, notifies the physician and communicates the salient facts, and documents the activity in the patient record. The physician should support the nursing staff by giving covering orders for this and anticipated future interventions.

POTENTIALLY VIOLENT SITUATIONS

Many health care professionals agree that assaultive behavior can result from fear, anger, self-destructive activity, psychosis, antisocial activity, and organic states. Nursing staff should become familiar with all of these in order to develop intervention techniques.

Assaultive behavior associated with fear may occur for several different reasons. The individual may perceive a threat to self-image or self-esteem. The patient often fears an attack by other patients or staff. These fears may be based on real or imagined danger. Anxiety associated with change such as admission, transfer, or impending discharge frequently causes fear in individuals. A fearful individual may wish to escape from the ward. Conversely, assaultive behavior may result when the patient realizes he or she will have to remain on the unit.

Physical or verbal assaultive behavior may result from anger. Anger often arises from depression or psychotic symptoms such as paranoia. Individuals with impulse control problems, such as personality disorders or those with primitive emotional make-up, may also express their anger through assaultive behavior. Self-destructive activity also may be a release for anger, and self-destructive individuals can become assaultive when they are not allowed to harm themselves.

Individuals having a functional psychosis may display assaultive behavior including that related to random agitation. The agitation may be associated with treatment, for example, with medication, the use of seclusion, or the initial admission procedure. Assaultive behavior can also be associated with delusions or hallucinations caused by psychosis. These are especially noted in patients with schizophrenic symptoms, depressive symptoms, paranoia, and/or grandiose feelings.

Antisocial activity also is associated with assaultive behavior. Individuals may purposefully harm others for their own pleasure or gain. They may utilize assaultiveness for exploitation of the staff or other patients, for example to make the staff afraid. It can also be a method to obtain escape from police holds, commitment procedures, and the like.

Individuals with organic CNS disease or injury also may be assaultive at times, often in an attempt to protect themselves. In this group assaultive behavior can result from paranoia, hallucinations, disorientation and confusion, medication reaction, high fever, electrolyte imbalance (often due to poor nutrition), impaired renal functioning, or neurologic disorders such as temporal lobe epilepsy, organic brain syndrome (OBS), or drug or alcohol toxicity. Drug or alcohol usage may be noted on admission or on return from pass or the patient may be ingesting the substance on the unit.

PREVENTION OF ASSAULTIVE BEHAVIOR

The best nursing methods for managing assaultive behavior are anticipation and prevention. In order to make best use of these methods, nursing staff need to draw on both basic theory and their own experience with violence. In their training programs, psychiatric nurses are taught the fundamentals of anxiety, anger, and aggression. Understanding these basics is necessary when assessing a patient's behavior.

At least once a year nursing staff should attend a hospital in-service program that describes preventive methods and the policies and procedures for dealing with assaultive behavior. Preventive methods for nurses include knowledge of anxiety theory, self-awareness, patient history, careful observations of usual behavior, communication techniques, and respecting the patient's dignity. Review of the hospital's policies and procedures is important to outline the specific intervention techniques recommended (or allowed) and to clarify any revisions.

Nursing theory regarding anxiety has been clearly defined by Peplau.[5] Four levels of anxiety can be easily visualized on a continuum ranging from mild, moderate, severe, and ending with panic. Understanding the differing levels of anxiety and the signs and symptoms of each will allow the nursing staff to assess behavior and to intervene at an early stage, thereby preventing the patient from resorting to violence.

The patient in the fourth level, panic, should be observed closely for assaultive behavior. At this level the anxiety so overwhelms the individual that intellectual processes are almost eradicated; learning cannot be expected to occur. This individual can not communicate or function effectively. Feelings of anger and/or helplessness may emerge explosively. This level of anxiety can not be tolerated over a long period of time without danger of physical or emotional exhaustion. Since the patient is so uncomfortable, a "fight or flight" reaction can occur. Warning signals that may be observed when "fight" is chosen include clenched fists, walking briskly, continuous pacing, throwing items, an exaggerated response to annoyance, yelling, pressured and curt speech, quivering of the lips, rigid muscle tension, biting, and scratching. When nursing staff observe these signals, interventions should be initiated.

Kelly states that the ability to intervene in violent or assaultive behavior depends on a sensitive awareness of one's own usual response pattern.[3] Intuition and personal maturity are important correlates to experience and example. Pisarcik concludes that one is likely to feel ill at ease with the patient who has a disturbed affect, although one may feel, "I can't quite put my finger on what's bothering me."[6] The nurse may have a "gut-level" feeling of uneasiness, perhaps feeling the patient has a "chip on his shoulder," is "walking on eggs," or is "sitting on a powder keg." These feelings have a basis in one's past experiences, although their source may be unclear. When they occur it is wise to increase one's caution until more is learned about the patient.

The patient who has used violence in the past is likely to do so again. On admission the nurse should thoroughly question the patient regarding a past history of assaultive behavior. Ask the patient what methods he or she has used in the past to relieve anger or stress. The nurse should also ask the family and/or significant others how the patient expresses anger. The patient may not be a reliable predictor of his own violence.

Communication is very important in the preventive stage. Both verbal and nonverbal communication to the patient should convey calmness, reassurance, and support. Nursing staff members should use their voices as tranquilizers, maintaining a confident manner and speaking softly and slowly. Loud, rapid speech is likely to agitate the patient further. An authoritarian posture by staff (often arising out of fear) may make the patient feel pressured or trapped. It should be remembered that in the panic stage, the patient's thought process is fragmented and learning can not occur. Therefore directions given to a panicking patient must be simple, concrete, and specific. If there are options available to the patient, they should be explained clearly.

Nursing staff should help the patient to recognize and verbalize what he or she is feeling. Examples of phrases to open communication are, "It must be very frustrating to feel this angry," and "Your actions show you're really upset. You probably have a good reason."

As the patient explains what he or she feels is happening, the nurse must be an active listener, showing interest by facial expression and encouraging comments. Sincere concern about the patient's feelings and a willingness to help him or her express them decrease the chance that physical action will be necessary for either party. Some therapists feel one should express his or her fear to the patient, for example with a statement such as "I don't know if you realize you're making me afraid right now. . . . You don't have to do that."[6] It is often reassuring to tell the patient that help with self-control is nearby, perhaps by saying "I am here to help you. I will not let you hurt yourself or anyone else."

Touch is important in communication, but staff must remember that it is often misinterpreted by the assaultive patient. Maintaining a degree of physical distance lessens the patient's misconception of attack or sexual advance. Nursing staff members must continually reassess the amount of physical distance necessary to maintain the safety of everyone involved.

The patient's dignity should be maintained as much as possible, consistent with the safety of the patient, other patients, and the staff. The self-esteem of the patient should be protected. Nursing staff can show respect for the patient through a genuine, warm, caring attitude. This often decreases the patient's need for violent action.

INTERVENTION DURING VIOLENT SITUATIONS

Hospital policy should define for the nursing staff those situations in which seclusion or restraint is acceptable and the procedures which will be followed. Specific nursing responsibilities for patient assessment, physician notification, intervention, and postseclusion (postrestraint) management should be outlined. Some examples are given elsewhere in this chapter. Techniques for handling agitated patients safely and effectively should be taught in in-service training programs, as should the rights of patients and staff.

In most hospital settings the nurse is the first health care professional to observe behavioral deviations in a patient. The nurse should be able to recognize actions that may require seclusion or restraint and be prepared to intervene. Decisions regarding physical or chemical management of the patient are made by the physician, although most agitation or violence occurs without warning. The nurse, therefore, often will be required to make a nursing judgment about the patient's need for seclusion and/or restraint; physician notification often follows stabilization of the situation. Both male and female nursing staff should be trained to deal with potentially violent situations.

When making shift assignments, the charge nurse should assign an easygoing, mature, experienced nurse to care for a potentially violent patient. Such a nurse is likely to be more alert to warning signals and to use preventive interventions. The importance of not placing onself in danger should be stressed; one should never attempt to manage violent behavior alone.

Threats, rudeness, sarcasm, yelling, and gossip are all forms of verbal assaultiveness. Nursing staff can assist the patient to express this anger constructively. For example, while sitting in the day room with a group of patients, one patient jumped up, walked briskly across the room to a staff member, and screamed, "If you don't stop watching me, I'm going to hit you." Staff should always take such threats seriously and not make light of the patient's statements. It is important not to challenge or provoke the patient. This may cause the behavior to escalate and encourage physical assaultiveness.

While threats must be taken seriously, they should rarely be taken personally. At times, the expression of anger connotes the patient's comfort with the staff, a feeling of acceptance without danger of rejection when true feelings are expressed. Techniques of reflection or validation, such as the simple statement "You feel like I've been watching you?" can help the patient maintain control and avoid feeling "backed into a corner." They also help the patient to become aware of his behavior and to identify the underlying causes.

When controlling assaultive behavior, limit-setting techniques are essential. One should clearly define acceptable and nonacceptable behavior, and the consequences of the nonacceptable. The limits may give direction ("One of the rules of this unit states you may not hit other people.") or to exact discipline ("You are not in control of your actions at this time. You will have to go to the seclusion room."). Limits may help the patient explore alternative channels for expressing feelings ("You may not hit other people, but I can go with you to the gym to punch the punching bag."). The patient should feel the right to be angry and to express it in a constructive, acceptable manner, while being protected from going out of control.

The patient may need a reduction in environmental stimuli to decrease anxiety and allow time for regaining self-control. The nurse may decide to take the patient to his or her room. Nursing staff should not isolate themselves with the assaultive patient. When working with the patient in the room, the door should be kept open and one should not turn his or her back on the patient. Staff can also accompany the patient to an area where he or she can run, shoot baskets, punch a punching bag, or otherwise physically dissipate energy and feelings. The following is an example of the need for reduction in stimuli:

Case Study 16-1

While on an outing at the park, a male patient impulsively grabbed a tree branch and began threatening a staff member with it. He began smiling and his voice became louder as he saw the others watching him. The staff member immediately stepped back and began talking to the patient in a slow, soft manner. Two staff members stood by to deliver assistance and the other staff removed the remaining patients to another area. Due to these quick, nonviolent interventions by the staff, the patient regained control of his impulsive behavior within a few minutes and was escorted back to the hospital setting.

A reduction in stimuli is also useful to maintain the patient's privacy and dignity. After the patient has regained control, he or she may be embarrassed or anxious about what has happened. It is comforting to know that one does not have to explain one's actions to numerous individuals.

If possible, other patients should not be allowed to witness the assaultive behavior. They may become fearful for their safety or they may encourage the behavior. One staff member can attend them and assure them that they will not be hurt. Later an informal group discussion can be held with these patients to allow them the opportunity to explore and ventilate their feelings regarding the situation.

Occasionally the previously mentioned interventions do not prevent physical violence. When a patient becomes overtly assaultive, the staff must take immediate action. In these situations, safety of patients and health care personnel is of utmost importance. The hospital's policies and procedures should define the steps staff should take to organize a team to assure this safety.

When a team is organized to assist a patient to seclusion, one member must always be designated the leader. It is crucial that the team members follow the leader's directions. The leader will determine the number of team members and degree of force necessary to control the violence. The team members should apply the force in such a way that will assist the patient to become calm rather than provoke further aggression.

When teams are utilized certain staff assignments are important. An individual can be assigned to take each of the patient's limbs and another to support the patient's head and prevent biting. Before approaching the patient, staff should be reminded to remove anything from their clothing or possession that could be snatched by the patient and used as a weapon. This would include pens, jewelry, keys, name tags, and ties. Long hair should be pulled back to prevent its being grabbed. As staff approach the patient, they should grasp the limbs at a major joint. This will reduce the patient's leverage and also reduce the possibility of fracture or dislocation. If the patient is still struggling, the staff can take him or her down to the floor. This further reduces the patient's leverage and makes it difficult for him to lash out or injure anyone. Only the team leader should speak during the intervention. The leader should use his voice as a tranquilizer to explain clearly to the patient what is happening.

Occasionally, during assaultive situations, the patient will have a weapon. When this happens, two staff members carrying mattresses can approach the patient from two sides until the patient is sandwiched between them. The patient can then no longer lash out, the weapon can be safely removed, and the patient subdued without injury to anyone. These and the following techniques should be taught *and practiced* before they are needed.

Since no one has the ability to deal with every instance of assaultive behavior, all health care professionals should feel comfortable in requesting assistance. Security personnel will occasionally be asked to participate in the restraint process. They may be used as a back-up team for assistance if the situation becomes uncontrollable, or for times when a "show of force" is needed. For some patients the security officer's uniform will have a calming effect. The uniform may represent law, order, and control. It is important to remember that security personnel *must remove their guns before entering* an inpatient unit. The presence of firearms escalates the violent situation rather than calms it, and increases the risk of a tragic outcome.

After the decision has been made to use seclusion, the leader must decide whether the patient can walk or needs to be carried. If walking is chosen, two staff should take the patient between them. If the patient refuses to walk, the staff can grasp him or her firmly by the arms and walk the patient *backward*, while the staff members walk forward. The staff should stay close to the patient, making it more difficult for him to kick or get leverage. It is important for the staff to maintain body alignment to prevent injury.

One must always check the seclusion room before placing a patient in it. Safety features are important.

Case Study 16-2

Once, while in a hurry, the staff placed a male patient in the seclusion room and locked the door. In five minutes, when the nurse checked the patient, she saw him wrapping a cord around his neck. The team had to be reorganized to remove the cord.

The cord must have been in the room when the patient was placed there. This situation could have been prevented if someone had cleared the room before placing the patient in it.

When the patient is in a locked seclusion room, a compromise is obtained between safety and patient respect. For safety reasons, the patient should be placed in a hospital gown. Staff (of the same sex) will assist the patient in removing his or her personal clothing and dress in the hospital gown. The patient's belts, ribbons, jewelry, wigs, bobby pins, and glasses* also need to be

*Note that removal of glasses may lead to further confusion or disorientation.

removed. The patient could use these items for self-injury or to injure others. When PRN medications are necessary, the staff should explain to the patient that the medications will have a calming effect and help him or her to regain self-control. It is also helpful to explain to the patient that he or she can return to ward activities as soon as he or she regains self-control. If the patient is very agitated or dangerous, the staff can lay the patient face down and pull the patient's arms behind his or her back as they prepare to leave the seclusion room. Then one person can hold the patient while the others leave the room. As the last staff member leaves the room, the door is locked. Duration of seclusion should be as short as possible, and should be consistent with safety and therapy, *not punishment*.

One should not enter the seclusion room alone. If the patient is in seclusion at mealtime, see that the food is served on a paper isolation tray. The staff should offer the patient fluids frequently, monitoring the intake. The patient's toileting needs should be attended every two hours. When escorting the patient to the toilet, two staff members should be present. For example, one staff member felt she could control a secluded patient's behavior and proceeded to escort her to the toilet alone. Suddenly, the patient slammed the aide against the wall and ran off the unit. This event may have been prevented if two staff members had been present.

The use of mechanical restraints is a controversial issue, and they should be avoided when possible. If the hospital's policies and procedures allow for mechanical as well as chemical restraints, the seclusion room may (or may not) contain a hospital bed. One should remember that restraints frighten patients and their use lowers patients' self-esteem. The staff must thoroughly explain what they are doing to the patient and that the restraints will be removed as soon as the patient regains control. Tell the patient that the staff realize the restraints are uncomfortable and then assist the patient with relaxation techniques. One should use the least restrictive restraints necessary for control of potential dangers, judging when the patient needs four-point restraints or when waist restraint will be sufficient. Next, the patient is positioned comfortably in bed and the restraints applied, allowing for some mobility. It is important to secure the restraints to the bedframe, as it is more stable than the siderails. When using the frame the side rails can be lowered without causing injury to the patient. The restraints should be applied snugly. One should be able to slide two fingers between the skin and the restraint. At this time the padding should be checked—it should be thick enough to prevent skin breakdown.

As with the seclusion room, intensive care is needed when restraints are used. The patient should be checked every 15 minutes (or continuously monitored). The restraints are removed or loosened every two hours to assure circulation and prevent skin breakdown. The restraints are removed one at a time to allow the patient to perform an active range of motion exercises, or the nurse to perform passive exercises. The patient's vital signs are frequently evaluated, especially if medications have been given. Allow the patient to reposition regularly. The patient's field of vision can be increased by elevating the head of the bed. A staff member should remain in the room if the patient is smoking.

Mediction can be an effective measure to prevent and/or control violent behavior. Chemical restraints are often considered more acceptable than mechanical ones, may be better tolerated by the patient, and may help to protect self-esteem. Proper dosages of medication and wise use of PRN drugs decrease the patient's chances of becoming assaultive. PRN medications are usually prescribed for brief sedation or to decrease anxiety, not for continued sedation. Parenteral administration should be used only when the need is acute and when oral medication is refused or felt to be insufficient. Anders states that the most desirable injection site is the upper outer quadrant of the gluteal region.[1] It can be given by laying the patient in the prone position and loosening his or her clothing.

Patients should not have visitors while they are confined in seclusion. Even though they can not visit, the patient's family may be informed when seclusion and/or restraints are being used. In some hospitals notification is required. The family often does not understand the procedures, and, like the patient, is frightened by them. One should explain the purpose of the procedure and answer any questions the family may have. Assure the family that the patient is checked frequently and will be removed from seclusion and/or restraints as soon as the need abates and safety can be assured.

POSTINCIDENT MANAGEMENT AND TREATMENT

Immediately after secluding the patient, the team should meet to discuss their interventions. The need for improvements should be assessed. If certain aspects of the intervention were unsuccessful, possible reasons should be explored and modified responses suggested for future incidents. The leader or charge nurse should give the team a chance to deal with their feelings. Were they comfortable or uncomfortable? Are there any additional comments? The team leader should always remember to thank the team members. The staff have risked their own safety and should be cited for their quick assistance. Support from peers and supervisors is necessary. Gair states that the nursing staff need to know that they can also count on being supported by the physician, in whose delegated authority they act.[2] This is essential to staff morale.

The unit staff members also need to review their actions at the time the incident began. Staff might consider the following: did they provoke or worsen the incident; did they argue, challenge, or back the patient into a corner; was there a problem with staff–patient communication before or during the incident; was the staff inattentive to early warning signals; did they allow the patient's anxiety to increase without trying to assist the patient with problem-solving methods to decrease it; what were the positive aspects of staff intervention; were the staff supportive to one another; what about staff morale—was it good, fair, or poor? When there is poor morale or conflict between staff, patients can often sense it and act it out.

Individual hospital policies and procedures will define the staff duties necessary to assure quality care for the secluded patient. Procedures for monitoring the patient's activities, vital signs, food intake, and elimination should be quite specific. They must also explain whom to notify regarding the incident (for example, the physician, relatives, or police).

Entries in the medical record are an important part of the overall management of an episode of patient violence. There are clinical and legal needs to document the presence of an emergency, acute intervention techniques, seclusion or restraint procedures, injuries or damage, and regular evaluation of the secluded or restrained patient. Physician's orders, descriptions of the behavior of patient and staff, names of involved personnel, and the like must be legibly recorded. The notes should make it clear that quality nursing practices—consistent with safety, patient care, and hospital policy—were carried out. This may be done graphically, by means of a flow chart such as that in *Figure 16-1.*

The process of termination of control modalities must be considered as carefully as the original decision to seclude and/or restrain. One must carefully and frequently evaluate the patient's behavior to determine the earliest time for safe termination of seclusion or restraint. Rosen and DiGiacomo list the folllowing general criteria as a guide: decrease in restlessness and anxiety; stabilization of mood; increased attention span and orientation; and improvement in reality testing and judgement with a decrease in hallucinations, delusions, and/or violent impulses.[7] The physical parameters to evaluate include regularization of food intake and sleep patterns, and the normalization of pulse and blood pressures.

Whaley and Ramirez state that a gradual release with continuous discussion is needed.[8] They claim that a too-hasty removal exposes the patient to potential failure, suggests confusion on the part of the therapist, and/or reinforces the belief that restraints were used as a form of punishment.

When the patient is released from seclusion, the staff should review the assaultive incident with him or her. The patient may feel guilty or fear that someone may have been hurt. Reviewing the incident may help alleviate those feelings. One should discuss how the incident happened and explore alternative actions the patient might use should he or she become anxious and/or angry in the future.

Patient Identification

Date: _____

Time of day:																	
Orientation:																	
Person																	
Place																	
Time																	
Behavior:																	
Crying																	
Yelling																	
Laughing																	
Standing																	
Pacing																	
Sitting																	
Hitting wall																	
Hitting door																	
Lying																	
Sleeping																	
Nutrition:																	
Meal Served																	
Fluid intake																	

Elimination:

Urine _____ | | | | | | | | | |

Stool _____ | | | | | | | | | |

Restraints:

Chemical—PRN _____ | | | | | | | | | |

—routine _____ | | | | | | | | | |

Physical—loosening and ROM* (every 2 hours) _____ | | | | | | | | | |

—checked for padding _____ | | | | | | | | | |

Vital Signs:

every shift _____ | | | | | | | | | |

Hygiene:

Oral _____ | | | | | | | | | |

Smoking:

with staff present _____ | | | | | | | | | |

Other: _____

Nursing Staff Signature:

_____ 7:00–3:00

_____ 3:00–11:30

_____ 11:00–7:30

*ROM = range of motion

Figure 16-1. Flow chart for recording an episode of patient violence. Specific behaviors displayed are indicated by a check mark beside the behavior in the appropriate column for time of day.

237

STAFF INJURIES

Injured staff are victims. The hospital administration must be supportive of staff who are injured and should investigate workmen's compensation policies to determine the coverage they provide. The victims often benefit from crisis intervention therapy, either formal or informal. The institution might also provide therapists to assist victims or pay the bill when injured staff seek out such assistance. These resources are very important.

The possibility of filing suit or criminal charges against the patients who injure others should be considered. This is done in some institutions, especially when careful documentation of the patient's behavior indicates that he or she was responsible for his actions. Discharge or transfer to a more appropriate facility may be another alternative.

SUMMARY

Dealing with assaultive behavior is one of the many responsibilities and duties of the psychiatric nursing staff. It is a challenge for both the staff and the patient. Nursing judgement is a key factor when dealing with assaultive behavior, which can be prevented in most cases. Nursing staff must continually assess the patient's level of anxiety, interactions, and any deviations from routine behavior. When deviations occur, the staff must decide whether to utilize intervention techniques and, if so, which ones. The staff may be able to proceed through a series of steps beginning with verbal intervention, or may need to immediately proceed to the use of the seclusion and/or restraint process.

REFERENCES

1. Anders RL: Management of violent patients. Critical Care Update, 7:5–15, 1980
2. Gair DS: Limit-setting and seclusion in the psychiatric hospital. Psychiatric Opinion 17:15–19, 1980
3. Kelley EM: The client who generates fear, in Haber J, Leach AM, Schudy SM et al. (eds): Comprehensive Psychiatric Nursing. New York: McGraw-Hill Book Company, 1978, pp 247–262
4. Penningroth PE: Control of violence in a mental health setting. Am J Nurs 75:600–609, 1975
5. Peplau HE: Process and concept of learning, in Burd SF, Marshall MA, (eds): Some Clinical Approaches to Psychiatric Nursing. New York: McMillan Company, 1963, pp 333–336
6. Pisarcik G: Facing the violent patient. Nursing 81 11:63–65, 1981
7. Rosen H, DiGiacomo JN: The role of physical restraint in the treatment of psychiatric illness. J Clin Psychiatry 39:228–232, 1978

8. Whaley MS, Ramirez LR: The use of seclusion rooms and physical restraints in the treatment of psychiatric patients. J Psychiatr Nurs 18:13–16, 1980

ADDITIONAL READINGS

Anders RL: When a patient becomes violent. Am J Nurs 77:1144–1148, 1977

Burd SF: Effects of nursing intervention in anxiety of patients, in Burd SF, Marshall MA (eds): Some Clinical Approaches to Psychiatric Nursing. New York: McMillan Company, 1963, pp 307–320

Clark J: Nursing interventions into the aggressive behavior of patients, in Burd SF, Marshall MA, (eds): Some Clinical Approaches to Psychiatric Nursing. New York: McMillan Company, 1963, pp 199–205

Convertino K, Pinto RP, Fiester AR: Use of inpatient seclusion in a community health center. Hosp Community Psychiatry 31:348–350, 1980

DiFabro S, Ackerhald EJ: Teaching the use of restraint through role play. Perspect Psychiatric Care 16:218–222, 1978

Fitzgerald RC, Longo I: Seclusion in the treatment and management of severely disturbed manic and depressed patients. Perspectives in Psychiatric Care 11:59–64, 1973

Graves HH and Thompson EA: Anxiety: A mental health vital sing, in Longo DC, Williams RA, (eds): Clinical Practice in Psychosocial Nursing: Assessment and Intervention. New York: Appleton-Century Crofts, 1978, pp 87–104

Guirguis EF: Management of disturbed patients, an alternative to the use of mechanical restraints. J Clin Psychiatry 39:295–299, 1978

Gutheil TC: Observations on the theoretical basis for seclusion of the psychiatric patient. Am J Psychiatry 135:325–328, 1978

Hays DR: Teaching a concept of anxiety to patients. Nursing Research 10:108–113, 1961

Hays DR: Anger: A clinical problem, in Burd SF, Marshall MA (eds): Some Clinical Approaches to Psychiatric Nursing. New York: McMillan Company, 1963, pp 110–115

Kerr N: Anxiety: Theoretical considerations. Perspect Psychiatric Care 1:36–46, 1978

Knowles RD: Dealing with feelings: Managing anxiety. Am J Nurs 81:110–111, 1981

Kronberg ME: Anxiety assessment and interventions, in Norris JF (ed): *Mental Health-Psychiatric Nursing: A Continuum of Care*. New York: John Wiley and Sons, Inc. in press.

Lion JR: Evaluation and Management of the Violent Patient. Springfield, Illinois: Charles C. Thomas, 1972

May R: The Meaning of Anxiety. New York: The Ronald Press Company, 1950

Misik I: About using restraints with restraint. Nursing 81 11:50–55, 1981

Moritz DA: Understanding anger. Am J Nurs 8:81–83, 1978

Peplau HE: A working definition of anxiety, in Burd SF, Marshall MA (eds): Some Clinical Approaches to Psychiatric Nursing. New York: McMillan Company, 1963, pp 323–327

Perry SW III, Gilmore MA: The disruptive patient or visitor. JAMA 245:755–756, 1981

Redmond FC: Study on the use of the seclusion room. Quality Rev Bull 6:20–23, 1980
Sullivan HS: The meaning of anxiety in psychiatry and life. Psychiatry 2:1–13, 1984

Paul H. Soloff

17
Seclusion and Restraint

Violence and assaultive behavior are part of the working reality of the modern psychiatric milieu. Despite advances in dynamic and pharmacologic treatment, assaults within psychiatric facilities persist with alarming frequency. A survey of university affiliated psychiatrists working in a wide variety of settings revealed that 42 percent had been assaulted by their patients at some time in their carrers.[18] Whitman found that 24 percent of therapists including psychiatrists, psychologists, and social workers were assaulted during one calendar year by one or more patients.[36] Among psychiatrists, 24 percent were physically attacked—15 percent on more than one occasion. A threat of personal harm was reported by 43 percent of therapists while 79 percent reported at least one incident in which a patient threatened someone else. Within hospital settings, the true incidence of assaults is widely underreported. Lion found that the number of assaults on staff in a state hospital as reported in the daily nursing notes was five-times greater than the number of assaults in the official incident reports.[16] In the same study an estimate of 1108 assaults annually was made for a hospital with 1500 patients and 800 nursing staff.[16]

The frequency of assault on staff makes this oldest of problems a major focus of concern in contemporary psychiatric treatment.

This chapter addresses the management and treatment of violent and disruptive behavior in the acute treatment setting. The discussion will emphasize the intelligent use of seclusion and restraint as legitimate and effective treatment modalities for the management of assaultive and disruptive patients. The theoretical and empirical bases of this treatment will be reviewed in an effort to define proper indications and guidelines for use, especially in the prevention of assault. Finally a pragmatic guide to physical technique will be described to enhance the utility of this discussion. For the purpose of this presentation, we assume that violence occurring in the psychiatric treatment setting is related, at least in part, to one or more psychopathologic symptoms including impairment of reality testing, perceptual distortions, loss of control over affect or impulse, severe psychodynamic conflict or cortical dysfunction. The management of willful, malicious violence—although occasionally a fact of life in the mental hospital—deserves in-depth consideration elsewhere.

Recent Controversy on Seclusion and Restraint

Physical restraint and seclusion persist in the modern psychiatric milieu because they are needed to deal with the clinical realities of violence, agitation, and assault. Within the field, physical controls are viewed, at best, with embarrassment, at worst, as an unacceptable anachronism. Little is written or taught of the practice. Were it not for psychiatry's legal critics, seclusion and restraint in the modern treatment milieu most certainly would have remained unstudied. The practice of seclusion in mental hospitals came under judicial scrutiny as a natural sequel to reviews of administrative segregation in prisons,[11] the use of seclusion in hospitals for the criminally insane,[22] and the retarded.[37] In each case the court defined legal safeguards governing the application of physical controls. In *Rogers* v. *Okin*[25] (formerly *Rogers* v. *Macht*), the issue was extended to the use of seclusion in a state mental hospital where seclusion was part of the treatment plan for patients exhibiting disruptive behavior. Attorneys for the patient-plaintiffs argued that forced seclusion was not a legitimate form of treatment but rather a "cruel and unusual punishment" imposed arbitrarily, on poorly defined indications, for unspecified durations, and without due process rights of the patient. In the case in point psychiatrists on a university unit of Boston State Hospital were charged with the use of seclusion in nonemergency situations—in apparent violation of Massachusetts law governing restraint. The legal question centered around the issue of whether seclusion represented restraint of violent behavior or treatment of underlying illness, with no recognition of the unity of the two in most cases. In defense the Massachusetts Psychiatric Society, as *amicus curiae*, stated that seclusion was "a highly respected form of treatment, of great value to many severely disturbed patients and essential to the preservation of order and safety during psychiatric emergencies."[25] Seclusion was defended as a treatment for the illness predisposing to behaviors requiring emergency restraint. From the legal perspective behaviors warranting restraint were divorced from underlying cause, negating any treatment considerations in the use of seclusion. In ruling against the psychiatrists, the presiding judge chose to view the use of seclusion on nonemergency indication as an administrative sanction requiring regulation by the court.[9]

Following this judicial review Gutheil and Rosen detailed the theoretical indications for seclusion and physical restraint as forms of treatment for disruptive or violent patients.[8,26] The therapeutic principles of this intervention include containment of disruptive impulse, isolation from the demands of interpersonal relatedness and decrease in sensory input. For the patient who loses control over internal impulse, seclusion or restraint represents a measure of external control assuring both patient and staff that self-injury and injury to others will not occur while the patient is out of control. An external limit is placed on the painful and frightening loss of ego boundaries. Isolation from relationships minimizes the distortions and fearful projections which make social interaction intolerable. Destimulation prevents further disorganization of attention and cognition by lessening the sensory overload that overwhelms the psychotic patient. As treatment for symptomatic relief of underlying illness, seclusion may be a preventive measure, used to abort predicted outbursts of aggression or excitation in many disorders. Seclusion has been recommended for "disturbed, unpredictable psychotics,"[5] violent schizophrenics, manic or brain damaged patients, and for patients with personality disorders with episodic dyscontrol or who are intoxicated. Arguing for clinical flexibility, Bursten describes the use of physical restraints on request of nonpsychotic patients to assure control over disruptive and frightening impulses or to set limits to diffuse ego boundaries.[4]

The concern of psychiatry's critics and the resulting judicial reviews have prompted renewed interest in systematic studies on the use of seclusion and restraint in the modern treatment milieu. A review of studies conducted in a wide variety of clinical settings will define the current pattern of use, indications, and contraindications, and will provide empirical support for the legitimacy and efficacy of this treatment modality.

SYSTEMATIC STUDIES

Empirical guidelines for the use of seclusion and restraint as methods of treatment may be derived from studies of the incidence of seclusion, demographic and diagnostic characteristics of secluded patients, and behaviors precipitating seclusion. To be a legitimate form of treatment, a clear relation-

Table 17-1
Review of Seclusion/Restraint Experience in Acute Treatment Settings

Author	Method	Incidence of Seclusion/Restraint (Percent)	Setting	Frequency of Precipitants (Percentage of Total Seclusion/Restraint Experience)
Soloff PH. 1978	Chart Review	3.6	Two acute inpatient units (51 beds) of a large military teaching hospital	Violation of community or administrative limits, 35.1 Nonspecific rationale (e.g. patient escalating, unable to control his behavior, inappropriate, etc). 16.2 Physical attack or threat to staff with physical contact. 14.4
Wells DA. 1972	Chart Review	4.0	Short-term university unit with a mixed clinic and private population	(Not Studied Quantitatively)
Mattson MR. Sacks MH. 1978	Chart Review	7.2	Private, voluntary psychiatric division (104 beds) of a general hospital	Behavior disruptive to therapeutic environment, 34.4 Assaultive to others, 25.1 Other, 18.0
Soloff PH. Turner SM. 1981	Prospective	10.5	2 inpatient units (41 beds) in a university-operated psychiatric hospital "with extensive catchment area responsibility"	Physical attack on staff with physical contact, 34.6 Patient escalating, unable to control behavior, inappropriate behavior, etc. (as a preventive measure), 24.3 Verbal threat toward staff with no physical contact, 10.3
Plutchik R et al. 1978	Chart Review	26	University affiliated large municipal hospital (4 wards, 100 beds)	Agitated, uncontrolled behavior, 21.1 Physical aggression toward other patient(s), 15.3 Loud noisy behavior 9.7
Schwab PJ. Laymeyer CB. 1979	Prospective	36.6	Psychiatric unit (24 beds) in a university general hospital	Destimulation, 28 Agitation or acute excitement, 17 Poor impulse control, 15
Binder RL, 1979	Chart Review	44	Short-term crisis intervention unit (11 beds) in a university psychiatric hospital with catchment area responsibility	Agitation. 16 times Uncooperativeness, 14 times Anger, 12 times
Wadeson H, Carpenter WT. 1976	Retrospective	66	NIMH acute schizophrenia clinical research unit	(Not Studied Quantitatively)

ship must exist between the theoretical principles underlying the treatment and the clinical indications for which the treatment is actually used. While differences in research methods, clinical settings, and treatment philosophies make comparisons between studies difficult, the investigation of who is secluded and why allows a test of legitimacy of physical controls in the modern treatment setting.

Incidence

Six retrospective and two prospective studies have systematically studied the use of physical controls in acute treatment settings (Table 17-1). The incidence of seclusion varies directly with the clinical population and treatment philosophy of the unit. In acute treatment settings physical controls are used least in private, voluntary, prescreened populations. Soloff reported the lowest incidence (3.6 percent) of patients requiring the use of physical controls during admission to a military teaching hospital serving a well-disciplined active duty population.[28] Wells found an incidence of 4 percent in a small psychiatric unit of a noted university hospital serving a mixed private and clinic population.[34] The private, voluntary division of a general hospital in New York City, with 7.2 percent secluded, may be contrasted with a large university-affiliated municipal hospital in the same city, in which 26 percent of all patients required physical controls during admission.[19, 24]

The "acuteness" of the clinical population is a critical factor in determining the need for seclusion or restraint. Binder reported the need for seclusion in 44 percent of admissions to a short-term crisis intervention unit, where half of the patients were brought in by police.[2] In sharp contrast Tardiff described a low rate of 1.9 percent secluded in a traditional custodial care state mental hospital, where 71 percent of the patients had spent more than 10 years in the hospital.[32]

Philosophy of care appears to be the critical variable responsible for the 36.6 percent secluded in Schwab and Lahmeyer's study of a small (24-bed) psychiatric unit in a university hospital.[27] As a matter of policy, patients admitted to this unit were kept free of medication for a prolonged period of clinical observation. A 66 percent incidence of seclusion was reported by Wadeson and Carpenter on a NIMH (National Institute of Mental Health) clinical research unit for acute schizophrenics, where medication was withheld as part of a research strategy, and patients were managed through interpersonal therapies.[33]

A historical comparison serves to place these findings in perspective. Following a survey of 40 American mental hospitals in 1880, Daniel Tuke reported that 5.4 percent of the 40,992 patients were found in restraints—varying from camisoles and muffs to straps, ball, and chain.[14]

Demographic, Diagnostic, and Behavioral Variables

The issue of who is secluded and why is answered in part through comparisons of demographic, diagnostic, and behavioral variables in the seclusion process. In general, the young and psychotic schizophrenic or manic is at highest risk for seclusion. Again, the setting and "acuteness" of the clinical population bias all comparisons.

Schizophrenics account for 46.7 percent of secluded patients in the Wells study,[36] 63 percent in Mattson's sample,[21] and 64 percent for Plutchik et al.[24] Schwab and Lahmeyer reported a higher incidence for manic patients with no significant difference between secluded and nonsecluded schizophrenics.[27] In the chronic population of the state mental hospital, patients with mental retardation and nonpsychotic disorders were responsible for the greater proportion of seclusions, through the largest absolute number secluded were schizophrenic.[32]

In a prospective study Soloff and Turner related the incidence of seclusion to the mental status of the patients at the time of seclusion. Although patients judged to be psychotic were responsible for 68.9 percent of all episodes, this rate was not proportionately or significantly different from the experience of nonpsychotic patients.[30] Psychotic patients are generally secluded early in their hospital course, before medication and milieu can exert maximal beneficial effect. In contrast, nonpsychotic patients show no significant preference, implying little therapeutic effect of the treatment setting over time.[28] While the incidence of seclusion is related to diagnosis in most studies, the frequency of seclusion is not. Controlling for the time-at-risk, (the length of hospital stay), Soloff found no significant difference in frequency of restraint between psychotic and nonpsychotic patients.[28]

Chronicity and committed status are both correlated with increased incidence of seclusion. The hopelessness and futility pervading the care of chronic patients, staff resentment at noncompliance with previous treatment efforts, and the advanced state of decompensation found in such patients increase staff readiness to use seclusion. The committed patient comes to the unit burdened by an attribution of violence, dyscontrol, or inability to care for himself. He is presumed dangerous—by definition—until proven otherwise. Soloff and Turner found that the precipitating events leading to seclusion of committed patient did not differ objectively from secluded voluntary patients in regard to violence of precipitant. committed patients are secluded as much for their status as for their acts.[30]

Race and sex bear no relationship to seclusion practice. Where trends appear, the question of systematic bias should be entertained.[30]

The Purpose of Seclusion and Restraint

Seclusion and restraint are used to contain violent or disruptive behaviors which are not responsive to less restrictive verbal, chemical, or physical means of control. While actual violence or assault is the most dramatic indication for physical controls, behaviors dangerous to self or others are not the leading precipitants to seclusion or restraint in five of six studies where prcipitating factors were noted. The more complex indication of "behavior disruptive to the social milieu" is the predominant rationale given for the use of physical controls. No question has been raised of the legitimacy of physical controls in the management of dangerous behavior; however, the use of seclusion and restraint to control disruptive behavior warrants careful definition and close examination.

The poor impulse control, regressed and bizarre behavior of psychotic patients is a legitimate indication for seclusion and restraint. In such cases, treatment is for "destimulation," containment of psychotic impulse, or control over potentially dangerous agitation. Seclusion and restraint may abort imminent physical assault. Physical controls also play a critical role in preventing decompensation and progressive psychomotor agitation—independent of the threat of violence. One need only to consider the psychomotor drive of an escalating manic patient or the fecal smearing of a regressed schizophrenic to retain perspective on the use of physical controls in containing disruptive impulse. A review of actual precipitating factors leading to seclusion and restraint indicates the widespread use of physical controls to contain such disruptive, albeit nonviolent, behaviors. In the large municipal hospital described by Plutchik et al., "agitated uncontrolled behavior" was the principal reason for seclusion, accounting for 21.1 percent of all reasons cited.[24] Mattson and Sacks found "behavior disruptive to the therapeutic environment" precipitating 34.4 percent of seclusion episodes.[19] "Destimulation" (28 percent), "agitation or acute excitement" (17 percent) "poor impulse control" (15 percent) were leading causes of restraint and seclusion in the Schwab and Lahmeyer study.[27] In the prospective study of Soloff and Turner, a nonviolent precipitant, "patient escalating, unable to control behavior, inappropriate behavior, etc. (as a preventive measure)," was scored by nursing staff as the determining indication for the use of seclusion in 24.3 percent of episodes.[30]

A review of precipitants also reveals the occasional use of seclusion as an administrative sanction. Seclusion for "verbal abuse," "refusal to participate in activity," or "refusal to take medication" raises the issue of whether seclusion "at times is used as a weapon of retaliation and control."[2] Binder noted that the two longest seclusions in her study involved incidents "in which staff's dignity was affronted; in one case urine and in the other case water was thrown at staff."[2] The use of seclusion or restraint as a punishment, divorced from the treatment interests of the patient, can not be justified and indicates a serious mismatch between the needs of the patient and the treatment setting.

Duration

The duration of seclusion varies widely among studies and is a complex variable which correlates with age, sex, and psychosis at the time of seclusion. In a large municipal hospital Plutchik reported a mean duration of 4.1 hours[4] while Binder reported a mean of 15.7 hours for a crisis intervention unit.[2] In the prospective study of Soloff and Turner, the mean duration of seclusion episodes was 10.8 hours, with a median of 2.8 hours, and a range of 10 minutes to 120 hours.[30] Patients less than 35 years old spent more total time in seclusion during their hospital stay compared to older secluded patients. Similarly, patients who were psychotic at the time of seclusion spent more total time in seclusion during their hospital stay compared to nonpsychotic secluded patients. Men had longer discrete seclusion episodes than women. Specific diagnoses, precipitating factors and number of prior episodes were not related to the duration of seclusion. In fact, there was no significant change in average length of seclusion with repeated episodes using each patient as his own control. The independence of precipitating cause and duration may be attributable to a number of clinical or staff issues related to the patient's illness such as poor response to medication, unpredictable episodic outbursts (conditioning staff caution), or ward factors delaying release of potentially disruptive psychotic patients. From a purely legal perspective, the wide disparity in seclusion times and the independence of duration from precipitating behavior and diagnosis raise the unpleasant question of arbitrariness in determining duration; a needlessly prolonged seclusion is a punitive sanction. In actual practice, ward factors independent of the patient often must be considered before termination of seclusion. Staff may require time to settle a troubled ward before reintegrating a vulnerable patient. Under some circumstances reintegration is most successful when the patient's primary nurse is available to spend time with the patient. Similarly, reintegration of a minimally controlled patient may await sufficient staff to allow safe transition from locked seclusion to the less restrictive isolation of a single bedroom. The legal argument gains validity only when seclusion is used to isolate the patient for excessively long periods purely as a convenience to staff.

These systematic studies indicate the widespread use of physical controls in a variety of clinical settings. Most importantly, they emphasize the use of seclusion and restraint in the treatment of disruptive behavior as a preventive measure; that is, to contain progressively decompensating behavior which could result in gross disorganization or overt assault if not aggressively treated.

The seclusion of such patients serves a dual function: the intensive care of their underlying illness and defense of the therapeutic milieu. It is a basic assumption of this discussion that seclusion is a treatment for disruptive and assaultive patients, not primarily an administrative sanction to maintain social order. When the preventive use of seclusion serves only to preserve decorum, there exists a profound mismatch between the patient's clinical needs and the treatment setting.

Staff attitudes and treatment philosophy are intimately related to the use and abuse of physical controls. To define the proper use of seclusion and restraint in the prevention of assault, we must first examine the role of staff and patients in provoking violence.

STAFF CONTRIBUTIONS TO PATIENT VIOLENCE

Staff Attitude

From the earliest days of "moral treatment," it was recognized that the way in which a patient was received and treated by staff made a major impact on the violence of his behavior. Conolly noted that the use of force and punishment to deal with the insane only aggravated the underlying illness such that the patient's condition seemed "more the product of ill-treatment than of mere malady."[5] Bearing witness to the same truth in modern times, Barton observed that "a frightened but docile person who is accosted in a hostile and aggressive manner can be turned into a barracaded battler." The attitude of staff toward the potentially violent patient may convey threat or, conversely, the assurance of help. Barton further states, "Most disturbed people who are already standing their ground and making threats, can be rendered quickly cooperative by someone who is trained and who knows what he is doing."[1]

A psychodynamic approach to the potentially combative patient has become standard practice in most acute care settings. The attitude of the dynamically trained staff generally reflects the belief that "the patient's aggressive behavior represents a defensive stance against overwhelming feelings of helplessness and fragility."[15] Lion holds that "the main principle of intervention and treatment should always be to help the violent patient control those aggressive impulses which he himself finds frightening."[15] Staff are taught to show confidence in dealing with the disruptive patient and convey an expectation that the patient will behave well. Patients are reassured that staff wishes to help them contain the disruptive impulses they experience and master their frightening perceptions and beliefs. The patient is encouraged to verbalize feelings instead of acting out, uncover specific targets of aggression and deal with issues such as fear of helplessness, dependency, and abandonment. The dynamic approach is more applicable to patients with character disorders, borderline syndromes, or mild distortions of reality testing. In actual practice, however, many patients brought to the emergency room in crisis are already beyond the reach of verbal controls.

The approach of "talking down" the potentially violent patient assumes that the patient can perceive the same causal reality as the clinician and, indeed, that verbal communication is meaningful at all. In the severely agitated psychotic and in the delirious or drug intoxicated patient, these preconditions to communication may not be met. While the psychodynamic philosophy has great appeal and efficacy in working with nonpsychotic or marginally psychotic (borderline) characters in crisis, its utility with decompensated psychotics must be tempered by the facts of the patient's actual behavior. In so far as the psychodynamic approach distracts the examiner from behavioral realities, it delays preventive action and lulls the clinician into a sense of false security. The occasional loss of life that has resulted from a physician's attempts to "talk down" violent patients serves as a stark reminder of our limited understanding of violence and the need to closely monitor behavior as the only reliable key to action.

Behavioral predictors of violence in the crisis setting include the patients' muscle tone (poised for fight or flight), the content of his speech (loud or profane), escalation of motor activity (restless and pacing) and finally, ambivalence in confronting or avoiding the clinician (approach avoidance). The angry, loud patient pacing the halls is at imminent risk for violence and requires immediate attention. Within each clinical setting where disturbed and potentially assaultive patients are seen, the staff must have clearly defined behavioral limits beyond which forceful intervention is used to abort actual assault. A therapeutic attitude of understanding the potentially violent patient must be coupled with preventive action based on observed behavior.

The attitude of staff toward the assaultive patient is dominated by fear and anger. Lion observes that staff perception of danger may be derived, in part, from projection of their own anger at the potentially combative patient.[17] These countertransference reactions may lead to defensive denial on the part of the clinician or, conversely, a violent overreaction. A sustained state of anxiety and fear among staff is intolerable and invariably leads to a forced resolution. The "dangerous patient" may actually be encouraged to "act out" his potential, justifying staff retaliation and discharge of tension into action. The use of strict behavioral guidelines for instituting physical controls tempers the role of countertransference anger.

The Ward Atmosphere

Staff attitude, enthusiasm, and morale are critical to the successful outcome of psychiatric care in any treatment setting. This is especially true in dealing with severely disturbed or assaultive patients. The therapeutic significance of every interaction with the patient was emphasized by Greenblatt in his effort to reduce patient violence and the use of seclusion at the Boston Psychopathic Hospital in 1946.[6] The key to converting this custodial care facility to a modern therapeutic hospital lay in the attitude of staff. A concerted effort was made to educate and enlist the ward attendants in the therapeutic process since it was they—not the senior medical staff—who embodied the tone of the institution, and through their behavior, provoked or prevented patient violence. Their fears of the disturbed patient and anger at administrative change were vented in group meetings with supportive senior staff. The ward attendants were taught that patient violence was related to the way the patient was treated, and that seclusion was often used out of fear and as punishment for disruptive behavior. Under an enlightened administration, the attendant came to play a critical role in the treatment process, converting custodial to therapeutic attitudes. As a result of this effort, patient hours in seclusion dropped from nearly 1000/year to 40/year within three years.

In recent years the therapeutic impact of the treatment milieu has been systematically studied to identify aspects of attitude, philosophy, and composition of staff that relate to treatment outcome. Approaching the study of treatment environments from an epidemiologic perspective, Moos developed an attitude inventory designed to assess ward atmosphere through the eyes of patients and staff.[20] The Ward Atmosphere Scale was applied to wards in 55 VA hospitals with a total of 1680 patients and 590 staff respondents. On the Ward Atmosphere Scale, Moos found that increased amounts of disturbed behavior on a ward correlated with decreases in perceived patient autonomy and loss of adult status. On "disturbed wards" patients perceive greater degrees of staff control than in other wards, while staff feels less control. Disturbed wards are characterized by little involvement of staff of patients in common ward efforts and little practical concern for patient's social adjustment after hospitalization. Staff express a lack of program clarity while paradoxically encouraging the exploration of patients' personal problems and expression of anger and aggression. These wards stimulate affect while neglecting order and organization. Klass et al. have shown that effective treatment wards, those with the longest community tenure rates postdischarge, are characterized by high degrees of order and organization and little encouragement of angry affect.[13] Using the Ward Atmosphere Scale in a survey of 431 patients on 21 long- and short-term wards, (with an 89.7 percent schizophrenic population), these investigators concluded that psychotics do better after treatment on a ward stressing order and organization over the free expression of anger.[13] Moos, Shelton, and Peety described effective programs as those high in systems maintenance (order and organization, program clarity, and staff control), relationships (patient–staff involvement, support, and spontaneity), autonomy, and practical orientation—but with less emphasis on patients' personal problems and the open expression of patients' anger and aggression.[21] Perhaps the most revealing finding was a correlation between disturbed behavior on a ward and lack of agreement between patient and staff perception of ward atmosphere. Recalling the disturbed behavior was found where patient autonomy was low, it is not surprising that the greater the degree of adult status that patients perceived themselves to be accorded, the less disturbed and the greater the agreement between staff and patients on the attitude survey.[21]

Staff Group Dynamics

In addition to epidemiologic considerations of ward atmosphere and function, the study of staff group dynamics has contributed greatly to our understanding of patient violence. Stanton and Schwarz first described the phenomenon of patients' overtly acting out the covert, but forbidden, wishes of staff.[31] A dramatic example of this dynamic was reported from the Massachusetts Mental Health Center (formerly the Boston Psychopathic Hospital) during a period of institutional crises precipitated by the sudden and unexpected resignation of the superintendent of the hospital, a powerful and charismatic leader who had directed the hospital for over a decade. In the absence of effective leadership, the hospital was directed by state mandate to begin a far-reaching reorganization of its patient care delivery system, a change affecting the working conditions of a majority of staff. In a climate of administrative crisis, there was a dramatic increase in physical and verbal patient assaultiveness culminating in an epidemic of fire setting that involved 13 fires within a four-month period. The four patients involved had no prior history of fire setting and were expressing the sentiments of a loyal staff that felt abandoned and vulnerable following the loss of their leader.[3]

Staff Splitting

At the level of intrastaff dynamics the phenomenon of "staff splitting" is responsible for provoking violent "acting out" of patient conflicts. This phenomenon is best illustrated in patients with the borderline personality disorder. These primitive character types maintain split images of their internalized self and object representations, separating "good" from "bad" self percepts and "good" from "bad" object representations. In an uncanny manner, the patient seduces staff into assuming roles in one or more of these partial self-object dyads (e.g., good self–good object, bad self–bad object, and so on). The patient presents him- or herself to selected staff in one of the split-self modes, encouraging the development of the corresponding part object response from staff. Just as the split internal self and object dyads represent discrete and separate aspects of the patient's personality (in interaction with another), the staff comes to view the patient from many separate perspectives. A poll of staff opinion will reveal widely divergent attitudes and behavior toward the patient.

A clash between the recipients of the "good" and "bad" object roles acts out the internal conflict. The result may encourage violence.

Individual Factors

Although not widely studied, it is apparent that certain personality styles among staff engender a violent patient response. Repetitive incidents of assault or threat on specific staff members usually reveal a personality that is controlling, rigid, authoritarian, and intolerant. The nurse most likely to be battered can generally be identified by patient (and staff) complaints long before an actual assault occurs. By tone of voice, physical demeanor, or actual threat, these staff members convey an intimidating authority to patients that provokes violent defense of self-esteem. Other staff note their intolerance of criticism, arrogance, and inability to cooperate in a team effort. Since the "Battered Nurse Syndrome" represents the staff members' pathology more than the patients', these nurses should be counseled out of the mental health setting for their own good.

SOME PATIENT FACTORS PROVOKING VIOLENCE

Cultural Issues

In the debate over the origins of patient violence, theories of causality generally sway, according to the fashion of the moment, between hospital factors and patient's contributions. The truth is a complex mix of both. The patient's contribution includes—in addition to the obvious facts of psychopathology and history of violence—the patient's cultural attitude concerning violence. Guenther notes that "violence as a way of life is imported to the mental health hospital where it becomes the dominant mode of adaptation for patients from that background."[7]

Within our violent society attitudes toward violence vary widely with socioeconomic status and subculture. Kalogerakis attributed a sharp increase in assaultive episodes at Belleview Psychiatric Hospital between 1964 and 1970 to social attitude changes in the community from which the patients were admitted.[14] Serving an urban ghetto, where racial tensions ran high in the 1960s, racial hatred accompanied the patients to the hospital and provoked conflict between black patients and white staff. In this survey Kalogerakis noted that all of the serious assaults were on white staff members by black patients, although there were many blacks in authority positions on the ward. Racial prejudice justifies expression of hostile feelings regardless of their origin. The racial difference encourages depersonalization and projection of fantasy on the victim. This prejudice operates in both directions, as illustrated by the study of

Flaherty and Maegher who showed a systematic bias in the treatment acorded black and white schizophrenic inpatients in a teaching hospital.[5] Black patients were given more PRN medication, were more likely to be secluded or restrained, and less likely to receive recreation therapy, occupation therapy, or higher privilege levels. Soloff and Turner also noted a trend toward increased use of seclusion for black patients admitted to a university psychiatric hospital.[30] An attribution of violence and a presumption of dangerousness follows the projection of cultural fear of the black patient by the predominately white staff. A readiness to act on this projection coupled with a real difficulty in emphathic understanding sets the stage for social bias and violence in patient care.

Dynamic Issues

Conventional wisdom teaches that violence is often a defensive response to externally perceived threat or internally perceived helplessness. A prevalent and dangerous variant of this principle is the dynamic of pseudohomosexual panic. The symbolic expression in sexual terms of perceived threat to one's cultural sense of manhood has been termed "pseudo" homosexual anxiety.[25] Following a humiliating loss, confrontation or threat, the patient feels that his sense of "masculine self-esteem" is threatened and, following the classic unconscious equation: "I am not a man = I am a homosexual," responds with a violent protest, the pseudohomosexual panic. Soloff has described the presentation of acute psychosis precipitated by this dynamic in a military basic training program.[29] A violent outburst signals an effort at restitution of masculine power as well as a defense against fantasized sexual abuse. The absence in these patients of true homosexual orientation, or even "latent" homosexual concerns, differentiates the phenomenon dynamically from true homosexual panic despite similar consequences.

The Nonpsychotic Patient

When the nonpsychotic patient presents with violent or threatening behavior, a complex set of medical and legal issues must be raised. Foremost among these is the issue of responsibility, i.e., a determination of whether violence is willful and malicious or defensive and "irresistable." A dynamic psychotherapist may hold the patient responsible for both expressions of aggression, yet from a medico-legal perspective, some judgment must be made concerning degrees of responsibility and subsequent treatment. At the extremes such distinctions are clear. Patients who strike out as a final desperate response to intolerable conflict—perhaps feelings of helplessness or frustrated dependency—may be successfully engaged in a therapeutic program leading to relief of intolerable and ego dystonic impulse. The structure of the hospital milieu may relieve the external threats (or deprivations) that provoke violence in the conflicted patient. Conversely, the patient who is violent without anger, whose aggression is almost a casual response to mild frustration, brings to the hospital setting a deeply ingrained proclivity for violence. Individuals who are intolerant of authority and discipline in their own lives will most certainly bring willful violence into the hospital setting. This behavior should not be tolerated or treated in an inpatient psychiatric setting. Whether such patients should be admitted to mental health facilities at all is a legitimate administrative question. In cases where such distinctions can not be made at the time of admission, staff must clearly advise the patient of the consequences of willful violence. In some particularly enlightened hospitals patients may be held responsible for aggression as part of ongoing therapy. Gutheil and Rivinus include "the cost of breaking windows" in the price of hospital care where such costs are incurred through willful violence.[10] In spite of possible adverse publicity, some hospitals have pressed charges against patients for such violence and have insisted on the common-sense approach that responsibility is therapeutic.

A second problem emerges in the treatment of the nonpsychotic aggressive patient once staff has determined to treat the root causes of the presenting violence. How should staff manage disruptive behavior that emerges symptomatically during the course of treatment? To present the paradox most clearly, let us assume that the nonpsychotic patient is *voluntarily* admitted for treatment and that the use of forced medication or seclusion in this setting is allowable only for involuntary patients and only upon well-defined urgent need. Given these common legal constraints on the use of physical controls, how does one treat the escalating disruptive behavior of a nonpsychotic, voluntary patient?

In the acute, emergency circumstance, staff must act to abort or contain violence. A court order (temporary commitment) may be obtained after the fact to justify the use of force. More important, however, is negotiation with the patient that returns him or her to voluntary care (or results in discharge). In order to return to voluntary treatment, the patient must participate in negotiating a behavioral contract with staff in which the limits of tolerated behavior are defined, the consequences of violence are outlined, and the rewards for personal control are clearly stated. Such an agreement may call for "time out" periods of defined length for progressive agitation, the taking of PRN medication or even a brief period of seclusion (without undue force) as part of an etablished treatment plan. It also specifies the privileges available for compliance in a hierarchical ranking. The behavioral contract, as a formal treatment plan, represents a therapeutic alliance that is binding on both patient and staff. It defines the terms of treatment, including the use of physical controls, and by-passes legal entanglements in treating aggressive but nonpsychotic patients on a voluntary basis. Without such a treatment plan the use of force not only exceeds legal limits but raises the ethical issue of seclusion used in the service of social control or as punishment instead of treatment.

The Incompetent Patient

The complex relationship between civil commitment, competence, and informed consent to treatment is at present a topic of great legal controversy. A conflict arises between the patient's "right to treatment" and his "right to refuse treatment" when the treatment in question involves the forced use of medication, seclusion, and restraint. While no court has challenged the emergency use of physical controls as restraint, i.e., in self-defense, the use of seclusion and restraint to treat underlying illness or in the service of behavior modification have been strongly contested. In the case of the voluntary patient, informed consent to such use is essential. Pending the outcome of cases arguing the right to refuse treatment, the use of physical controls as *acute* treatment in committed patients remains accepted practice regardless of actual competency. Special attention should be paid, however, to the specialized use of seclusion or restraint in the systematic behavioral management of chronic symptoms in incompetent patients. The use of physical controls as negative reinforcers in long-term behavioral programs to shape behavior is qualitatively different from its use in treating acutely ill psychotic patients. This specialized use of seclusion and restraint in behavioral therapy generally is limited to retarded or severely regressed psychotic patients who generally are not competent to understand the treatment of give fully informed consent. For this specialized use in non-competent patients, legal safeguards should be provided to prevent abuse.

One legal model currently under consideration by the Florida legislature establishes administrative review of all methods of behavior control used with incompetent patients, in this case, patients of the Division of Retardation. A peer review committee, composed of "highly regarded professionals trained in applied behavior analysis," rules on the acceptability and efficacy of proposed procedures, while a lay review committee, the Committee on Legal and Ethical Protection, judges "the appropriateness of the behavior proposed to be strengthened or weakened and on the ethical propriety of the means to be employed." The purpose of this elaborate administrative model is to balance the noncompetent patient's "right to treatment" and "right to refuse treatment."[37]

SECLUSION IN DEFENSE OF SOCIAL MILIEU: RESTRAINT VERSUS TREATMENT

Seclusion-as-Restraint

Among psychiatry's critics the use of physical controls to maintain social order in the treatment milieu arouses the greatest concern. This was apparent in the judicial review of seclusion in Boston State Hospital. The presiding judge created a legal distinction between the use of seclusion-as-restraint, to control a violent episode in progress, and seclusion-as-treatment, for disruptive behavior. The restraint of assaultive patients in self-defense was considered legitimate, while the modification of disruptive behavior and intensive treatment of underlying illness through seclusion were not allowed. The distinction between seclusion as treatment and as a punitive tool of social control was not clear enough to satisfy legal standards. In clinical practice restraint, treatment, and defense of the milieu are inseparable components of seclusion, though each element varies in importance in relation to the patient's need. It is our contention that the use of physical controls in defense of the therapeutic milieu is justified only to the extent that the patient's treatment needs also are met.

In contrast to seclusion-as-restraint, where control of a momentary violent impulse is the goal of intervention, seclusion-as-treatment is the intensive care management of underlying psychosis. Seclusion-as-treatment is used to deal with patients who show such adverse behavior as smearing feces or drinking urine, continual yelling obscenities, or abnormal posturing. Severely regressed psychotic patients often require seclusion as the optimal treatment. The need for containment of impulse, destimulation, and a controlled environment for aggressive pharmacotherapy define the treatment indications. The duration of seclusion for the treatment of agitated, regressed behavior is gauged by the patient's mental status and gross behavior. As the underlying psychosis comes under control, the patient's behavior becomes more amenable to interpersonal approaches and less influenced by hallucination and delusion. The duration of seclusion is proportionate to the clinical response to treatment. It is important to note that potential dangerousness is not the sole determinant of duration when seclusion is used as treatment rather than punishment.

PRACTICAL MANAGEMENT OF THE DISRUPTIVE PATIENT

Isolation, Attention, and Medication

When confronted with a progressively disruptive patient, every effort should be made to contain the patient's behavior without resort to forceful seclusion or restraint. These methods include progressive isolation of the patient, increased (or decreased) personal attention, and PRN medication.

To a great extent the physical structure of the ward determines the feasibility of progressive isolation. The therapeutic intent of this maneuver is to reduce disruptive stimulation, provide a contained, well-defined space for mastery of ego boundaries or for reassurance of protection and defense. Although the specific method must be tailored to the patient's acute psychotic dynamics, the quiet back-of-ward or the patient's own (single) room most often are used. In an isolated, quiet area, the manic patient is less stimulated, the psychotic less disorganized and the paranoid less frightened. Isolation progresses from back-of-ward, to patient's room to open seclusion as needed, while personal contact and PRN medication contribute an additive pacifying effect.

Medication must be viewed as the mainstay of nonviolent restraint of the disruptive patient; however, without interpersonal rapport and cooperation, the administration of medication may become the first forceful confrontation with the agitated patient. Because of the time delay in the pharmacologic response, PRN medication should be used early in the treatment plan, along with progressive isolation and interpersonal attention. Oral medication generally is preferred to intramuscular (IM) when the needle would be viewed as an assault. Again, the method used depends on an understanding of the patient's dynamic response and the amount of time staff is willing to wait for a response. The objectives of intervention with medication must be clear from the onset. Staff may choose a level of response ranging from simple sedation on a one-time basis, through rapid neuroleptization to intravenous narcosis. The clinical condition of the patient, risk of violence, and time needed are the critical parameters in this decision. Where the urgency of time is predicted in hours (before escalation proceeds to uncontrolled violence), rapid neuroleptization with high potency agents (e.g., haloperidol) should be considered. Here the treatment goal is control over disruptive anxiety and the psychotic process itself. When an urgent clinical need is measured in a shorter time frame, the sedating neuroleptics may be indicated. In an extreme emergency situation a violently combative patient may require intravenous narcosis (e.g., sodium amytal) for control. It is important for staff to understand that all violent behavior can be brought under control acutely with medication, (e.g., with narcosis) but that the risk of the patient forces consideration of physical controls to "buy time" for less aggressive and safer pharmacologic approaches.

Seclusion Procedures

The proper application of seclusion as a treatment for disruptive or violent behavior requires the coordinated effort of all responding staff. It is sobering that half of all assaults on staff reported by Lion occurred during the process of restraining or secluding a disruptive patient or during management of the seclusion.[3] This risk can be minimized through proper technique. Once staff decide to seclude the patient, the physician, head nurse, or staff member responsible for instituting physical controls quickly assigns roles to participating staff. Special attention should be paid to selection of the seclusion leader and a seclusion monitor. The seclusion leader should be well known to the patient and, ideally, have a preexisting relationship which will encourage compliance. Dynamic factors must also be considered, e.g., one would not choose a male seclusion leader when a homosexual panic is the cause of the disruptive behavior. In general, the least intimidating staff member is to be preferred over the most authoritarian. The seclusion leader will direct all stages of the procedure. The seclusion monitor is not involved in the physical action but clears the area of other patients and physical obstructions to entering the seclusion room. The monitor then notes and records the progress of the seclusion so that an accurate critique can be made after the fact.

In the urgent but nonemergency situation, sufficient manpower must be present to guarantee safe but certain physical control over a potentially resistive and combative patient. This show of force must be apparent to the patient from the beginning of the confrontation. The seclusion leader addresses the patient in clear but nonthreatening terms, states the reasons for the seclusion ("your behavior is getting beyond your control," and so on), and requests the patient to move voluntarily to the seclusion room. It must be made clear to the patient that the time for discussion has passed and seclusion will be instituted by force if necessary. The attitude and demeanor of staff at this point greatly influence outcome. Every effort must be made to appear nonthreatening but clearly in command of the situation. Patients' response to intimidation almost invariably is defensive violence. Conversely, a nonthreatening, even deferential, request by a staff nurse may preserve self-esteem sufficiently to allow the patient to comply without humiliation. The decision to seclude the patient must be made quickly and should span seconds rather than minutes. Perhaps the greatest error in seclusion procedure is a last minute attempt to negotiate, reason, or interpret dynamics with an escalating disturbed patient. Prolonged dynamic negotiation at this point is more a function of staff need to justify the use of force and is superfluous to the patient. Rather than calming an agitated patient, a prolonged confrontation generally increases the patients' anxiety and confuses the staff's intent. (Now the patient must "understand" as well as comply.) After waiting a few seconds in silence for the patient to comply, the seclusion leader gives an unambiguous verbal command instituting the physical restraint of the patient. By this point, each staff member should be in a position to physically seize and control movement in one extremity. The patient is brought to the ground with a backward movement (protecting the head) while staff restrain the legs at the knee. Physical control is complete when the patient is lying on his back with staff controlling each extremity. In the emergency case where one or two staff have successfully brought a disruptive patient to the ground, primary attention is given to restraining arm movement. This is accomplished by forcefully holding the patient's arms crossed on top of the head and using the upper arms as a vise to control head motion. The staff member crouches low behind the patient's head to avoid being kicked by movement of the knees. When help arrives, the legs are controlled by force at the knee.

Once physical control is secured, the patient is moved to the seclusion room. Sufficient manpower should be present to allow the patient to be physically lifted in the recumbant position with arms pinned to sides, legs wrapped, head controlled and lift applied to the back. Inside the seclusion room the patient is dressed in a hospital gown; street clothes are removed, with special attention paid to rings, watches, belts, shoes, or other potentially destructive objects. Medication is given (PO or IM depending on compliance) and the patient is given final instructions in clear concise terms. Exit from the seclusion room should be a coordinated maneuver. The patient lies on his back with his head toward the open door and feet in the opposite direction. Control of the arms and head are switched to one staff member using the crossed arm maneuver. The lower extremities are released first, with each staff member exiting quickly. The last staff member releases the patient's arms and backs out of the open door, which is quickly secured. All seclusions require the continuous presence of a staff member who remains just outside the seclusion room.

Following each seclusion a debriefing should be conducted by the seclusion monitor in an effort to critique procedure and allow staff to deal with their feelings. Periodic reviews should be conducted of staff technique and preparedness to perform these physical maneuvers.

Release from Seclusion

The patient's ability to control disruptive impulses is assessed when staff enter the seclusion room to feed, bathe, medicate, or toilet the patient. Each entry is preceded by a request that the patient sit down away from the door and cooperate with the procedure. The seclusion room is always entered in an orderly fashion and in force, with security personnel preceeding medical staff on entry and following on exit. In the earliest contacts when the patient is most agitated or violent, each seclusion entry must accomplish multiple purposes to minimize the number of visits. In the most violent cases, where restraints are not in use, each entry may require physically restraining the patient with all the attendant risks of injury. Later, longer periods of time are spent with the patient and mental status and history are updated. The patient's ability to cooperate for longer interviews and for all procedures leads to a decision to "wean" him or her from seclusion. The patient is fully advised that his or her progress is determined by the ability to control impulse and cooperate with directions. The seclusion door is opened for progressively longer periods allowing more direct interaction between the patient and the nurse who has been in attendance throughout the seclusion episode. Finally, the patient is moved to a single room in a quiet area of the ward. Integration into the patient population follows continued control of behavior. Any loss of control results in return to increased security, such as open or locked seclusion or restraint, as needed.

The patient should have an opportunity to discuss the impact of the seclusion room experience. Acknowledging the patient's thoughts and feelings about seclusion helps the staff reintegrate the patient into the therapeutic process of the milieu. One of the most subtle and pernicious effects of the seclusion process is an altered staff perception of the patient. The secluded patient becomes a management problem to be handled in an objective efficient manner to prevent violence. The underlying causes or psychodynamic issues are often forgotten even after the seclusion has ended. Listening to the patient "debrief" the seclusion experience addresses these issues and often corrects distorted perspectives.

A Note on Instrumental Restraint

The use of mechanical restraint by "wet pack" or four-point leathers presents a final level of physical control and should be used whenever the patients' self-destructiveness presents a risk in locked seclusion (e.g., head banging) or whenever the threat of violence accompanies each staff contact with the patient. The ability to freely approach the patient without fear is the greatest advantage of mechanical restraint over locked seclusion. Where locked seclusion may deteriorate into isolation and neglect, the use of four-point leathers in the modern treatment facility enforces staff contact with the patient, if only to minister to the patient's comfort and needs. Feeding, bathing, and toileting the patient all require intimate contact which establishes interpersonal rapport that is not available through the locked door. The cultural humiliation of being bound and the physical risks of constraint must be weighed against the advantage of accessibility in each case. There is little justification for the use of mechanical restraint as a routine, nonintensive treatment. The camisole or hobbles which allow the patient freedom of the ward exact too high a psychological toll of humiliation to justify their use in the service of "prevention" of assault or elopement. In our experience these partial constraints provoke more conflict than they prevent. *Seclusion and restraint are intensive care treatments. The use of mechanical restraints for less than intensive care is symptomatic of subjective distortions in patient–staff relationships.*

CONCLUSION

Seclusion and restraint are indicated for the treatment of violent and disruptive behavior which is not responsive to interpersonal, chemical, or less restrictive physical interventions. They are useful in three related treatment strategies:

1. As restraint, in the emergency and acute control of violence
2. As treatment, for mental disorders underlying aggressive and disruptive behavior
3. As limit setting procedures ("time out") or negative reinforcers in systematic,

long-term, behavioral treatment programs (given the appropriate legal safeguards)

Seclusion and restraint are intensive care treatments and should not be used as a substitute for less restrictive therapeutic interventions or as a convenience to staff, as a form of punishment, or to exclusively serve social control without clear benefit to the individual patient.

Seclusion and physical restraint remain important treatment techniques in the care of violent and disruptive patients. The great advances in psychodynamic and pharmacologic management of violent patients have not relieved us of the need for these methods. There is a genuine need to relearn and refine the theory and practice of seclusion and restraint as they apply to the modern treatment milieu. It is equally important to relearn the "evils" inherent in the method since abuse of physical controls erodes the very foundations of humane care of the mentally ill. Through constant vigilance, we hope to avoid the overroutinization of use, the emphasis on procedure rather than on person, and the loss of interest in the basic psychologic needs of the patient that accompany abuse of physical controls. Through intelligent use, we hope to safely manage and prevent violent and disruptive behavior in the psychiatric treatment setting.

REFERENCES

1. Barton W cited in Glasscote R (ed): The Psychiatric Emergency. A Study of Patterns of Service. The Joint Information Services of the APA and the National Association for Mental Health, Washington, D.C., 1966, p 30
2. Binder RL: The use of seclusion on an inpatient crisis intervention unit. Hosp Community Psychiatry 30:266–269, 1979
3. Boling L, Brotman C: A fire-setting epidemic in a state mental health center. Am J Psychiatry 139:946–950, 1975
4. Bursten B: Using Mechanical restraints on acutely disturbed psychiatric patients. Hosp Community Psychiatry 27:757–759, 1975
5. Flaherty JA, Meagher R: Measuring racial bias in inpatient treatment. Am J Psychiatry 173:679–682, 1980
6. Greenblatt M, York RN, Brown EL: From Custodial to Therapeutic Patient Care in Mental Hospitals. New York, Russell Sage Foundation, 1955
7. Guenther AL: Conference report: Handling the violent patient in the hospital. Hosp Community Psychiatry 29:463–476, 1978
8. Gutheil TG: Observations on the theoretical bases for seclusion of the psychiatric inpatient. Am J Psychiatry 135:325–328, 1978
9. Gutheil TG: Restraint versus treatment: Seclusion as discussed in the Boston State Hospital case. Am J Psychiatry 137:718–719, 1980
10. Gutheil TG, Rivinus TM: The cost of window breaking. Psychiatr Ann 7:72–76, 1977
11. Holt v. Sarver 309F. Supp. 363 (1970)

12. Kalogerakis MG: The assaultive psychiatric patient. Psychiatr Q 45:371–381, 1971
13. Klass DB, Growe GA, Strizich M: Ward treatment milieu and post hospital functioning. Arch Gen Psychiatry 34:1047–1052, 1977
14. Knopf WF: Modern treatment of the "insane." An historical view of nonrestraint. New York State J. Med 60:2236–2243, 1960
15. Lion JR: Evaluation and Management of the Violent Patient. Springfield, Ill, Charles C. Thomas, 1972, p 73
16. Lion JR, Snyder W, Merrill GL: Underreporting of assaults on staff in a state hospital. Hosp Community Psychiatry 32:7, 497–498, 1981
17. Lion RJ, Pasternak SA: Countertransference reactions to violent patients. Am J Psychiatry 130:207–209, 1973
18. Madden DJ, Lion JR, Penna MW: Assaults on psychiatrists by patients. Am J Psychiatry 133:422–425, 1976
19. Mattson MR, Sacks, MH: Seclusion: Uses and complications. Am J Psychiatry 135:1210–1213, 1978
20. Moos RH: Evaluating Treatment Environments: A Social Ecological Approach. New York, John Wiley and Sons, 1974
21. Moos R, Shelton R, Peety C: Perceived ward climate and treatment outcome. J Abnorm Psychiatry 82:291–298, 1973
22. Negron v. Preiser 382F. Suppl. 535 (1974)
23. Oversy L: Homosexuality and Pseudohomosexuality. New York, Science House, 1969
24. Plutchik R, Karasu TB, Conte HR et al: Toward a rationale for the seclusion process. J Nerv Ment Dis 166:571–579, 1978
25. Rogers v. Okin (Rogers v. Macht) Civil Action No. 785-1610T in the U.S. District Court for the District of Massachusetts
26. Rosen H, DiGiacomo JN: The role of physical restraint in the treatment of psychiatric illness. J Clin Psychiatry 39:228–233, 1978
27. Schwab PJ. Lahmeyer CB: The use of seclusion and restraints on a general hospital psychiatric unit. J Clin Psychiatry 40:228–231, 1979
28. Soloff PH: Behavioral precipitants of restraint in the modern milieu. Comprehensive Psychiatry 19:179–184, 1978
29. Soloff PH: Pseudohomosexual psychosis in basic military training. Arch Sex Behav 7:503–510, 1978
30. Soloff PH, Turner SM: Patterns of seclusion: A prospective study. J Nerv Ment Dis 169:37–44, 1981
31. Stanton AH, Schwartz MS: The Mental Hospital: A Study of Institutional Participation in Psychiatric Illness and Treatment (ed 1). New York, Basic Books, 1954
32. Tardiff K: Emergency control measures for psychiatric inpatients. J Nerv Ment Dis 169:614–618, 1981
33. Wadeson H, Carpenter WT: Impact of the seclusion room experience. J Nerv Ment Dis 163:318–328, 1976
34. Wells DA: The use of seclusion on a university hospital psychiatric floor. Arch Gen Psychiatry 26:410–413, 1972
35. Wexler DB: Mental Health Law: Major Issues, vol. 4 in Sales BD (ed): Perspectives in Law and Psychologies Series. New York, Plenum Press, 1981

36. Whitman RM, Armao BB, Dent OB: Assault on the therapist. Am J Psychiatry
     133:4, 426–421, 1976
37. Wyatt v. Stickney 344F. Supp. 387 (1972)

Barry J. Nigrosh

18

Physical Contact Skills in Specialized Training for the Prevention and Management of Violence

THE NEED FOR SPECIALIZED TRAINING

The prevention and management of violence deserves thorough attention as a specialized subject for staff training in clinical psychiatric settings. Such training properly includes the physical contact skills of self-defense and restraint with clinical intervention. The psychological consequences of poor prevention and poor handling of violence are serious enough to warrant such attention. However, the element of physical danger to others as well as to the patient distinguishes the problem of violence from other areas of psychiatric concern and makes it particularly important. Yet, despite its high emotional

The suggestions concerning training methods and content found in the last section of this chapter are based on the author's experience providing training on violence prevention and management in a variety of mental health treatment settings. I wish to acknowledge my collaboration on several occasions with William Paul, Ed.D., of the Social Science Program, San Francisco State University, San Francisco, California 94132. Dr. Paul's expertise in nonviolent self-defense, humane restraint, and physical contact skills training methodology is strongly reflected in the training suggestions presented in this chapter.

and physical costs, violence as a training problem has in many settings been virtually neglected.

In contrast, other kinds of physical danger are treated with the utmost respect in health care settings and other facilities which serve the public. Emergency safety programs aimed, for example, at fire prevention, evacuation, first aid, cardiac emergency care, and water safety receive a great deal of special planning regulation, training, drilling, and testing. Indications are, however, that in some psychiatric facilities assaults may be the leading cause of injury.

Mounting evidence shows that the incidence of assault- and violence-related injury is much greater than previously assumed.[15, 18] Even if the number of cases were lower, their overall cost, measured in the several different terms described below, must be viewed as great.

Financially, violence creates a significant expense to some hospitals. In 1980 the facility in which the author works suffered 160 employee days of lost work attributable to patient assault, making an average for that year of about 0.6 days per worker. The hospital pays twice for this loss since not only does the worker receive compensation benefits for time off the job but overtime wages must often be paid to replace him or her.

Occupational Safety

There is labor–management friction over violence as an occupational safety issue. Workers perceive, with justification, that in this area there is a lack of programmatic commitment to protect their interests, in comparison for example, with industrial work-sites. Following an investigation in response to charges made by hospital workers, the California Occupational Safety and Health Administration agreed that the workers were not receiving adequate protection from violent patients.[14]

Hospitals face a relatively high rate of job-related injury, but they also bear the burden of most investigations and prosecutions when patients are hurt. Staff members feel that they are easily sacrificed when the exigencies of policy or staffing are in fact more at fault. The physically larger male staff members complain that they are frequently singled out to work in potentially violent situations, then criticized because the record shows them to be involved in a disproportionately high number of violent incidents and injuries. Sometimes direct care workers will seek criminal charges against assaultive patients. But courts look unfavorably on complaints by individual staff, citing the doctrine of "assumption of the risk" by those who accept employment in mental hospitals. In short, a fair amount of resentment toward administration accrues among staff who feel they shoulder danger and liability without concomitant supervisory support. In an era of "patients rights," hospital labor organizations are becoming exquisitely sensitive to their own legal positions.

Clinical Concerns

The cost of violence illustrates the critical need to prevent or minimize the occurrence of violence, but certainly for psychiatric facilities we would *not* add to this "by any means necessary." After all, with sufficient use of force, intimidation or drugs it would be possible to subdue any ward. Our long-range clinical objectives as well as our immediate humane desires should dictate very specific and careful methods of intervention. These methods are among the most difficult and time consuming to learn. They stem from theory, not from convenience, and can not be expected to emerge from staff without benefit of training.

The patient's deficits in internalized control and the potential of these deficits to lead to dangerous behavior are often a primary reason for inpatient treatment, especially involuntary treatment. As a result of developmental failure or complication by organic pathology, these patients are prone to express themselves through socially unacceptable and sometimes dangerous action. Our goal is not to control the patient—though it is a necessary first step—but to strengthen his ability to control him- or herself so that when the patient is discharged he or she is less likely to act dangerously. This is not simply a responsibility to society at large, for we believe that people feel better when they control their own action rather than relying on others to do it for them.

While there is a legitimate prophylactic use of medication for limiting violence,[28] the repeated use of chemicals on an emergency basis to quell violent behavior clearly does not aid in the development of self-control. The use of behavior modification programs which manipulate environmental contingencies may also have value in limiting ward violence.[15] It is extremely difficult, however, if at all possible, to "export" the modified behavior from the treatment setting to the environment that may have spawned the disorder.[13] The control, rather than being internalized as "self-control," remains bound to the stimuli of the treatment environment. Even the extreme punishments and controls used in prisons have never clearly been shown to deter violence after release.[31]

The goal of fostering self-control is best served when staff interventions are informed by a shared understanding of the underlying dynamics of the patient's violence. Although the etiology of violence is complex and multidetermined, and many theoretical persuasions compete to explain it, certain useful generalizations can be made which cut across functional and organic diagnostic categories. These generalizations, if carefully illustrated in terms of daily experience on the ward, can be understood and confirmed through the staff's own experience. A generalized etiology of violence then can serve as a premise to guide intervention enabling the staff to respond creatively to varying situations, rather than proceding by rote.

Attributes of Violence

The Subjectively Threatened Self

Most violence, excepting the purely instrumental kind, is a response to events that expose the vulnerability of the perpetrator. Such events include attacks, threats, losses, frustrations, and insults.[25] In ego psychological terms this can be viewed as defense against narcissistic injury.[24] Social learning theorists view it as response to aversive events.[29] The cognitive theorist calls it a reaction to "assault on the personal domain."[3] Consciously or otherwise, the raised weapon or the violent assault offers the assailant a brief experience of power and momentary relief from feelings of passivity, helplessness, or ignominy. Though the defensive purpose of the act often is not achieved, and afterward individuals may feel remorse or humiliation, many report feelings of boundless strength, however briefly, during explosive moments. The more repetitive an individual's violence, the more likely we are to uncover personal histories of childhood abuse or humiliation contributing to chronically poor self-esteem. Although the insecurity and hurt that underlies most violence may seem obvious, often the truth is obscured for staff by countertransferential fears. The first step, therefore, in dealing with angry, potentially violent, or violent patients is to protect his injured self-image as much as possible in order to avoid escalating his motivation toward destructive action. This includes, for example, acknowledging the patient's power to hurt, allowing certain victories, supporting the urgency of a grievance, offering choices instead of simply ordering, and addressing the patient as a dignified adult.

Loss of Control

Violent patients fear and are threatened by loss of self-control.[16] This point is known by experience to most health care workers who witness the many direct and indirect ways that potentially violent people seek to be controlled. A patient's plea for medication or restraint to "stop me before I do something", an adolescent resident's limit-testing destructiveness before the watchful eyes of staff, or a murderer's lack of attempt to escape detection, all are indications that violent individuals on some level do not wish to go unchecked. This can be understood on two levels. First, developmental theoreticians have observed an apparent motivation toward the mastery of self-control, i.e., to bring behavior under conscious control so that action is purposeful and effective.[12, 30] Lapses in the ability to control one's actions are a painful and humiliating throwback to a helpless, infantile state of development. Second, in the process of socialization the developing child internalizes society's values concerning aggression as they are represented by the parent and enforced through limit setting. Violent transgressions recall punishment and guilt and awaken anxiety by threatening the sense of security and self-worth that originates in the sustenance and approval once given by the parent. Although it may seem contradictory that violent action promises an individual a feeling of power yet stirs anxiety over loss of control, that is exactly the point which the staff member must understand; the patient is in conflict over competing internal demands. The worker must attempt to protect the patient's self-esteem and must also give assurance to the patient that the staff can provide the necessary external controls where the patient's internal controls fail. Just as in child development, the foundation for limit setting is the staff's ability to provide complete physical control[7] though infrequently required. The patient must be able to view the staff as in control of itself, organized, professional, and disciplined, yet still unconditionally supportive of the patient's self-worth. Viewed in this light, the proper management of a physical confrontation with a patient is every bit as much a clinical therapeutic intervention as the proper management of an interview and as such is an equally important subject for training.

Levels of Self-Control

Violent behaviors are on a continuum with harmless minor acts against inanimate objects at the low end and homicide at the high extreme. An element of self-control can be seen in the displacement of violence on property rather than person. Some potentially violent patients may need only the calming attention of a staff member, the reassurance of safety, or the removal of dangerous objects from their presence to maintain self-control. Others at times may need the presence of several staff, an unlocked quiet room, voluntary medication, or the suggestions to lie on their beds. For others more complete external control such as seclusion, mechanical restraint, or physical holding may be required. The point here is that the degree of external control exercised should be enough to supplement whatever remaining controls exist in a patient at any given time and not more. The patient should be told of the staff's intent to replace the patient's missing controls only so much as and as long as necessary.[23]

The primary clinical reason to avoid using more staff initiated control than is necessary is to protect the patient from overreliance on others for control. Repeated use of overly restrictive measures to control behavior demonstrates to the patient the expectation that he is not capable of controlling himself. In addition, if the patient can see that the staff members are overreacting and not in control of themselves, his or her confidence in their ability to help with his or her problem may be undermined. Another problem with overly restrictive measures is that the patient obviously will view the intervention as punative, further insulting his or her damaged self-esteem. One should remember that the more extreme control interventions have special risks of physical and psychological complications. For example, seclusion may cause some patients to direct violence against themselves. It may create conditions of sensory deprivation which can exacerbate perpetual distortion in psychotic patients or encourage certain unfortunate wary phenomena such as "seclusion envy."[9] Chemical restraint contains the hazard of side effects, especially hypotensive reactions.[28] Any control interventions that require transport to special rooms entail risk of physical injury to staff and patient in the process.

It should be noted that the touching of patients by staff without the patients' permission is not termed illegal battery on the condition that the touching is in the interests of the patient and his fellow patients. The limit on permissable physical contact is usually defined by the standard of "least force necessary" which coincides with the clinical standard we have discussed. In Massachusetts, for example, regulations govern the use of mechanical and chemical restraint and locked-door seclusion (Massachusetts, Department of Mental Health Regulations, 104 CMR 312). The regulations state that the staff must first demonstrate attempts to use lesser measures before resorting to these more restrictive measures.

The training problem involves helping staff to find the right degree of control for each incident of violence. It is possible to err by intervening too weakly or too late just as it is possible to err by acting too forcefully. The first skill requirement is the ability to assess the patient's type and degree of self-control at a given time. The next is to have available a range of control-supporting measures from which to choose. All too often staff members will briefly attempt to engage in conversation with an upset patient, then, finding no immediate effect, will resort to physical restraint without attempting to find creative intermediate measures. Even when the patient must be physically moved, there is still a range between "soft" escorts (e.g., staff at patient's arm guiding him to objective) versus immobilization holds (e.g., four or five staff carrying the patient face down). The staff's ability to modulate the use of external controls can be enhanced through training and practice under simulated conditions.

Diminished Capacity to Think and Speak and the Potential for Violence

Not every insult to self-esteem ends in violence because normally a variety of mental mechanisms aid in channeling or modulating the motivation toward violence. Some mechanisms involve the capacity to imagine or foresee the likely consequences of an act, especially the sanctions of society as represented by police, jail, ostracism, and the like. Others involve the ability to use words or fantasy rather than action for the gratification of "getting even," i.e., devaluing the object so as to elevate self-worth by comparison. The experience of empathy, of understanding the other's position, or recognizing mutual characteristics exerts an inhibitory influence on violence, as does the ability to plan more effective and less self-injurious alternative response to violence. These capacities all involve the use of cognitive representations in mental events that are interposed between provocation and (violent) response. They provide a means of releasing tensions and solving problems through thinking rather than through action.[4] These processes also take time and thusinterpose a delay between impulse and act which may be of critical importance in the outcome of an incident.

Forming a Therapeutic Alliance with a Potentially Violent Patient

Forming such an alliance requires an understanding of the peculiar limitations on the patient's capacity to have a relationship. Staff tendencies to make two common types of errors must be overcome. The first and most dangerous error involves confusing the need to provide controls with confrontation. The origin of this error is easy to see, since in society the control of one person over another's behavior generally occurs in the context of the exercise of authority and often involves aggressive postures and stern warnings or threats. The obvious danger, previously discussed, is that an overpowering approach will compound the injury to the patient's self-image. Another danger, more to the point, is that the staff person will become a target of the patient's anger, eliminating the possibility of a working alliance. The second and opposite sort of error stems from recognizing the patient's injury and approaching it with too much expressed empathic and supportive concern characterized by statements such as "I know how you feel and I'm here to help you." This mistake also is easy to understand, because much of the emphasis in beginning clinical training is on the development of a supportive empathic approach. This attempt at securing a working relationship often backfires with the patient turning on the staff person, insisting that his or her feelings can not be understood and that the staff person is part or all of the patient's problem.

These methods of attempting to engage the angry patient fail to account for an important aspect of anger, i.e., the mechanism of projection. Like violence, the anger which often preceeds it serves a defensive purpose. In an attempt to ward off the attack on his or her self-worth, the angry person externalizes the attack and focuses insult and flame on others. In a state of acute arousal, this focus may be rather indiscriminately displaced on convenient objects in the patient's perceptual field.

Gutheil and Havens[10] have provided us with useful suggestions on forming a "situational alliance" with patients who use projection as a major defense, and Havens has amplified this by describing the therapeutic technique of "counter-production."[11] The goal of the situational alliance is to quickly form a relationship that minimizes patient's projection on the helper. In contrast to more traditional forms of therapeutic alliance, counterprojection seeks to draw attention away from the clinical relationship, so that "The situation resembles that of two strangers witnessing some disaster on the street."* A counterprojec-

---

*Reprinted with permission from Havens LL: Exploration in the uses of language in psychotherapy: counterprojective statements. Contemp Psychoanal 16:53-67, 1980.

tive intervention has three parts. First, "It must point 'out there,' because in part protection follows attention."* This is why skilled interviewers do not stand face-to-face with angry or paranoid people. Instead they stand obliquely or at the patient's side symbolically facing what the patient faces. Likewise, in contrast to traditional therapeutic interactions, the skilled interviewer will avoid eye contact since it draws attention to him- or herself and thus invites projection. Second, the counterprojective intervention should center on the figures that concern the patient, as if "on a protective screen before the patient and therapist."* For example, if the patient complains, "That nurse said I'm too disturbed to go to the dance!" a simple declaration such as "What a drag!" will be a much more effective statement than "I can see how you must be upset by that," because the second statement draws discussion back to the patient and staff person. Likewise, interpretations, since they show the staff person's concentration on the patient's mind, should be avoided. Interpretive statements such as "You're really angry because your mother cancelled her visit" directly attack the patient's projective defense and are bound to increase his disturbance. Third, "Some part of the patient's feelings about those figures must be expressed by the therapists . . . The therapist joins the patient for a moment in the patient's attitude towards the figures because his standing aloof would reinvite the projections."* Thus, the staff person's approach must not be too controlled and clinical, but rather should show some affect approaching the patient's own. Exclaiming, "That stinks!" is more likely to form instant rapport than saying, "Sometimes such situations are difficult to tolerate," because the first statement places the staff person on an emotional plane much closer to the patient's, providing a basis for affiliation.

PHYSICAL INTERVENTION AS CLINICAL INTERVENTION

Training Programs

Just as there is danger in ignoring contact skills training, there is a corresponding pitfall in rushing to teach physical skills without a comprehensive clinical training program. The training of physical contact skills outside the context of clinical theory reinforces the attitude that when action starts clinical concerns are dropped. Instituting common martial arts or self-defense training classes is the most serious error of this kind. Such systems do not belong in psychiatric settings for several reasons. The types of unarmed combat taught to police, armed forces, or for self-protection on the street take advantage of pain for the purpose of control. They overlook the fact that pain may stimulate

---

*Reprinted with permission from Havens LL: Exploration in the uses of language in psychotherapy: counterprojective statements. Contemp Psychoanal 16:53–67, 1980.

increased resistance and instead count on the ability to completely overwhelm the opponent. Blows, kicks, jointlocks, and unsafe takedowns should not be used in a clinical setting for obvious psychological reasons and because of their high potential for injury and abuse. There is a great deal of romantic sensationalism in the American perception of Asian martial arts which is incompatible with the attitude we wish to promote among staff, yet in the minds of staff such sensationalism often emerges as the first response to the mention of training in physical contact skills. Many martial arts systems feature aggressive fighting stances accompanied by cries and other sounds calculated to intimidate opponents. Moreover, they often do not address questions of safety such as protecting the opponent's head and avoiding fracture. Skills required for safe escort and transport, and problems involved with multiple team assists are not dealt with. Most importantly, the concept of modulating force to match the patients' need for control is ignored.

In recent years training consultants specializing in contact skills for health care settings have begun to appear. Although to a great extent the systems they teach are based on existing schools of martial arts, they have drawn on the martial arts selectively and have attempted to overcome the shortcomings mentioned above. Some have succeeded more than others, and instructors vary in the degree of aggression they communicate to their trainees. Nonetheless they represent a significant advance in bringing technology and discipline to bear on this previously haphazardly managed subject. Facilities considering initiating such training would do well to shop around among programs, to scrutinize the curriculum, and watch instructors in action. Some institutions have the entire program previewed by human rights committees. Avoid programs that promise to accomplish a great deal in just a few hours or a day, because rapid acquisition of such skills is impossible. Audiovisual programs that do not allow for practice under supervision are also of questionable value and may lead to faulty development of motor coordinations.

It is of the utmost importance for the physical contact skills training system to be carefully integrated into a larger training program that puts physical intervention in proper clinical perspective. The ability to make sound judgments about how, when, with what degree of intensity, and for what purpose to intervene physically is more important than the physical skills themselves. Such judgments can not be made without a basic understanding of dynamic principles such as those previously described. Additionally, the use of physical intervention along with verbal intervention should be discussed and practiced at length. It is critical for staff groups to develop protocols for team interventions so that members of a team know how to call for help, how to assemble, who should speak, who should be in charge, and how decisions should be made. Staff needs to understand how team intervention should be used to promote talking when possible, rather than to replace talking. Then, in cases where physical intervention is required, staff must learn through supervised rehearsal to coordinate and assist each other in an expeditious manner. Ample opportunities to explore countertransferential problems pertaining to the use of force must be allowed. Legal questions concerning the use of force must be addressed and the proper documentary justification for physical intervention should be studied and practiced.

An indication of the "state of the art" in Massachusetts is offered by the results of a survey conducted in 1980.[27] Six training programs were found to be receiving funds from the State Department of Mental Health. The oldest program was three years old, and the average age was less than two years. Four of the programs were for the mentally retarded. Of the two that were aimed at a mentally ill population, one was developed for adolescent group homes and one for state psychiatric hospitals. The six programs ranged from 4 to 40 hours in length and averaged about 22 hours each. The trainer-to-trainee ratio ranged from 1:4 to 1:20.

All placed some emphasis on understanding and preventing violent behavior but this varied widely in quality and degree. All had some discussion of assessment, *warning signs*, or *cues*. One, the program for the psychiatric hospital, provided analysis and role play of interview and noncontact techniques. This program also was the only one to provide analysis and role play of noncontact and contact team interventions, although all programs devoted some discussion to *team building* questions. The approach to teaching contact physical skills fell into two categories. Four had primary emphasis on discrete, situation-specific skills such as "release from hair pull," "arm grab controls," and "standard therapeutic hold." Two programs provided practice in situation-special skills but gave more emphasis to general abilities such as "evasive maneuvers," "safe approach and engagement," and "deflection and neutralization of blows." All had some mention of legal issues and documentation. Several programs were instituting periodic retraining and testing at the time of the survey. Evaluation procedures, where conducted at all, varied widely and could not be considered rigorous.

Barriers and Resistances to Training

Clinicians often express the belief that the problem of violence in psychiatric facilities, once serious, has now been solved. It is taken on faith that modern medication and therapeutic milieu management have eliminated violence. The passing of the use of extreme and prolonged methods of restraint is seen as evidence of the passing of the problem. Yet the fact that few facilities have useful data collection procedures on this subject indicates that clinicians have avoided asking the simple questions that would confirm their beliefs, and this, viewed against the medical and psychotherapeutic gravity of the question, implies a measure of denial.

The countertransferential response to anxiety elicited by violent patients is one of the chief sources of denial. Lion and Pasternak have discussed the therapist's anxiety that his or her own urges may be awakened in the face of violence, and lead the therapist to ignore obvious signs of dangerousness.[17] In a related discussion Adler and Shapiro mention withdrawal from the patient and counterphobic denial of danger in response to the projections or to real threats of violent patients.[2] Guilt about involuntary physical control of patients also may be a contributing factor, especially among clinicians who feel embarrassment on behalf of their profession for the mishandling and abuse of physical restraint in previous eras.

Not only are unexamined aspects of the clinician–patient relationship likely to play a part in denial, but psychological factors between the clinician and staff may contribute to the clinician's avoidance of the problem. On some level clinicians may be aware that they have failed to support ward staff. Often clinicians can walk away from ward violence but ward staff can not. Guilt about this may in turn lead the clinician to minimize the problem, or to rationalize it in terms that justify removing him- or herself. Viewing the issue as one of safety management rather than therapeutics provides such an excuse, defining away leadership in violence control as "not part of my job." This avoidance may be further bolstered by stereotypes of the staff as somehow better equipped by experience, origin, or physical capacity to handle the task. Ward staff may collaborate in this process, taking advantage of an area where they may distinguish themselves as being more capable than clinically trained leaders.

Clinicians may fail to see the management of violence as a clinical concern because management includes physical contact, and traditional psychotherapeutic training and practice excludes "touching." Only the most experimental and "fringe" schools of therapy include body contact between therapist and patient. Access to the patient is gained through the mind or sometimes the bloodstream but not the body. In essence there is no precedent in the clinician's training for physical contact. To overcome this separation clinicians will be called on to enter a previously excluded territory. Development of a refined technology for physical intervention in violence will require collaboration with experts outside the field of psychotherapeutics, especially in physical education. An interesting example of such collaboration can be found in the emerging field of sports psychology, where perhaps the glamor and profitability of modern sports have induced clinicians to venture outside their traditional domain. In addition, other disciplines such as social psychology and anthropology may make valuable contributions on subjects such as interactional factors, nonverbal communication and "body buffer zones."

THE DEVELOPMENT OF TRAINING STANDARDS

Because training in this area has been slow to develop, there is little consensus on how to go about it, creating yet another roadblock. There are few accepted training standards and little research on the safety and effectiveness of intervention methods. To some extent every facility that undertakes such training today is engaging in a pioneering activity. In the past few years several papers describing efforts made by individual facilities have been published.[1,8,14,22] All of these offer brief descriptions of curricula that include physical intervention. All use some form of role playing and discussion to highlight basic clinical ideas. Three discuss administrative steps, including the formation of study committees, taken as part of the program development.[1,8,14] These articles provide encouragement and a starting point but make it clear that for the present each facility must develop its own standards and methods of training. The lack of an authoritative body of knowledge, especially for the training of physical intervention, is itself a barrier to the spread of training. It means that the administrators or clinicians who sponsor such training must take full responsibility for methods that may be alleged at some time to be the cause of injury.

Perfecting and standardizing the technology and training methods for this area, which has to date received so little study, will require much effort. Lest it seem overwhelming, let us briefly examine some comparable problems that have been handled successfully.

Although we have stressed that violence prevention and management training should not be regarded simply as a form of safety training, examples from the field of safety and emergency medical care provide a model of how organized and standardized of training can be developed.

Until the 1960s numerous methods for attempting to revive people suffering cardiopulmonary collapse have been practiced. The quality in each form of training varied, and for many interested persons captioned illustrations were the only source of information. In 1966 the National Academy of Sciences-National Research Council sponsored a conference on Cardiopulmonary Resuscitation (CPR) that recommended CPR training for medical, allied health, and paramedical personnel and stimulated a wide variety of private and governmental agencies to contribute research, organization, and training on the subject. In 1973 a conference cosponsored with the American Heart Association led to the standardization and promulgation on a national basis of CPR and Emergency Cardiac Care Training. Today we know this to be a tremendously effective life-saving program.[26] Similarly during the same period, the Department of Public Health spearheaded the development of Emergency Medical Technician (EMT) Training which led to national training and certification of a corps of paraprofessional emergency responders and began to make order out of chaos in emergency medical transportation. A third example can be found in the area of water safety where the American Red Cross, in 1915 began to demonstrate life-saving techniques and succeeded in improving, standardizing, and disseminating life-saving training. The nation's drowning rate was cut by more than half, and today virtually no public swimming places operate without certified Red Cross Lifesavers in attendance.[5,6]

A comparative survey on these three examples of national training programs was prepared by the Human Services Training and Development Consortium.[21] The survey found that all three provided standards in the following ways. Curriculum content is prescribed by the central body and distributed to local approved instructors with training guides. Standardized Training Handbooks are periodically revised to accommodate new research findings and technology. Training duration and time distribution is specified as is the acceptable ratio of trainers to trainees. The training design, methods, and the nature of the training practicum is specified in detail. Training facilities and equipment also are specified. Entry requirements for trainees including medical restrictions, minimum physical skills and capacities, and prerequisite training are described. There are established criteria for certification including attendance, standardized written examinations, and most importantly performance on prescribed practical exams. Lastly, there are criteria and methods for periodic training and testing for recertification.

Instructor training is also strictly prescribed along lines similar to the basic training. The method for selection and certification of instructors, however, differs among the three programs. The American Heart Association delegates this authority to local committees, EMT instructors are selected and certified centrally by the Department of Public Health, and the American Red Cross empowers centrally approved instructor-trainers to certify local instructors.

The high degree of effectiveness that these programs demonstrate is attributable to their large scale. Although they drew on the experience of local programs, the sponsorship of prestigious national bodies and the mandate to serve the national population allowed for a degree of development that never could have been achieved on a local scale. Progress in the area of violence prevention and management might be served best by a similar national approach. Since staff turnover and the need for periodic retraining require that training be a continuous process, most facilities will wish to have certified instructors among their own staff. This suggests that the training should be disseminated mainly through the certification of instructors at a central or regional institute. If one considers the needs of other types of facilities in addition to psychiatric hospitals—such as psychiatric community residences and outpatient centers—as well as nonpsychiatric facilities that might benefit— such as juvenile and adult corrections facilities, general hospital emergency rooms, and even schools—it becomes clearer that a centrally organized training effort is the most economical and helpful approach.

As we have seen the prevention and management of violence requires the combination of therapeutic skills such as assessment, interviewing, and milieu management with the physical contact skills involved in the neutralization and containment of violent action.

TRAINING METHODS AND CONTENT

Noncontact and Contact Skills

A simple first step in promoting the integration of noncontact and contact skills involves the time distribution of the elements of training. Ultimately the trainer wishes to have both types of skills discussed and applied simultaneously in combination. Initially, however, the fundamentals of both classes of skills must be learned separately. Rather than modularly structured teaching— presenting, for example, interviewing techniques one day and self-defense maneuvers the next—one- to two-hour periods of each technique should be interspersed in alternation throughout the early parts of training until the staff is sufficiently well versed in both, and the techniques can be combined. This teaching method serves several purposes. Practically speaking, it avoids boredom by providing physical exercise to breakup potentially wearing mental exertion, and conversely it creates rest periods to forestall physical exhaustion. Some staff may come to the training motivated only to learn physical contact skills. Delays in providing some of what they are seeking may encourage resistance to material which they may perceive as more traditionally academic. The most important reason for proceeding as described is to show by example the program's commitment to the belief that both verbal and physical intervention are inseparable parts of a unified and balanced approach to the management of violence. The order of the curriculum suggestions presented below is an example of how such an integrated presentation can be achieved.

The first exposure to physical contact skills should cover two sorts of basic principles. First, through demonstration and practice the trainer should illustrate important fundamentals of body mechanics concerning, for example, balance, force deflection, where power is best generated, protective postures, footwork, and safe falling. Safety in dress should be discussed. Second, the transactional aspects of physical intervention should be illustrated. Important points about nonverbal communication can be shown experientially if the trainer physically approaches trainees in various ways leading to discussion about nonaggressive postures and minimizing threat cues. This is also a good time to illustrate the nonverbal correlates of the "counterprojective" position showing how, for example, approach from the side and "facing with" rather than confronting can reduce adversarial expectations and support a "situational alliance" and minimize conflict.

The trainer's next step is to sharpen the staff's assessment skills and to impress staff with the importance of early intervention to increase the likelihood that the incident can be managed on a verbal rather than physical level. Experienced staff usually are quite able to discern warning signs, so a good approach is to draw on their experience by having trainees meet in small groups to compare and record their observations. Then in the large group the trainer can build master lists based on contributions from the small groups under headings such as "observable behavior," "speech content," "organic conditions," "ward environment," and "history." Such lists can be used to stimulate discussion which further understanding of theoretical principles. It is particularly important for staff to be instructed in assessing the patient's levels of available self-control. It is also useful at this juncture to discuss attributes of the ward environment that may cause or exacerbate violence.

Staff should be taught basic required motor skills in pairs. At the outset clear rules of discipline should be specified regarding conduct during training. One very important rule, drawn from martial arts instruction requires a "ready" or "greeting" sign such as bowing which shows mutual respect between opponents before each engagement. The trainer should start with simple "core" skills on which others will be built. These skills should be drilled initially in stylized "slow motion" so that the instructor has an opportunity to correct faulty moves before basic motor coordinations are formed. Gradually the speed and intensity of the moves should be increased.

The specific contact skills to be mastered can be divided into two categories, defense and restraint. A good start on defense ability will have been made under the fundamentals already discussed. Now is it time to practice releases from different holds, blocks for different kinds of blows and kicks, weapons controls and the like. When in subsequent segments the required competence in defense is evidenced, the instructor should turn to basic restraint maneuvers including making the opponent off balance controlling limbs, conducting safe takedowns, standing partial restraints, and immobilizing on the ground.

Because staff may be insecure about their competence as interviewers, the trainer must be careful at first to minimize anxiety and protect staff self-esteem. For unsophisticated audiences it may be unwise to begin with role plays. A good beginning method is for the trainer to present vignettes or situations for group discussion. For example, he or she can say; "I'm a patient. If I stormed into the nurses' station and shouted 'I'm sick of all your rules!' How would you begin talking to me?" or "What would you say if I said, 'I feel I'm going to explode and do something?'" Once the comfort level of the group arises, role plays can be staged in pairs. The trainer can instruct the patient actor to: "Threaten to hurt that staff person unless she grants you a privilege," or "give an indirect warning by asking how many staff will be left on the ward at dinner time." To make the dramatizations more real and to allow for more specificity of intervention, the trainer should introduce the events to be enacted by describing the location, the ward conditions, and the preceding occurrences. Some role plays will be more useful if they are accompanied by a description of the patient's pathology and descriptions of his or her history for behavior under different kinds of circumstances.

A side benefit of role-play techniques is that they provide the trainee with the opportunity to experience the patient's dilemma, thus expanding empathic ability. This becomes more significant as training progresses and role plays eventually include extreme control measures. The trainee who is actually restrained, transported, or secluded receives a first-hand lesson concerning the physical and emotional response to these events.

The subject of interviewing may require several training segments because there are many important points to cover. Some examples include: making broad declarative openings; the appropriate level of affect to express in order to meet the patient's own; acknowledging a patient's grievance; acknowledging his or her power to hurt and otherwise supporting the patient's strength; ressuring the patient that staff will provide external control as needed; dealing with displacement; diffusion and protection; expressing limits in most face-savings ways; what to say when confronted with weapons and threats; and, intervention in interpatient arguments. At this point it is also logical to introduce discussion about the pros and cons of "cathartic" activities (e.g., punching bags), when if at all, these can be used, and how they should be structured. Certain statements used to begin verbal interventions or to respond to typical patient's comments may arise repeatedly during practice sessions. At times the trainer may worry that he or she is leading staff members to rely on "magic words." It is the author's belief that an assortment of "pat" phrases that become part of staff members repertoire is not a bad thing because in anxiety-provoking interactions their use may avoid awkward speechless moments and provide needed time to plan what to say and do next. To the extent that trainees arrive at a useful understanding of the theoretical objectives of intervention, they will be able to expand their repertoires and adjust them to suit their personal styles.

For contact and noncontact skills alike, one of the trainer's main jobs is to aid staff in coping with the anxiety inherent in violent situations. To some extent this is achieved through understanding dynamics, developing empathy, and rehearsing interventions. However, the most powerful method for strengthening the trainee's ability to manage stress is through a gradual desensitization to anxiety-provoking stimuli under controlled conditions. This behavioristically inspired method, similar to the "stress innoculation" described by Novaco[19] involves the successive approximation to real conditions through stimulation. Once the fundamentals of verbal and physical skills are established, the practice of each should follow a pattern of increasing affective intensity with more realistic yelling and threats and more forceful touching. Eventually, the interactions should become random and unpredictable, so that those who are in the role of staff will not be prepared for what is to come and will have to make quick judgments about what to say and do. In contact skills segments this will take the form of spontaneous "sparring." The processing of these exercises in group discussion should allow ample time for staff to discuss their feelings in response to these dramatic and life-like pressures and to receive support from each other.

Group Intervention

Initially the subject of group intervention should be divided into non-contact and contact segments, in accordance with the previous format. This is important because we want to overcome the common staff belief that assembling several staff is always for the purpose of physical restraint. The trainer should emphasize the use of the group as a technique to reduce the need for contact intervention by providing an intermediate level of control. This involves exploring the value of group presence as a containment factor, and the ways in which a group can extend the possibility of "talking" solutions. Once again we appeal to role play to draw out the important principles of group coordination. One method that the author has found useful has been to deliberately stage chaotic scenes by coaching the actors to talk simultaneously and take opposing approaches. Asking "What's wrong with this picture?" leads to stimulating discussion on the effect of group disorganization on the patient. It also highlights the need for leadership. Then dramatic situations can be set up in which the "patient" is instructed to approach, but not cross, the line between verbal accessibility and the need for physical control. Some of the important questions to be discussed include: When should team intervention begin? How to get help to the scene? How can staff communicate and make decisions in front of the patient? Who should be in charge? Who should talk? What if a team member disagrees with a group decision? How can the patient's anxious fantasies about what the group might do be dealt with? How do team members know where to position themselves? A good goal for this segment is for the training group to come up with a written proposal for a protocol to answer these questions. This is important because strategies for team coordination are of little use unless known and shared by all individuals who may be called on to function together within or across wards in a facility.

After the methods of team coordination have been discussed, a segment or more on group contact skills is required. As with all previous maneuvers, these maneuvers should be presented first in slow motion, then with increasing intensity. The skills treated under this heading should include: assisting an assaulted staff person, two-person standing escorts, full immobilization on the ground, and full involuntary transports. In addition, if seclusion, emergency medication, or mechanical restraint are used in the treatment setting, then proper methods for conducting these procedures should be discussed and rehearsed at this time.

Simulating Ward Incidents

The culmination of training is the combination of noncontact and contact skills in intense and random simulations of all kinds of incidents. These are set up as much to perfect the trainees' judgment as to provide for intervention practice. The trainer should organize the simulations in such a way that the trainees who are chosen to intervene will not know what to expect. As on the ward, their job will be to assess the patient's controls and the specific nature of his or her problem. They will then have to make judgments about whether one-on-one verbal intervention should be attempted or if group intervention or physical restraint is required. They may have to decide, for example, whether to restrain or transport a patient. Which of the following, if any, is indicated; escorting the patient to his or her own bed or using an open room, locked seclusion, mechanical restraint, or intermuscular injection? Training exercises requiring such judgments serve to increase the staff member's flexibility and broaden his or her range of response to varied situations. An equally important virtue of this design is that it allows study and rehearsal of verbal interventions to be used in conjunction with physical interventions. Questions for discussion under this heading include: How and when to explain the purpose, method, and duration of restraint interventions to a patient? What, if anything, should be said to a restrained patient? What can you say to a struggling patient? What should be said after a restraint is completed?

The value of recreating life-like simulations can be extended by using them to improve understanding of statutes and regulations as they apply to violence management. Questions relevant in Massachusetts, for example, would include the following: Did the staff person have a "duty to retreat" rather than intervene with force? Does this intervention represent the "least force necessary?" What evidence is there that the patient's behavior reflected "a substantial likelihood of imminent bodily harm" and thereby justified use of involuntary emergency "chemical restraint," seclusion, or mechanical restraint? These questions most often will not have definitive answers, but the trainer will find that staff members appreciate the opportunity to have important terms defined and to clarify the intent of the authorities who set down the rules which staff must follow.

Not all staff members are suited for duties which include interacting with potentially violent and violent patients. Some may need special help; The training format which we have described provides a good occasion for evaluation by the trainer. Observing trainees under simulated conditions enables the instructor to spot special problems. Some trainees may be too anxious and timid, others may demonstrate their anxiety by refusing to be serious and disciplined, while still others may be overly "macho" and unable to give up aggressive, authoritarian styles. A certain number will be physically unable to learn or perform particular skills. For some, remedial counseling or coaching may be helpful. The trainer may find it necessary to recommend that others be channelled into services where the violence potential is lower. Because of the clinical and safety importance of competence in this area, facilities should not pass up this valuable opportunity for screening staff.

Methodological Considerations

A training program as comprehensive as that described can easily run a total of forty hours. Trainee groups with higher skill levels may require somewhat less time. The fact remains, however, that this is probably a more time-consuming endeavor than usual training events. This raises the questions of whether the training should be "massed" or "distributed" over time. In the author's experience there is special value in distributing sessions, usually half days once or twice a week. This is probably the best way to consolidte learning the physical skills. A more important advantage arises from the fact that a program such as this has a training effect that occurs outside the classroom as well as in. It generates much peer discussion and "raises consciousness" about issues related to other aspects of clinical performance. Spacing apart the training sessions extends the period of lively debate. It also allows for a greater number of actual incidents to arise in daily ward life, providing more case material for analysis.

The training program's credibility will be enhanced if the trainers are drawn from ranks similar to the trainees. Except with very small groups it is best to have more than one trainer because the training job is demanding and trainees benefit from individualized attention, especially with contact skills. Multiple trainers allow for multidisciplinary representation. A major effort should be made to include women as trainers. Because of the nature of the subject, there is a tendency for men to dominate and prevent women from deriving as much value as possible from the training. Female trainers demonstrating competency with physical skills serve as encouraging models for female staff and also provide a useful lesson in important performance attributes for men. An instructional team of female and male trainers is an excellent solution since it can create an example of mutual respect and cooperation.

The best trainee group normally works together in staffing a particular area. This creates certain staffing problems by stripping a ward of "regulars" so that they can train together. If this problem can be overcome by providing appropriate relief it is of significant advantage. When a staff group goes through the training experience together there is an excellent opportunity for "team building." They can establish a shared understanding of theory, learn to use subtle forms of communication, know each other's strengths, and support each other in dealing with anxiety and countertransferential problems. With regard to more practical issues, they can develop plans and policies that may help lower the violence potential inherent in their particular environment. Some facilities have found it helpful to include all levels of staff in the training so that direct care staff, clinicians, and administrators gain a first-hand appreciation for the realities of each other's concerns.

REFERENCES

1. A program for the prevention and management of disturbed behavior. Hosp Community Psychiatry 27:724–727, 1976
2. Adler G, Shapiro LN: Some difficulties in the treatment of the aggressive acting-out patient. Am J Psychother 27:548–556, 1973
3. Beck AT: Cognitive Therapy and the Emotional Disorders. New York, International Universities Press, 1976
4. Carney FL: Treatment of the aggressive patients, in Madden, DJ, Lion JR (eds): Rage, Hate, Assault and other Forms of Violence. New York, Spectrum, 1976, pp 223–248
5. Commodore WE: Longfellow—Water Safety Crusader, American Red Cross pamphlet, 1964
6. Dulles FR: The American Red Cross—A History. New York, Harper and Row, 1950
7. Gair DS: Limit setting and seclusion in the psychiatric hospital. Psychiatr Opinion 17:15–19, 1980
8. Gertz B: Training for the prevention of assaultive behavior in a psychiatric setting. Hosp Community Psychiatry 31:628–630, 1980
9. Gutheil TG: Observations on the theoretical bases for seclusion of the psychiatric inpatient. Am J Psychiatry 135:325–328, 1978
10. Gutheil TG, Havens LL: The therapeutic alliance: Contemporary meaning and confusions. Int Rev Psychoanal 6:467–481, 1979
11. Havens LL: Exploration in the uses of language in psychotherapy: counter-projective statements. Contemp Psychoanal 16:53–67, 1980
12. Hendrick I: The discussion of the "instinct to master." Psychoanal Q 12:561–565, 1943
13. Hersen M: Limitations and problems in the clinical application of behavioral techniques in psychiatric settings. Behav Ther 10:65–80, 1979
14. Learning to manage assaultive behavior. Innovations 6:35–36, 1979
15. Liberman RP, Barringer MD, Burke, KL: Drug and environmental interventions for aggressive psychiatric patients, in Stuart RB (ed): Violent Behavior: Social Learning Approaches to Prediction, Management and Treatment. New York, Brunner Mazel, 1981, pp 227–264
16. Lion JR: Evaluation and Management of the Violent Patient. Springfield Ill, Charles C. Thomas, 1972
17. Lion JR, Pasternak SA: Countertransference reactions to violent patients. Am J Psychiatry 130:207–210, 1973
18. Lion JR, Snyder W, Merril GL: Hosp Commun Psychiatry, (in press)
19. Novaco RW: A stress innoculation approach to anger management in the training of law enforcement officers. Am J psychol 5:327–346, 1977

20. Pinderhughes CA: Managing paranoia in violent relationships, in Usdin G (ed): Perspectives on Violence. New York, Bruner-Mazel, 1972, pp 109–140

21. Promoting the Provision of Quality Training in the Prevention and Management of Violence: Suggested Procedures. Unpublished manual prepared for the Human Services Training and Development Consortium, Office of Manpower Planning and Development, Department of Mental Health, Cambridge, Mass., 1980

22. Ramirez L, Bruce J, Whaley M: An educational program for the prevention of disturbed behavior in psychiatric settings. J Continuing Ed Nurs 12:19–21, 1981

23. Redl F, Wineman D: Controls from Within; Techniques for the Treatment of the Aggressive Child. Glencoe, Ill: Free Press, 1952

24. Rochlin G: Man's Aggression; the Defense of the Self. New York, Dell, 1973

25. Staub E: The learning and unlearning aggression: the role of anxiety, empathy, efficacy and prosocial values, in Singer JL (ed): The Control of Aggression and Violence: Cognitive and Physiological Factors. New York, Academic Press, 1971, pp 94–124

26. Standards for cardiopulmonary resuscitation and emergency cardiac care. JAMA 227:833–868, 1974

27. Training in The Prevention and Management of Violence: A Survey of Massachusetts Programs. Cambridge MA, Human Service Training and Development Consortium. Prepared for Massachusetts Department of Mental Health, Office of Manpower Planning and Development, 1980

28. Tupin JP: Management of violent patients, in Shader R (ed): Manual of Psychiatric Therapeutics: Practical Psychopharmacology and Psychiatry. Boston, Little, Brown, 1975, pp 125–136

29. Turner CW, Fenn MR, Cole AM: A social psychological analysis of violent behavior, in Stuart RB (ed): Violent Behavior: Social Learning Approaches to Prediction, Management and Treatment. New York, Brunner Mazel, 1981, pp 31–67

30. White R: Ego and reality in psychoanalytic theory, Psychol Issues 3:1–210, 1963

31. Zimring FE: Perspectives on Deterrence. Rockville, MD, National Institute of Mental Health, Center for Studies of Crime and Delinquency, DHEW Publication No. (ADM) 74-10, 1971

John R. Lion

19
Special Aspects of Psychopharmacology

The topic of medication invariably arises when a violent patient is presented at a clinical conference. The question "What is the patient on?" usually is heard. This query is an interesting one, for there is an implicit belief that medication and only medication is the most important intervention in preventing assault. Indeed, when it is learned that the patient is still aggressive, a change in medication often is mandated with the hope that one or another drug will correct the behavior, as though the behavior could not be influenced by the milieu, by a behavior modification plan, or by simpler verbal interventions. This chapter will comment on the rational use of medication with the premise that pharmacologic agents alone are not the answer to violence. Thus, psychodynamic considerations of drug use will be discussed briefly as well. The reader is referred to a previous larger work on this subject.[9, 10]

ANTIPSYCHOTIC DRUGS

Antipsychotic drugs are the most widely used to control combative and assaultive patients within institutional settings. Because of extensive literature describing the rapid neuroleptilization technique[4] utilizing haloperidol

(Haldol), this drug has been seen as a drug of choice for aggressive patients. Other medications such as fluphenazine hydrochloride (Prolixin) can be used with equally efficacious results, but the body of clinical experience with this drug is not quite as great as that with haloperidol. Rapid neuroleptilization is in effect simply the repetitive administration of small amounts of parenterally administered medication until behavioral quiescence is reached. Although a medication such as haloperidol should in theory be used only for assaultiveness of "psychotic" proportions (i.e., stemming from a psychotic patient's behavior), it is used in a more nonspecific fashion to control belligerent alcoholics, agitated character disorders, or organic syndromes. Use of high-potency antipsychotic drugs such as haloperidol has largely replaced previous use of chlorpromazine, which is more cardiotoxic.

Administration

Utilizing neuroleptic techniques is an art. This author is constantly surprised how few physicians know how to use a syringe and delegate the task of injection to a nurse while aides restrain the patient. Attitudes may have to be revised in this matter. It is unrealistic for a clinician to think that his or her control over a patient is optimal if, in effect, other people are treating the patient with a host of unpleasant procedures. This author favors the clinician's giving the medication and offering the necessary reassurance. This means that the clinician must have the cooperation of a team and should have rehearsed the skills in restraining the patient to make the injection safe. The best place to inject is in the buttocks; absorption is somewhat quicker from the deltoid because of increased blood flow but use of an extremity is riskier.

It is demeaning to jab a violent patient in the body with a needle without a word of explanation. Even flagrantly psychotic patients can comprehend the events around them and should be told what medication they have received and what results are expected. If the patient has been violent enough to require restraining, parenteral medication, and seclusion, he or she needs more care, not less. This means that staff, including those who took part in the subjugation, should spend time with the patient immediately as the behavior subsides after the event. All too often, the patient is hurled into a special room, medicated, and left alone.

Offering oral medication to a patient often precludes the need for parenteral drugs. The patient can be told that he could take something to calm down. Undermedication is the rule, and such patients can be told that the drug may not work in which case the dose will be increased. If the clinician predicts excessive sedation or the patient hears the phrase "knocked out," he or she is apt to become more violent. This is particularly true for paranoid patients who value hypervigilance and are wholly intolerant of lethargy unless it is self-induced with alcohol or other drugs.

Table 19-1
Format to Document Evaluation of Medication Used to Treat
Aggressive Symptoms

Drugs	Maximum Dose Used	Exposure (Days)	Effect (Described)
Haldol (haloperidol)	60 mg	7 days	minimal change
Cogentin (benz-tropine mesylate)	1 mg		
Navane (thiothixene)	15 mg	14 days	moderate improvement
Cogentin (benz-tropine mesylate)	1 mg		

List all regimens of jointly used drugs but specify dosages for each.

The matter of practicing restraint and seclusion cannot be overstressed (see Chapter 17). A good team approach to a violent patient does more to preserve a milieu and prevent future outbreaks of violence than all the medication in the world.

The use of antipsychotic medications outside the emergency room situation is more a function of the clinician's preference and the patient's medication history. It is logical to get a good history of drug exposure from the patient and the family before deciding which medication will work and which medication will not. A common expression heard in the management of assaultive patients is that "he has been tried on everything." This remark usually means that the patient has received innumerable medications for very short lengths of time in inadequate dose ranges. It is thus useful to construct a medication table as outlined in Table 19-1. Documenting dose, exposure, and outcome helps avoid the notion that the patient has indeed been tried exhaustingly on various regimens of drugs.

Dosage

Most clinicians ask what dosages to use in an assaultive patient. The answer has to do with several factors including the degree of psychosis, the size of the patient, and the clinician's familiarity with dose ranges beyond control of the acute case. This author has seen more mistakes made from underdosing than from overdosing. There is a tendency to view the dosages cited in the *Physician's Desk Reference* (PDR)[17] as the medico-legal limit in medication when in fact these are simple guidelines; dosages in excess of PDR limits can be given as long as the specific rationale and indication for the excess is mentioned in the chart. Nonetheless, a 100-mg dose of haloperidol is commonly considered "massive," while in fact it is merely the upper limit of the PDR-recommended dose. ("Megadoses" are dosages 100 times greater than those conventionally used in the U.S.) If the patient is beginning to respond to 60–80 mg of haloperidol and shows no adverse affects of toxicity, it might be logical to go to 100 or 110 mg to see if there are any changes while documenting the rationale for the larger dose and recognizing PDR guidelines. The mistake is in "calling it quits" too soon. At a time when acute hospital stays are common, this author generally urges residents to start a patient on a reasonable amount of medication such as 10 mg of haloperidol. They can double the dose each third day until a PDR maximum is approached. If no effect is seen, and noncompliance or poor absorption can be ruled out, the drug should be discontinued, and another antipsychotic agent should be tried. The clinician needs to remember that no dose works overnight and that a several-day minimum exposure is required to see behavioral changes. It must be recalled, incidentally, that assaultive patients may become less assaultive but remain quite delusional; thus the target symptoms of hallucinations and delusions will require more aggressive pharamacologic treatment.

Overmedication occasionally is an issue, particularly when it causes sedation and lethargy and worsens the delusion and subsequent behavior by inducing an organic brain syndrome. Taking patients off medications when this is suspected sometimes demonstrably improves conditions. This author has often seen the "snow phenomenon" whereby a patient is viewed as exceedingly dangerous and assaultive, given large amounts of medication, and secluded and put in what is tantamount to sensory deprivation.[1] Fearful of being in a locked room, the patient's behavior escalates and becomes loud and boisterous. Nursing staff become more frightened and ask the doctor to prescribe more medication. The medication is administered parenterally without any verbal discussion, the patient's condition worsens leading to more medication, and a vicious cycle ensues. This situation can be reversed both by taking the patient out of seclusion and lowering his medication.

This author has no hesitation in trying an assaultive patient on four to five classes of antipsychotic drugs before deciding he is refractory. This would include a decent trial of phenothiazine, butyrophenone, loxapine, molidone, or some other chemical grouping. Perseverance is important.

Alternatives to Medication

Some patients benefit more from restraint techniques that enable them to mingle on a ward than from being medicated and placed in a seclusion room.

Creative uses of restraint garments, halters, and belts may enable assaultive patients to participate in group meetings and ambulate on the wards. Such devices, including the old straight jackets, are viewed with repugnance by many members of the profession. If used judiciously, however, with the aim of allowing the patient to benefit from the ward rather than exclude him, they are far more humane than placement in an isolated room with high amounts of psychotropic agents.

Ward personnel need to be fully familiar with the basic principles of behavior modification[14] and use simple paradigms for more chronic patients or even adolescent patients who test limits and are destructive and belligerent.

This author favors an outside opinion or consultation regarding any violent patient who does not improve within the hospital after a reasonable time. Feelings about these patients become highly polarized and a fresh opinion regarding both the milieu and medication are welcome.

Patients can not only be prescribed medication, they can be taught to ask for it specifically when they feel they are going out of control or becoming angry or violent. Such a tactic has the advantage of promoting affective awareness[8] and replacing chronic dosing with a PRN schedule. Less drug use occurs if the cumulative dose is monitored.

ANTIANXIETY AGENTS

An extensive literature, both professional and lay, now warns against the use of antianxiety agents unless there is a "pure" anxiety and unless dosages are time limited. While concurring with these principles of practice, this author has found that severe character pathology often warrants medication for less pure reasons and for longer lengths of time than is theoretically desirable. The target symptom for which one prescribes these drugs is not as clear cut as one might wish.

The antianxiety agents of choice presently are those of the benzodiazepine class such as diazepam (Valium) and chlordiazepoxide (Librium). These agents are useful for the nonspecific and more chronic anxiety seen in many severe personality disorders such as the paranoid personality, the obsessive-compulsive personality, or the labile antisocial personality or borderline personality.[12] The pervasive agitation in these people leads to labile reactions to stress at work, home, or in the hospital. When irritability is slightly dampened with an antianxiety agent, the tendency toward aggressiveness is reduced. Paranoid personalities are more tolerant of these drugs than of antipsychotic agents which inevitably produce side effects that worsen compliance. The more depressed obsessive-compulsive personality, when hospitalized, may be very difficult to manage on the ward because he or she is so perfectionistic and demanding; this type of person may react with anger and even physical violence to disturbances in routine and ritual or to the many imperfections that occur on a milieu. A small amount of diazepam such as 5–10 mg/day is a useful aid in helping the cause of patience.

These drugs are also useful for behavior disorders seen in organic brain syndromes or in patients exhibiting mental retardation. Some geriatric patients who are belligerent and assaultive may benefit from short-acting forms, which have no metabolites and short half-lives, such as oxazepam (Serax) and lorazepam (Ativan).

It is as illogical to combine antianxiety drugs with antipsychotic drugs as it is to combine a variety of antipsychotic agents. One drug at a time is the rule.

"Paradoxical rage reactions" have been described as associated with the administration of benzodiazepines in some patients.[7] In this author's experience no such findings have occurred when these drugs are given to violent patients.[11] The rage reaction is a disinhibitory phenomenon more ubiquitously seen with alcohol than with any other drug.

Lithium

A significant literature exists on the use of lithium for the treatment of aggressive patients and a variety of authors have used it to control assaultiveness. This author has used it to treat atypical affective disorders such as that in a mentally retarded adult who showed mood swings typified not by the usual depressive–manic cycle or despondency–hypomania pattern but by fluctuating levels of behavioral arousal.[13] This patient became aggressive during some weeks, quiescent during others. Lithium might be a logical choice in a nonpsychotic patient who is assaultive and shows some manic-like features with pressured speech, mood fluctuation, irritability or grandiosity. Lithium has also been used to control aggressiveness in mentally retarded patients[5] though the explanation for its effectiveness again is lacking. The most reasonable use of lithium to prevent violence in a patient is after longitudinal assessment of the patient's mood and lability, with the aim of extracting any evidence of cyclothymicity. If there is evidence of cyclic mood alterations or lability, and conventional treatments have failed, lithium is worth a try.

Lithium works well within the hospital but patients may discontinue it in the less-structured community. Thus it makes no sense to base the premise of use solely on its availability; one must also assess whether the patient is a realistic candidate for therapy after discharge. Behaviorally disordered patients or those with brain dysfunction often do not take their pills. Involvement of the family in therapy is helpful in overcoming this serious difficulty.

ANTICONVULSANTS

A variety of anticonvulsants have been touted as useful for aggressive patients including those who are assaultive. The current anticonvulsant of choice most described in the literature is carbamazepine (Tegretol). This drug has been found useful as an alternative to lithium for certain types of affective illness seen to stem from underlying limbic system kindling disorders such as temporal lobe epilepsy and for similar disorders in which violent behavior is the prominent symptom.[19]

On our inpatient service a good deal of carbamazepine is used in both clinical and experimental fashion for the control of patients who have "tempers." Diagnostically, these patients generally fall into the impulse control disorder groupings such as the Intermittent Explosive Disorder of DSM III. Some patients have superimposed character pathology, while others show atypical psychoses in which violent outbursts become prominent. The rationale for the use of carbamazepine in patients with impulse control disorders is that this drug reduces a temporal lobe seizure-like state that may underlie the behavioral outbursts of these patients.

The use of anticonvulsants requires that the clinician ascertain the existence of neurologic dysfunction, either by history, physical examination, or laboratory tests such as the EEG. Consultation with a neurologist for "soft" signs of minimal brain dysfunction may help to substantiate the diagnosis. Yet, even in the absence of much data, this author is still inclined to use the drug if there appears to be a strong "organic" component to the patient's violence. Sudden, abrupt-onset and recurring and paroxysmal violent outbursts with change of consciousness and CNS symptoms, including postictal changes such as drowsiness, may convince one to try the drug.

Not all clinicians have had exposure to the use of anticonvulsants to treat explosive outbursts or episodic behavior disorders,[15] and some clinicians seem to feel that the use of anticonvulsants lies more in the domain of neurology and should, therefore, be prescribed by specialists of that discipline. However, the number of neurologists who directly involve themselves in the therapy of aggressive behavior disorders is minimal, and the task of using "neurologic" drugs ultimately falls to the psychiatric clinician. Literature exists on the use of other anticonvulsants for the therapy of paroxysmal behavior, thought, and affective disorders.[6, 16]

One effect of prescribing anticonvulsants is to evoke the belief on the part of the patient, his or her family, and other patients and staff that a true seizure disorder is "responsible" for the patient's behavior, much as grand mal spells would result from the epilepsy by the same name. This can falsely exonerate the patient from taking responsibility for his or her acts. Anticonvulsants, if used, should be viewed as dampening the quality and quantity of violence, not removing the conflicts that gave rise to the act. Psychotherapy is still required and the diagnosis of an "epileptoid" condition, does not exempt the patient from participation in the hospital milieu.

INNOVATIVE AGENTS

Several drugs have been described as useful for the treatment of aggression but their use is still viewed as controversial or they have not been formally approved by the FDA. The first of these is the class of CNS stimulants in adult violent patients. Central nervous system stimulants are the drugs of choice for children with attention deficit disorders both with and without hyperactivity; the drugs do reduce aggressiveness secondary to their effect on the general syndrome. In adults their use is more innovative. The target population is somewhat at risk for drug abuse and drug traffic on an inpatient service is always a problem. Nevertheless, readers should be aware of a literature which documents, in more anecdotal fashion, the utility of these drugs.[2]

The progestational agents have long been used to control the aggressiveness that accompanies the heightened sexual drive state seen among paraphiliacs such as exhibitionists and also among rapists.[3] The drug has been used in this country but is still not approved by the FDA.

Less clinical experience surrounds the use of propranolol to control aggressiveness of hospitalized patients with irreversible organic lesions.[20]

The point to be made with the above description of innovative agents is that the clinician must document treatment failure on conventional regimens of therapy before using these agents. Only then is their use justified, assuming that consent is available, the family complies with treatment, and all parties are aware that the agent's use is innovative. Further technicalities such as the procurement from the FDA of an IND number (investigation of new drug) are beyond the scope of this chapter. The diverse variety of drugs to control violence should give hope to the practitioner. At the same time, it must be realized that the aim of pharmacologic therapy is not to completely suppress all aggression, but to control it and to help the patient control it. Violence in an aggressive patient can be controlled through complete sedation, but that is not an acceptable goal. The goal of drug treatment should be to curb the impulsivity and lability of the patient so that he or she thinks before acting and speaks while thinking, thus allowing for conflict resolution. This is a delicate task. The author has seen a profound depression develop in patients whose aggression was "quenched by drugs," and who were then, for interesting and complex reasons, unable to vent their anger but were forced to channel it inwardly.

CONCLUSION

Rare is the violent or assaultive individual who can not receive some benefit from a combination of intelligent milieu management and medication. To be sure, there are always in every state facility some intractably aggressive patients who have over the years developed behavioral life-styles with super-imposed organic deficits. These patients must be kept in virtual seclusion and might theoretically be candidates for psychosurgery, a problematic procedure in today's climate of informed consent. Most violent hospitalized patients, however, respond to the milieu, particularly when effort is made to identify at whom they are angry and at whom they are prone to become assaultive. Sometimes clear patterns emerge and victims can be identified such as the provocative teenager, the provocative geriatric patient, the provocative staff person. It is often assumed that patients are diffusely and randomly violent and destructive; on closer inspection, recurring trends can be seen, allowing for social interventions that complement the use of medication as a control measure.

REFERENCES

1. Appleton WS: The snow phenomenon: tranquilizing the assaultive. Psychiatry 28:88–93, 1965
2. Bellak, L (ed): Psychiatric Aspects of Minimal Brain Dysfunction in Adults. New York, Grune & Stratton, 1979
3. Berlin FS, Meinecke CF: Treatment of sex offenders with antiandrogenic medication: conceptualization, review of treatment modalities, and preliminary findings. Am J Psychiatry 138:601–607, 1981
4. Donlon PT, Hopkin J, Tupin JP: Efficacy and safety of rapid neuroleptization with injectable haloperidol. Am J Psychiatry 136:273–278, 1979
5. Dostal T, Zvolsky P: Antiaggressive effect of lithium salts in severely mentally retarded adolescents. Int Pharmacopsychiatry 5:203–207, 1970
6. Flor-Henry P: Schizophrenia-like reactions and affective psychosis associated with temporal lobe epilepsy: etiological factors. Am J Psychiatry 126:400–403, 1969
7. Lion JR, Azcarate CL, Koepke HH: Paradoxical rage reactions during psychotropic medication. Dis Nerv Sys 36:557–558, 1975
8. Lion JR: Evaluation and Management of the Violent Patient. Springfield, Ill, Charles C Thomas, 1972
9. Lion JR: Conceptual issues in the use of drugs for the treatment of aggression in man. J Nerv Ment Dis 160:76–82, 1975
10. Lion JR: The Art of Medicating Psychiatric Patients. Baltimore, Williams and Wilkins, 1978

11. Lion JR: Benzodiazepines in the treatment of aggressive patients. J Clin Psychiatry 40:70–71, 1979

12. Lion JR: Diagnosis and treatment of personality disorders, in Lion JR (ed): Personality Disorders Diagnosis and Management. Baltimore, Williams and Wilkins, 1974

13. Lion JR, Hill J, Madden DJ: Lithium carbonate and aggression: a case report. Dis Nerv Syst 36:97–98, 1975

14. Mann RA, Moss GR: The therapeutic use of a token economy to manage a young and assaultive inpatient population. J Nerv Ment Dis 157:1–9, 1973

15. Monroe RR: Episodic Behavioral Disorders. Cambridge, Harvard University Press, 1970

16. Monroe RR: Anticonvulsants in the treatment of aggression. J Nerv Ment Dis 160:119–126, 1975

17. Physicians' Desk Reference. Oradell, NJ, Medical Economics Co Inc, 1982

18. Sheard MH: Lithium in the treatment of aggression. Nature 230:113–114, 1971

19. Tunks ER, Dermer SW: Carbamazepine in the dyscontrol syndrome associated with limbic system dysfunction. J Nerv Ment Dis 164:56–63, 1977

20. Yudofsky S, Williams D, Gorman J: Propranolol in the treatment of rage and violent behavior in patients with chronic brain syndromes. Am J Psychiat 138:218–220, 1981

Manoel W. Penna

20
The Effect of the Milieu on Assaults

Case Study 20-1

A young man was admitted to a psychiatric unit after he presented himself in the emergency room with the chief complaint of experiencing the strong urge to approach women in order to engage in sexual activities. He was perplexed by the intensity of these impulses and was uncertain as to whether or not to carry them out. On examination he was found to have tangential thinking, auditory hallucinations, and paranoid ideas of reference. As a child he had been rather passive and had been beaten up by girls in street fights although in his adolescence he had successfully joined his high-school wrestling team. Following admission the patient was started on haloperidol (Haldol), which was progressively increased to 40 mg/day. His thought processes became better organized and he felt in better control of himself. He appeared sedated, however, and the dose of medication was decreased by half. A few days later the patient went home on a weekend leave to pursue a complex plan of extensive activities. He was not able to carry out this plan and aroused a great deal of concern among his family as he expressed the urge to fight with other people. When he returned to the psychiatric unit, it was noticed that his condition had worsened, and he was verbally expressing his difficulty in dealing with both aggressive and sexual urges. The staff listened to the patient and was aware of his predicament but no special intervention was made until the patient suddenly struck a female patient and was placed in seclusion. The following morning he was out of seclusion and attended a large community meeting in the ward during which he was restless and expressed paranoid ideas. The incident of the preceding evening was discussed and the patient was told by his doctor that violence was not tolerated on the unit and its recurrence would result in his discharge and transfer to another hospital. Immediately after the meeting the patient attacked the female patient again and his doctor felt obligated to carried out his admonition to the patient who was then transferred to another hospital.

This brief clinical vignette illustrates several aspects of the problem of managing and treating assaultive patients in the psychiatric hospital milieu. To be sure there are much more serious assaults occur in the milieu, sometimes resulting in extensive destruction of property or more severe physical injury to staff or other patients. Nevertheless, although such dramatic incidents arouse a great deal more interest and concern than an incident such as that in the case study, those incidents are much more rare than, and are usually preceded by, developments similar to this case. Assaultive behavior is only one of the elements in a complex chain of events that may start with the verbal report of experiencing uncontrollable impulses and move through various forms of aggressive behavior into full-blown assault. By the time the latter occurs as illustrated in our example, valuable opportunities have been missed for intervention that could very well have prevented the undesirable outcome.

Violent behavior certainly is not circumscribed to the hospital milieu and has aroused concern in a variety of clinical settings from the Emergency Room[8] to the patient's home.[13] Cultural variables seem to be important in determining the prevalence of violence; in the United States it unfortunately has acquired respectability as a serious clinical problem,[3] while other countries report relatively negligible figures.[4] Some suggest that shifts in social attitudes and policies, such as the emphasis on dangerousness as a behavioral attribute required for involuntary hospitalization, are actually making a large cohort of individuals prone to display violent behavior a legitimate subject of at least a psychiatric evaluation if not treatment. The likelihood of violent behavior occurring in the psychiatric hospital is thereby increasing.

To better understand the interactions between aggressive behavior and the psychiatric hospital milieu, two sets of variables need to be discussed: 1) the features of the milieu that are relevant to its functions of providing a context for behavior as well as for modifying it and 2) patient's characteristics such as the nature of individual psychopathology.

THE PSYCHIATRIC HOSPITAL MILIEU

The term milieu, as it applies to a psychiatric hospital, does not reflect a unitary, universally recognized concept. On the contrary, it reflects a variety of models—often proposed with a high degree of parochialism—stemming to a large extent from their origins in different therapeutic environments with different goals, serving different psychiatric populations, and following different staffing patterns. The organizational models derived from these different kinds of experiences are promulgated as an act of faith although they rarely can be completely extrapolated to a different setting. This is further complicated by the fact that the hospital treatment of psychiatric patients has historically been a fertile ground for ideological and political debate, perhaps more heated than in any other area of psychiatry. It is therefore necessary to emphasize that no single hospital milieu is entirely adequate or appropriate for the treatment of all kinds of psychiatric patients.

For the purpose of the present discussion, the milieu will be regarded as a context in which a wide variety of psychiatric treatments are deployed as long as certain principles are operatively maintained. The basic tenets include the following: (1) the psychiatric ward is a social matrix with a subculture of its own that is influenced by, but also shapes, the behavior of all its members— staff and patients alike; (2) the staff makes an ongoing, concerted effort to identify explicitly the underlying social processes; (3) and the staff directs these processes in a manner that increases patient participation, enhances growth and development, and facilitates a positive response to the whole treatment program of psychiatric inpatients. The resulting social organization must be a dynamic one so that as needs evolve and change the milieu may respond in kind. The successful milieu thus rests on a process that requires a great deal of flexibility and open communication, perhaps the only attributes of the community that need not change.[11]

A frequent source of chagrin to the members of the milieu is the impact of the community at large on the social processes of the hospital milieu. Although this immediately appears to be a predictable effect, it is not always clear to the staff engaged in the milieu's day-to-day operation. The prevailing issues and conflicts in the larger community, such as racial and sexual prejudices, filter through into the small community of the psychiatric ward. Of special interest to the specific problem of the interactions between the milieu and violent behavior are the ongoing debates regarding the issues of individual freedom versus involuntary confinement, and the doctrine of right to treatment as well as to refuse treatment. These issues affect the obligations and responsibilities of the hospital staff who are under an ambiguous charge of managing and providing treatment for aggressive patients while respecting their right to treatment.

The psychiatric hospital struggles to find a reasonable course tht makes possible the treatment of psychiatrically ill, potentially violent, and violent individuals among a diverse and at times contradictory set of expectations. Salient among them are the protection of the society versus the treatment of the individual, and the provision of adequate security versus the maintenance of an open-door policy. The latter extends beyond its literal meaning as it is translated into powerful and effective treatment strategies, such as less rigid controls, a greater reliance on open communication, increased patient participation, and the earnest development of clear expectations of patients' to maintain self-control and rational conduct.

Another source of strain in the milieu is the diverse mixture of patients which characterizes the population of most inpatient settings. The focus on the general needs of the group sometimes conflicts with the task of attending to the special needs of specific groups of patients such as the mentally retarded, adolescents, the alcohol or drug dependent, the antisocial, and so on.

The problems reviewed have the effect of generating tension in the milieu. Beyond a certain level such tension will disrupt the balance of the milieu which will in turn increase the likelihood that all sorts of aggressive behavior, including assault, will explode in the milieu. The regulation of this tension is always a basic concern of the psychiatric milieu.

Operation of the Milieu

Granting that the concept of a psychiatric milieu is not a unitary one, some consideration of the basic parameters that determine its various modalities is necessary. Perhaps the most important one is average length of stay. In an institution where stay usually is prolonged, especially beyond six months, the social processes of the milieu are intensified and readily lead to the development of a subculture of sufficient strength to powerfully influence the behavior of both staff and patients. This is the kind of phenomenon described by Jones as a therapeutic community.[7] It creates conditions highly favorable to a great number of patient's activities ranging from the production of ward bulletins and newspapers to a significant role in the decision-making processes, including a wide variety of patient governments. On the other end of the spectrum are acute treatment wards where the length of stay has been shortened to under four weeks. Here, the continuous turnover in the patient population produces rapid changes that are not conducive to these developments. As patients become more functional, they are quickly discharged and under these circumstances the maintenance of an active treatment milieu requires a great deal of activity on the part of the staff. For a number of years the trend in the United States has been toward a steady decrease in the length of hospitalization and a question has been raised whether the resulting strain on the psychiatric milieu could produce an increase in the incidence of assaultive behavior. Further research is needed in order to clarify this issue.

The social processes operative in the psychiatric milieu substantially contribute to determining whether or not aggressive and assaultive behavior will occur. The better the processes are understood the more effectively they can be directed as an essential aspect of the management and treatment program of violence-prone patients, and the greater the likelihood of successful early intervention to prevent violence. To be successful the staff must consider the full spectrum of behaviors that lead to assault as well as the impact of the milieu's social processes on behavior modulation and control. To understand this interaction more clearly, it is imperative that the psychiatric hospital milieu be viewed not as an abstract concept but as a specific form of a small society with individualized and often idiosyncratic characteristics. The following discussion thus will be more typical of the kind of milieu in an acute treatment psychiatric unit with an average length of stay of around four weeks that serves a diversified patient population with a variety of psychiatric diagnoses. It is hoped that such a narrowed focus, while enhancing clarity of presentation, will allow for the extraction of more general guidelines that can be rationally tailored to different therapeutic environments.

An orderly milieu in which the total community works harmoniously toward the common goal of alleviating suffering, resolving problems, and promoting the development of more effective interpersonal skills is a basic requirement for the creation of an atmosphere that discourages untoward manifestations of aggression. Since ultimate power lies with the staff, the success of the milieu depends on staff's ability to delegate responsibilities to the patients in proportion to the latter's capacity to assume them. This involves a complex assessment of the group as a whole as well as each individual patient with particular emphasis his or her strengths and functional weaknesses. Some patients are impaired to the point that they can function only in the context of structured daily activities, while others respond better to an adequately designed set of expectations with enough room for rehearsal and experimentation. Care must be exercised to avoid attitudes of paternalism, rigidity, and overcontrol but also not to raise unrealistic expectations that will tax an individual's repertoire of responses beyond his or her ability to perform resulting in demoralization and helplessness.

This individual variability is paralleled by group variability. The ever-changing character of the patient population will be reflected at times in a group capable of a high degree of autonomy and assertiveness in conducting the daily business of the milieu only to be replaced, in short notice, by a group characterized by disorganization, withdrawal, and inactivity. Maintaining the focus on the social processes of the milieu under the constraints of time-limited hospitalization and consequent dramatic changes in the character of the milieu demands a highly motivated and flexible staff. Staff must make a concerted effort to remain realistic and objective irrespective of their ideological orientation and beliefs. The importance of this matter is underlined by the existence of a series of basic assumptions not always made explicit in the operation of the psychiatric milieu. An example is the axiom that, although psychiatric disorders have multiple etiological determination, the ultimate responsibility for the patient's behavior lies with him- or herself. Other assumptions, in a list that is far exhaustive, include the following: patients always have the potential for getting better if not entirely well; they are capable of growing, maturing, and overcoming developmental gaps; they are capable of controlling their actions and of expressing their desires, wishes, feelings, and thoughts through verbal means; interpersonal conflict is an unavoidable vicissitude of the human condition that can be satisfactorily resolved through discussion and negotiation. Data may or may not be available to support these or other similar beliefs; in fact they constitute working assumptions, which—despite our ignorance of the etiology of behavioral disorders—maintain hope in the face of adversity and generate an expectation of success. When the outcome is unsuccessful, these assumptions may support the belief that the therapeutic limitations lie with the therapist rather than with the patient.

In practice the staff is engaged in an ongoing, objective assessment of changes in the functional capacity of the patient group. Staff must be prepared to assume and to delegate responsibilities in accordance with the perceived capabilities of the patient population without generating negative expectations of the patients' limitations. A critical aspect of the milieu's operation is early detection of norm-threatening processes, such as failure to resolve interpersonal conflicts by verbal means. Such transgressions call for immediate and effective intervention; hesitation at this point may generate disorganization and chaos, a state of affairs that will very likely increase the likelihood of various kinds of aggressive and assaultive behavior.

The early detection of milieu-threatening processes in preventing assault may be better understood in light of the fact that most patients requiring admission to a psychiatric unit have significant impairments in their ability to function within their social group. Ideally, the milieu will provide the support and structure needed to compensate for the functional difficulties while maximizing opportunities for patients to develop and exercise problem-solving skills. The strategy of early detection of conflict, in addition to its more general therapeutic role in promoting restitution of function and developing and consolidating additional coping skills, contributes to conflict resolution. To be effective the strategy requires that a high priority task in the work agenda of the hospital community should be to detect and highlight interpersonal conflicts. It is obviously important that the staff be able to resolve its own dissensions in a mature and effective manner—not only as a prerequisite for being perceived as adequate role models, but also for staff to develop an adequate level of morale, comfort, and satisfaction with their work to enable them to actively seek out indications of conflict within the ward. Denial or suppression of early signs of conflict is one of the most ominous developments in the milieu as it allows conflict to grow unattended and often to progress to a sudden, serious, and in many cases collective explosion of violence. Usually conceptualized as a form of resistance, the progression toward collective violence, if not denied by the staff, can always be anticipated in the patient group. When a large community meeting is the mechanism used to resolve conflict, such resistance may show remarkable resilience and effectively prevent the working through of the problem within the time allotted for the meeting. In this case the staff will need to determine whether the tension level has decreased sufficiently to allow the uninterrupted flow of activities until their next scheduled meeting provides another opportunity for the group to attain satisfactory conflict resolution. Otherwise, the problem at hand takes precedence over other needs of the milieu and additional meeting time must be allotted until a satisfactory solution is achieved. Such marathons can be time consuming and exhausting but must occur when needed; i.e., when the milieu faces the threat of imminent disruption and when serious acting out, including assault, is likely to occur. Unfortunately, error also may be made in the direction opposite denial; staff may become alarmed and overcontrolling. This is best avoided or corrected by staff monitoring and examining their own reactions.

Interpersonal conflict is an unavoidable development in the milieu. On the positive side, it provides both the material and the opportunity for the operation of therapeutic processes to restore function and develop problem-solving skills. However, the conflicts must be maintained within acceptable boundaries beyond which they will have a deleterious effect on the milieu, increasing the risk of acting out, aggression, and assault. A crucial aspect of delineating those boundaries is to be clear about the organizational structure, functions, and roles within the milieu. A common problem in this regard is whether the psychiatric unit here envisioned constitutes a democratic or an authoritarian social system. Obviously, when one group in an institution, i.e., the staff, has a great deal of power—including admission and discharge—over another group, i.e., the patients, that institution can not reasonably claim to be a democracy. This is true, however, only in the sense that ultimate responsibility for the welfare of the patients lies with the staff. It does not preclude the involvement of patients in deliberation about ongoing problems of the milieu or their sharing in a great deal of decision making in the unit. To make this integration truly operative, rather than a lip-servicing device, those areas where patients share responsibility with the staff must be clarified, keeping in mind that the capacity for independent functioning by the patient group is in a state of constant flux as a result of changes in the patient population. Although ideally one would want to see patients having total responsibility for directing their affairs in a psychiatric unit of the type described, such an approach would lead to disastrous consequences and would inevitably be regarded as staff abrogation of responsibility for patient care. When an individual needs psychiatric hospitalization, albeit voluntarily, the individual has exhausted the ability to cope and is entrusting his or her welfare to the hands of others.

Limit Setting

It is now clear that the effectiveness of the milieu in preventing and managing assaultive behavior in the psychiatric hospital depends on the staff's ability to detect and intervene in a variety of problems and behaviors that can be envisioned as precursors to assault. Limit setting is perhaps the most basic and the most common form of this intervention and, as such, needs a more complete discussion here.

A common feature of many psychiatric inpatients is the experience of actual loss of control or the disturbing fear that one is about to lose control. This may be manifested in major changes in mood, in overwhelming feelings of anxiety and panic, or in dyscontrol over one's responses to a variety of stressful situations. A common finding in adolescents is insufficiently developed internal controls usually associated with ineffective (frequently due to inconsistency) or even absent external controls. The problem may reflect a disruption of control mechanisms or a developmental deficit, but in either case the treatment of such individuals in the psychiatric milieu entails a shaping or reshaping of unadaptive (and often socially unacceptable) behavior into its more appropriate counterparts. Limit setting is one of the mechanisms the milieu uses to address this problem.

Effective limit setting requires a clear and shared delineation of the specific behaviors that need to be changed. In limit setting, it should be remembered that patients tend to reestablish within the hospital milieu the patterns of communication and interpersonal relationships that prevailed in the patient's original social environment. Poor communication among staff is almost a guarantee that staff will become split and be engaged by the patient in those unhealthy modes of interaction. Inconsistency, a major breeder of psychopathology, is another pitfall that can be avoided when implementing limit setting by designing a plan that is not only sensitive to the patient's strengths and vulnerabilities but is also workable; i.e., it can be carried out within the constraints of the milieu. Countertransference is a major obstacle in this respect and the patient can be unwittingly manipulated into the role of reenacting staff conflicts. Inexperienced members of the staff, such as students, are prone to error by failing to recognize pathology when it is present (for example, acting out in adolescents) and, conversely, by labeling as pathological those processes that are healthy quests for adaptation (for example, attempts at assertiveness made by passive patients). These problems and misperceptions need to be corrected for effective limit setting.

Individuals who have the potential to become assaultive often start early in the course of their hospitalization to test the resilience of the limits imposed by the staff. The recognition that the staff earnestly and cohesively enforces those limits provides an opportunity to air and, if necessary, correct his or her views of responsibilities, roles, and expectations, as well as of what is permissible or forbidden in the ward. Infringement of rules must be consistently met by clear and adequate sanctions; a process of early intervention has a salutary effect on many patients who might otherwise escalate their behavior into violence and assault.

Equally important as the needs of the individual are the welfare and safety of the group—both patients and staff—and the need to maintain an environment with sufficient stability for the therapeutic work to proceed without interruption. A wide range of behaviors can interfere with and disrupt this process. At the most simple level interpersonal conflicts among the community members are manifested through arguments that become increasingly heated. Unless an intervention is made—either by the staff alone or in conjunction with other patients whenever possible—the conflict usually moves to a nonverbal mode of expression, thus increasing the danger of a physical confrontation. This includes threatening gestures or postures, taking possession of another's belongings, destruction of objects, agitation, and, finally, assault. Depending on the character and gravity of the conflict, the staff has available a large repertoire of techniques to intervene for the purpose of setting limits and defusing the conflict. This includes meeting with the individuals involved to discuss the problem, separating patients in conflict, segregating them to different areas of the ward, restricting the level of their participation in the activities of the milieu, and, in the most extreme situations, resorting to seclusion and restraints.[5]

In general people experience discomfort in the face of violence, and a similar feeling is aroused by seclusion and restraint since they involve actual physical control of a patient. Seclusion continues to be a necessary and unavoidable form of intervention in the psychiatric milieu, and despite an age old search for more "humane" substitutes it is still fairly frequently utilized.[6,12] When used within a proper therapeutic framework and with adequate monitoring, seclusion is no less humane than other forms of limit setting.

Compared to seclusion, restraints are more rarely utilized but the staff of the psychiatric hospital must be prepared to apply them when necessary. It is difficult to describe specific criteria for their use, but Bursten proposes two conditions as guidelines: 1) when a patient is in the imminence of causing injury to himself or others, and 2) when the patient requests the restraints. Bursten adds that it is proper for the staff to offer restraints.[2] In practice, restraints are used when there are no other measures of effective control, as in the case of patients who will engage in self-mutilization as soon as they are let free.

INDIVIDUAL PSYCHOPATHOLOGY AND THE RESPONSES OF THE MILIEU

Countertransference is one of the major dynamic forces influencing the transactions of the milieu. It encompasses a wide range of feelings but fear is of paramount importance among them for the paralyzing effect it can have on the staff. In the presence of a violent patient, fear is a common reaction that must not be denied or rationalized away if violent behavior is to be effectively managed. Intense, paralyzing fear is far less common but needs to be taken into account because of the devastating effect is has in rendering the staff impotent. Sometimes the situation justifies intense fear, as was the case when an unusually strong patient suddenly broke out in a destructive rampage and threatened to strike out at people using an IV pole as a weapon while only two terrorized female staff members were present. More commonly this fear is an irrational response elicited, for example, by patients who verbalize aggressive and homicidal impulses in a manner that betrays little inhibition of primary process thinking. Such individuals usually have lifelong histories of severe behavior difficulties and deeply disturbed interpersonal relationships. On arrival on the psychiatric unit, they remain aloof and withdrawn and show poor tolerance for frustration. Their lack of adequate controls is manifested by verbal utterance with a highly aggressive content. Although these patients seldom display unprovoked physical violence on the ward, their perception by the staff as extremely dangerous individuals needs to be understood and resolved or these patients can not be successfully managed within the milieu.

The resources available to the staff constitute another element influential in determining whether or not assault will be a likely outcome of the social processes operative in the milieu. Staff quality which is a product of their training, experience, and level of sophistication, is of obvious significance in this regard. When the physical control of the patient becomes an issue however ready accessibility to sufficient security manpower is a dire necessity. In its absence the staff is vulnerable to intimidation, and an intimidated staff is hampered in the ability to intervene even at the earlier stages when the precursors of physical aggression such as mounting stages of agitation become manifested. A patient on the verge of losing control becomes frightened and more agitated as a consequence of the perception that his or her inadequate controls are not being supplemented or bolstered by external controls provided by the staff. Such resources are included in the design of the program in specialized units where potentially violent patients are expected to be present on a routine basis.

The policy of deinstitutionalization has produced a redistribution of the psychiatrically ill population. Larger numbers of potentially assaultive patients have been shifted toward settings, such as community hospitals, where patients are expected to be in better control over their aggressive impulses than patients in psychiatric institutions. The issue of whether or not a given hospital milieu has sufficient manpower to manage potentially violent patients is relative to the amount of care required by the total patient population at that period in time. Most units are prepared to deal with a certain amount of acting out, disorganized, agitated, or aggressive behaviors beyond which they may become overwhelmed. This factor, anecdotally referred to as "critical mass," is a real limitation to the idealistic notion that all psychiatric units are able to admit and treat any kind of patient at any time. Such a view undoubtedly rests on an assumption of homogeneity in the psychiatrically ill population, a notion that would not be entertained in relation to established somatic diseases, which have generated a complex system of specialized units as well as different levels of care. Although these two systems are not strictly comparable, they have sufficient similarities to suggest that the development of a rating system in terms of intensity of care may be useful in assessing the adequacy of the staffing of a given psychiatric unit. There is an unspoken recognition of this problem in the role of admitting officers who regulate the flow of patients between hospital units and the community at large. These matters are, however, seldom if ever clearly stated as a policy, and conflicts therefore always exist between the individuals generating the referrals and those in charge of admission.

Granting that enough resources are available, assault may occur in the milieu when the staff fails to identify signs that the patient's behavior is getting out of control. A typical example is the manic patient whose euphoria spreads rapidly throughout the milieu, and while everybody is smiling and laughing the community is gradually led into a major catastrophic experience. Constant evaluation of the milieu is necessary for the staff to strike a delicate balance between sharing and participating with the patients in the therapeutic transactions of the milieu and maintaining objectivity.

Staff interpretation of the patient's motivation for aggressive behavior shapes their attitude and reaction to the patient. Behavior that is perceived as a clear manifestation of treatable psychopathology usually meets tolerance and the staff is motivated to work on the resolution of the underlying condition. Under these circumstances it is likely that early intervention will interrupt the behavioral sequence that would lead to assault; if that fails the staff feels less ambiguous and reacts with greater promptness and efficiency in controlling the violence. On the other hand, behavior that is interpreted as an expression of personality traits under voluntary control evokes negative responses including the desire to get rid of the patient.

Of special relevance is the staff's interpretation of the patient's strengths, limitations, and vulnerabilities with particular regard to the patient's capacity to learn from experience and to develop insight into his or her behavior. Assessment of the condition as hopeless ordinarily shifts the approach from treatment to control, seclusion is more readily and frequently used, and the patient ends up transferred to a long-term institution. To counteract this process the milieu needs a mechanism to provide an ongoing analysis of the staff, the individual patients, and the milieu, including provisions to develop diagnostic and dynamic formulations to serve as a basis for continuously modified treatment plans. Accreditation requirements of written, multidisciplinary treatment plans are obviously inadequate to serve this purpose; while they are done to soothe bureaucratic scruples, the time consuming process of reevaluating and planning therapeutic strategies is but faintly relfected in the written documents of the milieu. Nevertheless, this process remains the basic instrument for anticipation of events in the milieu. When the possibility of assault is explicitly identified, the staff can search for the processes that are threatening a loss of control and design an adequate plan for preventive intervention without neglecting the possibility that violence could actually occur.

Certain psychopathological manifestations frequently associated with assaultive behavior are sensitive to the influence of the milieu. Psychomotor agitation is a common example. It can be precipitated by overstimulation of a psychotic patient who has difficulty filtering and processing information and is easily overwhelmed by the multiple demands of the milieu. Such patients may not be able to sit through the whole duration of a community meeting, and their participation in other activities may also need to be titrated to their level of tolerance. They may require frequent periods away from the group, either in their room or other areas of the unit. On the other hand, prolonged isolation is also to be avoided, so a balance must be struck between the two extremes. One-to-one contact with the staff is usually a necessity in such cases. Reality testing is regularly deficient in these patients but it can be bolstered by clearly articulating for the patient the identity and role of the various members of the community, what is being planned, why the patient is being approached, what is expected of him, the schedule of activities, and so on. This combination of controlled exposure to stimulation and clarification of events in the milieu may be sufficient to keep agitation under control. Otherwise, firm limits must be set and enforced, if necessary, by a show of force with sufficient manpower to ensure that the patient can be controlled.

Neuroleptics, of course, are commonly needed not only to control agitation in conjunction with what has been described but also to treat the underlying condition. Manic patients who are candidates for lithium carbonate may require neuroleptics in the earlier phase of hospitalization when they cannot be adequately managed in the milieu. Techniques of rapid neuroleptization are useful to develop adequate levels of medication in a short period of time. The rare patient, primarily with mania or catatonic excitement, may be agitated to the point of exhaustion, in which case electroconvulsive therapy (ECT) should be considered.

Patients suffering from persecutory delusions can strike out in response to a perceived threat to their welfare; this can also happen when command hallucinations with an aggressive content are present. These patients can benefit from the previously described techniques to prevent overstimulation and strengthen reality testing, but the patients often require limit setting in the form of clear and unambiguous statements that physical contact is not allowed in the milieu.

Mentally retarded patients with concomitant behavior problems of an aggressive nature are very difficult to manage and often undergo a series of exchanges between the mental retardation and the mental health systems. Their aggressiveness is usually of a chronic nature, and, while a given outburst of violence can be controlled, they do not benefit much from the psychiatric milieu. They are more likely to respond to a long-term program of behavior modification that is not available in the acute care psychiatric unit. In the acute care unit mentally retarded patients can usually be controlled but not treated, and the behavior patterns which led to admission remain operative on discharge.

Another group of patients carry a variety of diagnoses, from explosive disorder to borderline personality, and have in common low tolerance to frustration and a propensity for outbursts of anger sometimes leading to physical assault. Although they have poor control over their aggressive impulses, clarification and strict enforcement of the norms of the milieu in regard to violence is an essential aspect of their management. Elucidation of the particular conflicts that render them vulnerable and the development of awareness and appreciation for the components of their emotional responses, with particular emphasis on their experience of anger, can be effective therapeutic techniques. In some instances where anxiety plays a major role in triggering the violent response, benzodiazepines can be useful adjuncts to treatment. If the drug is not abused, the patient can learn to make judicious and effective use of the medication, but the possibility of a disinhibitory drug effect must be considered.

Perhaps the most difficult problem for the psychiatric milieu is the antisocial individual who, when frustrated, resorts to deliberate destruction of property or assault. These individuals can be, and are, successfully treated in specialized milieu programs designed exclusively for that purpose, and some are amenable to treatment in the ordinary psychiatric milieu. The difficulty lies primarily with those patients who disregard authority, show no concern for others, and are not committed to treatment. Their actions raise complex questions of responsibility and accountability, sometimes to the point of the staff trying to decide whether to view their behavior as an expression of psychopathology or a criminal act. Questions about the proper setting and the most effective response to antisocial patients ultimately lead to the issue of whether these patients belong in the psychiatric milieu or should be dealt with by the legal system. Often these patients are chronic offenders of the law but have not committed a crime punished by prolonged incarceration and, because of some obvious indicators of psychopathology, are repeatedly referred for treatment by the legal system. In the final analysis the psychiatric staff will have to face the fact that the existence of psychopathology per se does not make one a patient, and psychiatrists will have to come to terms with the limitations of their ability to engage antisocial individuals in a therapeutic contract. If such commitment is a tentative one, the staff needs to clearly define the conditions required for these individuals to stay in the hospital and should define the criteria for discharge. Failure to anticipate and act on these possibilities from the start will frequently lead to a major explosion of destructiveness or violence as a final determinant of discharge.

The issue of patients' legal responsibilities for their actions while living in a psychiatric unit has acquired a great deal of interest in recent times. In Canada a precedent has been set for legal charges against a patient for acts while undergoing treatment in a psychiatric hospital,[10] but no similar approach has been reported in the United States. Nevertheless, this is an intriguing question that will often be considered whenever a potentially violent patient enters the psychiatric hospital milieu.

REFERENCES

1. Almond R: Issues in milieu therapy. Schizophr Bull 13:12–26, 1975
2. Bursten B: Using mechanical restraints on acutely disturbed psychiatric patients. Hosp Community Psychiatry 26:757–759
3. Depp FC: Violent behavior patterns on psychiatric wards. Aggressive Behavior 2:295–306, 1976
4. Ekblom B: Acts of violence by patients in mental hospitals. Stockholm, Scandinavian University Press, 1970
5. Gair DS: Limit-setting and Seclusion in the Psychiatric Hospital. Psychiatric Opinion 17:11–19, 1980
6. Greenblatt M: Seclusion as a Means of Restraint. Psychiatric Opinion 17:13–14, 1980
7. Jones M: The Therapeutic Community: A New Treatment Method in Psychiatry. New York, Basic Books, 1953
8. Lion JR, Bach-y-Rita G, Ervin FR: Violent Patients in the Emergency Room. Am J Psychiatry 125:1706–1711, 1969
9. Lion JR, Pasternak SA: Countertransference reactions to violent patients. Am J Psychiatry 130:207–210, 1973
10. Scharz CJ, Greenfield GP: Charging a patient with assault of a nurse on a psychiatric unit. Can Psychiatric Assoc J 23:197–200, 1978
11. Shoenberg E: Therapeutic communities, the ideal, the real and the possible, in Sansen E (ed): The Therapeutic Community. London, Croom Helm Ltd., 1980
12. Wells DA: The use of seclusion on a university hospital psychiatric floor. Arch Gen Psychiatry 26:410–413, 1972
13. West DA, Litwok E, Oberlander K, et al: Emergency psychiatric home visiting: Report of four years experience. J Clin Psychiatry 41:113–118, 1980

INDEX

Page numbers followed by *t* indicate tables.